Antipsychotics

ANTIPSYCHOTICS

Drugs in psychiatry

Volume 3

ELSEVIER
AMSTERDAM · NEW YORK · OXFORD

Antipsychotics

Edited by

GRAHAM D. BURROWS
TREVOR R. NORMAN
and
BRIAN DAVIES

*Department of Psychiatry,
University of Melbourne,
Australia*

1985

ELSEVIER
AMSTERDAM · NEW YORK · OXFORD

ISBN Vol. 3 0-444-80635-0
ISBN Series 0-444-80490-0

PUBLISHED BY:

Elsevier Science Publishers B.V. (Biomedical Division)
P.O. Box 211
1000 AE Amsterdam
The Netherlands

SOLE DISTRIBUTORS FOR THE U.S.A. AND CANADA:

Elsevier Science Publishing Company, Inc.
52 Vanderbilt Avenue
New York, NY 10017
USA

Library of Congress Cataloging in Publication Data
Main entry under title:

Antipsychotics.

(Drugs in psychiatry ; v. 3)
Includes bibliographies and index.
1. Tranquilizing drugs. 2. Tranquilizing drugs--
Physiological effect. 3. Psychoses--chemotherapy.
I. Burrows, Graham D. II. Norman, Trevor R., 1946-
III. Davies, Brian, 1928- . IV. Series.
[DNLM: 1. Tranquilizing Agents, Major-pharmacodynamics.
W1 DR893T v.3 / QV 77.9 A633]
RM333.A57 1985 615'.7882 84-28664
ISBN 0-444-80635-0 (U.S.)

Printed in the Netherlands

Preface

This volume on antipsychotic drugs is the third of a series on drugs used in psychiatry. It was decided to attempt to cover the area from basic pharmacology to clinical applications. Frequently, volumes on this subject highlight one aspect only. We hope this volume will be suitable for the researcher, the specialist and the general practitioner. The next volume, and the final one of the series, will be on *Antimanics, Anticonvulsants, and Other Drugs in Psychiatry*.

We are grateful to the authors who have generously contributed from their valuable experience to this volume. We are also grateful to Mrs Gertrude Rubinstein for continued editorial assistance.

GRAHAM D. BURROWS
TREVOR R. NORMAN
BRIAN M. DAVIES

List of contributors

Thomas A. Ban 239
Tennessee Neuropsychiatric Institute and Vanderbilt University, Nashville, Tennessee, U.S.A.

Philip A. Berger 185
Norris Mental Health Clinical Research Center, Stanford University School of Medicine, Stanford, California, U.S.A.

Graham D. Burrows 3, 173, 253
Department of Psychiatry, University of Melbourne, Austin and Larundel Hospitals, Victoria, Australia

Magda Campbell 213
Department of Psychiatry, New York University Medical Center, 550 First Avenue, New York, U.S.A.

Stephen H. Curry 79
Division of Clinical Pharmacokinetics, College of Pharmacy, University of Florida, Gainesville, Florida, U.S.A.

Mamoun Dabbagh 147
Department of Psychiatry, Wayne State University School of Medicine, and Lafayette Clinic, Detroit, Michigan, U.S.A.

Brian M. Davies 3
Department of Psychiatry, University of Melbourne, and Royal Melbourne Hospital, Victoria, Australia

John M. Davis 57
Illinois State Psychiatric Institute, Chicago, Illinois, U.S.A.

Stephen I. Deutsch 213
Department of Psychiatry, New York University Medical Center, 550 First Avenue, New York, U.S.A.

David de Wied 27
Rudolph Magnus Institute for Pharmacology, Medical Faculty, University of Utrecht, The Netherlands

Meredith J. Dunn 185
Norris Mental Health Clinical Research Center, Stanford University School of Medicine, Stanford, California, U.S.A.

Samuel Gershon 147
Department of Psychiatry, Wayne State University School of Medicine, and Lafayette Clinic, Detroit, Michigan, U.S.A.

Leo E. Hollister 141
Department of Medicine, Pharmacology and Psychiatry, VA Medical Center, Miranda Avenue, Palo Alto, California, U.S.A.

H. Itoh 99
Department of Neuropsychiatry, School of Medicine, Keio University, Tokyo, Japan

Philip G. Janicak 57
Illinois State Psychiatric Institute, Chicago, Illinois, U.S.A.

Javaid I. Javaid 57
Illinois State Psychiatric Institute, Chicago, Illinois, U.S.A.

Y.D. Lapierre 115
Department of Psychiatry, University of Ottawa, and The Royal Ottawa Hospital, Ottawa, Canada

Odd Lingjaerde 163
Section of Clinical Psychiatry, University of Tromso, and Åsgård Hospital, Norway

Kay P. Maguire 71

Department of Psychiatry, University of Melbourne, Victoria, Australia

Stephen R. Marder 47

Veterans Administration Medical Center, Brentwood Division, and Department of Psychiatry and Biobehavioral Sciences, University of California at Los Angeles, California, U.S.A.

P.F. Marriott 173

Department of Psychiatry, University of Melbourne, Austin Hospital, Victoria, Australia

Philip R.A. May 47

Department of Psychiatry and Biobehavioral Sciences, University of California at Los Angeles, California, U.S.A.

Marcelle A. Mostert 57

Illinois State Psychiatric Institute, Chicago, Illinois, U.S.A.

R. Swami Nathan 11

Department of Psychiatry, University of Pittsburgh, Western Psychiatric Institute and Clinic, Pittsburgh, Pennsylvania, U.S.A.

Trevor R. Norman 71, 173, 253

Department of Psychiatry, University of Melbourne, Austin Hospital, Heidelberg, Victoria, Australia.

L.K. Oyewumi 115

Department of Psychiatry, University of Ottawa, and The Royal Ottawa Hospital, Ottawa, Canada

William M. Petrie 239

Tennessee Neuropsychiatric Institute and Vanderbilt University, Nashville, Tennessee, U.S.A.

Edmond H. Pi 129

Department of Psychiatry, Medical College of Pennsylvania, Philadelphia, Pennsylvania, U.S.A.

George M. Simpson 129
Department of Psychiatry, Medical College of Pennsylvania, Philadelphia, Pennsylvania, U.S.A.

Graeme J. Sloman 253
Department of Cardiology, Epworth Hospital, Richmond, Victoria, Australia

Michael Stanley 147
Departments of Psychiatry and Pharmacology, Wayne State University School of Medicine, and Lafayette Clinic, Detroit, Michigan, U.S.A.

Daniel P. van Kammen 11
Department of Psychiatry, University of Pittsburgh, and VA Medical Center, Highland Drive, Pittsburgh, Pennsylvania, U.S.A.

Theodore Van Putten 47
Veterans Administration Medical Center, Brentwood Division, and Department of Psychiatry and Biobehavioral Sciences, University of California at Los Angeles, California, U.S.A.

Jan M. van Ree 27
Rudolph Magnus Institute for Pharmacology, Medical Faculty, University of Utrecht, The Netherlands

Wim M.A. Verhoeven 27
Department of Psychiatry, Medical Faculty, University of Utrecht, The Netherlands

Contents

Preface v

List of Contributors vii

SECTION I. INTRODUCTION

Chapter 1. An introduction to the use of antipsychotic drugs – *Graham D. Burrows and Brian M. Davies* 3

SECTION II. BASIC RESEARCH

Chapter 2. Neuroendocrine effects of antipsychotic drugs – *R. Swami Nathan and Daniel P. van Kammen* 11

Chapter 3. Antipsychotic actions of the endorphins – *Jan M. van Ree, Wim M.A. Verhoeven and David de Wied* 27

Chapter 4. Prediction of response to antipsychotic drugs – *Theodore Van Putten, Philip R.A. May and Stephen R. Marder* 47

SECTION III. PLASMA LEVEL MEASUREMENT, PHARMACOKINETICS AND CLINICAL RESPONSE

Chapter 5. Antipsychotics: Plasma levels and clinical response – *John M. Davis, Javaid I. Javaid, Philip G. Janicak and Marcelle A. Mostert* 57

Chapter 6.	Plasma level measurement of phenothiazines and butyrophenones – *Kay P. Maguire and Trevor R. Norman*	71
Chapter 7.	Phenothiazines: Metabolism and pharmacokinetics – *Stephen H. Curry*	79
Chapter 8.	Butyrophenones: Plasma level and clinical response – *H. Itoh*	99
Chapter 9.	Thioxanthenes: Measurement, kinetics and clinical response – *L.K. Oyewumi and Y.D. Lapierre*	115
Chapter 10.	Clozapine and loxapine – measurement, pharmacokinetics and therapeutic levels – *Edmond H. Pi and George M. Simpson*	129

SECTION IV. CLINICAL APPLICATIONS

Chapter 11.	Choice of antipsychotic drugs – *L.E. Hollister*	141
Chapter 12.	New antipsychotic agents: Clinical studies – *Mamoun Dabbagh, Michael Stanley and Samuel Gershon*	147
Chapter 13.	Antipsychotic effect of the benzodiazepines – *Odd Lingjaerde*	163
Chapter 14.	The long-acting neuroleptic drugs and their treatment systems – *P.F. Marriott, Trevor R. Norman and Graham D. Burrows*	173
Chapter 15.	Tardive dyskinesia: The major problem with antipsychotic maintenance therapy – *Philip A. Berger and Meredith J. Dunn*	185
Chapter 16.	Neuroleptics in children – *Magda Campbell and Stephen I. Deutsch*	213
Chapter 17.	The use of antipsychotic agents in the elderly – *William M. Petrie and Thomas A. Ban*	239

Chapter 18. Adverse effects, cardiotoxicity and drug interactions of antipsychotic drugs – *Trevor R. Norman, Graeme J. Sloman and Graham D. Burrows* 253

Subject index 269

Section I

INTRODUCTION

Burrows/Norman/Davies (eds) Antipsychotics

Chapter 1

An introduction to the use of antipsychotic drugs

GRAHAM D. BURROWS

Department of Psychiatry, University of Melbourne, Austin Hospital, Australia

and

BRIAN M. DAVIES

Department of Psychiatry, University of Melbourne, Australia

Chlorpromazine (Largactil, Thorazine), first used in 1952 by the French psychiatrists – Delay and Deniker – was the first antipsychotic drug. Its use completely changed the management of disturbed patients and consequently psychiatric hospitals. It produced a tranquillization without impairing consciousness. While other antipsychotic drugs have become available, chlorpromazine is still widely used in the management of acutely disturbed patients.

The antipsychotic drugs now consist of several groups of chemically related compounds. The most important agents are phenothiazines (e.g. chlorpromazine) and butyrophenones (e.g. haloperidol). Another group, the thioxanthenes, are also antipsychotic drugs.

These drugs are used to quieten disturbed patients whatever the cause. In clinical practice they are used for disturbed patients with acute or chronic brain syndromes, mania, depression, severe anxiety and the group of illnesses called schizophrenia. It is in this last group of conditions that they have their main use; in the control of behavioural abnormalities, auditory hallucinations, and the thinking disturbances, that characterise this syndrome. Long-term treatment with these drugs is usually the most important aspect of the total management plan of patients with schizophrenia.

These drugs have been shown to act by interfering with dopaminergic transmission in the brain by blocking dopamine receptors. Consequently, extrapyramidal side effects are troublesome. Other side effects are caused by hyperprolactinaemia and the effects of the drugs on cholinergic, alpha-adrenergic and tryptaminergic receptors.

Tardive dyskinesia is the most important and troublesome side effect. This syndrome is discussed in detail in Chapter 15. It develops in a small percentage of patients, usually after some years of continuous treatment with an antipsychotic drug and most commonly after higher dose treatment. Once it develops, it may not remit, and there is no specific treatment. For these reasons antipsychotic drugs should not be used in low dosage for the treatment of chronic anxiety symptoms. The benzodiazepines are the drugs of choice for the symptomatic relief of severe or chronic anxiety.

Selection of antipsychotic drug

Table 1 gives a list of available antipsychotic drugs with their usual daily dosage. In practice, psychiatrists will choose from perhaps half a dozen regularly. The choice of drug depends upon whether a sedation effect is needed and upon the patient's susceptibility to extrapyramidal side effects.

As well as differences between drugs there is great variability in patients' response to side effects.

TABLE 1

Selected antipsychotic drugs and suggested doses*.

Phenothiazines	Recommended daily dose (mg)
Aliphatic	
chlorpromazine	Acute – 300 – 900
	Maintenance 100 – 500
trifluopromazine	20 – 100
promazine	150 – 300
acepromazine	50 – 300
propiomazine	10 – 40
Piperidines	
thioridazine	150 – 600
mesoridazine	100 – 300
pericyazine	7.5 – 90
piperacetazine	25 – 100
Piperazines	
prochlorperazine	25 – 150
trifluoperazine	10 – 30

TABLE 1 (*continued*)

Phenothiazines	Recommended daily dose (mg)
thiethylperazine	10 – 30
thioproperazine	10 – 40
butaperazine	30 – 100
perphenazine	12 – 24
fluphenazine	2.5 – 15
fluphenazine enanthate	12.5 – 25 each 1 – 3 weeks
fluphenazine decanoate	12.5 – 25 each 2 – 4 weeks
thiopropazate	15 – 30
methotrimeprazine	15 – 100
acetophenazine	40 – 80
carphenazine	40 – 400
Thioxanthenes	
chlorprothixene	50 – 300
thiothixene	10 – 30
flupenthixol	3 – 12
flupenthixol decanoate	20 – 40 every 1 – 3 weeks
Butyrophenones	
haloperidol	1 – 12
trifluperidol	1 – 3
benperidol	2 – 6
droperidol	5 – 20 i.v. (single dose for emergencies)
Diphenylbutylpiperidines	
pimozide	2 – 20***
fluspirilene	2 – 6 weekly
penfluridol	20 – 50 weekly
Benzamides	
sulpiride	600 – 1800
Dibenzoxazepines	
clozapine	150 – 300**
loxapine	50 – 250
Indole derivatives	
molindone	10 – 20
oxypertine	20 – 60

* Adapted from Table 6, pp. 123 – 129, in 'Drug Treatment in Psychiatry', by Trevor Silverstone and Paul Turner, 3rd edn., Routledge & Kegan Paul PLC, 1982.
** Higher dosages may be given (G. Simpson, personal communication).
*** Martindale 28th edn. 1982, W. Martindale, ed., Rittenhouse PA.

Editors' Note: The editors have consulted with the authors of chapters in the present volume, concerning apparent discrepancies for dosages in their chapters compared with this Table. It is suggested that although the dosages advised in this Table are based on findings reported in the literature, consideration should be given to adapting these doses, especially the upper extremes of dosage range, to clinical situations. Higher dosages may be required in the acute phase of illness. These should then be titrated downwards to the minimum effective dose. We thank Dr. Yvon Lapierre for this suggestion.

Classification of antipsychotics

Phenothiazines can be divided into three main groups.

1) An *'aliphatic'* group such as chlorpromazine and promazine. These drugs have pronounced sedative effects and moderate anticholinergic and extrapyramidal side effects.
2) A *'piperidine'* group including thioridazine, which has moderate sedative effects, but minimal extrapyramidal side effects.
3) A *'piperazine'* group including trifluoperazine and fluphenazine. These drugs have minimal sedative and anticholinergic effects but marked extrapyramidal side effects.

The *butyrophenones* and *thioxanthenes* are groups of drugs that tend to resemble the piperazine phenothiazines.

Compliance

Compliance is the most important clinical problem for long-term treatment in psychiatric patients. Everything that can be done to improve compliance must be part of clinical practice. Explanations should be given to patient and family and regular appointments with the same doctor or member of a team. The family doctor or primary care physician should be fully informed. Patients must be contacted if they fail to keep appointments. Despite the best precautions some studies have shown that noncompliance may be as high as 40%. Patients with chronic schizophrenia with paranoid thoughts who are associated with antidrug, antipsychiatry movements, are a particular problem in everyday clinical practice. They may remain ill and distressed for months or years while refusing available effective treatment.

In our clinical practice, chlorpromazine, haloperidol, thioridazine, trifluoperazine and fluphenazine decanoate are the most usually prescribed antipsychotic drugs.

Acute treatment with antipsychotic drugs

Chlorpromazine, available in tablet, syrup, suppository and ampoules for i.m. injection, and haloperidol available in tablet, drop, and ampoules for i.v. and i.m. injection are the drugs of choice to produce rapid tranquillization.

Chlorpromazine can be given by i.m. injection 25 – 50 mg every 6 – 8 hours. Equivalent oral dosage is 100 – 200 mg q.d.s. Dosage can only be learnt by clinical experience and some disturbed patients will need between 1000 and 1500 mg of chlorpromazine orally per day. Intravenous use is contraindicated. Despite lists of cautions and side effects given in textbooks, the drug is a safe one in everyday clinical practice. Hypotension is the main immediate problem in some patients.

Haloperidol is also used for acute management, 5 mg being equivalent to 100 mg of chlorpromazine. Intravenous dosage can be used and some groups recommend high dosage over the initial few hours of treatment, 10 – 30 mg every 6 hours i.v. or i.m. injection being the usual dosage.

This drug produces extrapyramidal and dystonic side effects in most patients. In adolescents and the elderly the dystonic symptoms (e.g. torticollis) can be very severe. Anti-parkinsonian drugs should be given routinely with injections of haloperidol to prevent these side effects. Its advantage over chlorpromazine is its relative lack of effects on the cardiovascular system.

Haloperidol drops are colourless and tasteless in water and are often useful in starting medication in both very distressed and manic patients.

Oral dosage should be substituted for injection as soon as possible whichever drug is used. It is best to use one antipsychotic drug only and not several together.

Antipsychotics for long-term management

Many schizophrenic patients need to have antipsychotic drugs for 2 – 3 years after the first episode of illness. The drugs are then gradually stopped and the patient observed. If symptoms return then long-term mangement with drugs is indicated. In such an instance drugs would be continued for another 5 years before a further attempt at ceasing medication.

For this regular medication, *if the patient is compliant*, oral medication with a piperazine phenothiazine or a butyrophenone, either haloperidol or pimozide, is usual.

To continue treatment in a patient suffering from schizophrenia who has been admitted to hospital for the first time and whose acute symptoms have been relieved with chlorpromazine over the course of 14 days, trifluoperazine is added 10 mg at night. This dosage is later increased to 20 – 40 mg and the chlorpromazine withdrawn. Anti-parkinsonian drugs might be necessary at the start of treatment, e.g. benztropine 0.5 – 2 mg nightly, or benzhexol 2 – 6 mg daily. Some clinicians prefer not to routinely prescribe anti-parkinsonian agents but wait for the onset of extrapyramidal symptoms.

Later this can be reduced. The eventual aim over the first few months is to get the patient to be compliant in regard to taking medication – one dose in the evening is best. Then to find the lowest dose of trifluoperazine that is needed to normalise the mental state and yet with minimal side effects that do not prevent everyday activities.

Haloperidol, or pimozide, or the thioxanthenes can be used similarly.

At this stage the patient and family would be told that the medication is necessary for at least 2 years. After 2 years the drugs are slowly reduced. If schizophrenic symptoms return the medication will need to be taken for say another 5 years.

For non-compliant patients, medication will need to be given by injection – usually fluphenazine decanoate. Details of this treatment are given in Chapter 14. Again, the aim is to find the optimal dosage then to continue treatment again for some years before seeing whether medication can be permanently withdrawn.

Tardive dyskinesia is fully dealt with in Chapter 15. It is important that overconcern about the risks of this unpleasant side effect does not prevent patients being given antipsychotic drugs regularly and at appropriate dosages.

In an ideal situation, one psychiatrist should see the patient in the acute illness and then see him regularly in out-patient or private practice. For the injectable drugs an actual day clinic is very helpful as described in Chapter 14.

It is not our intention to detail all the drugs and all the indications. We wish to emphasize three things.

1) Antipsychotic drugs are the most valuable drugs for the treatment of acutely disturbed patients from whatever cause, and for the treatment of the groups of illnesses called schizophrenia.
2) While many such drugs are available, psychiatrists should confine themselves to using half a dozen and learning their individual problems and values.
3) Individual doctors or team attention for the individual patient over many years is the cornerstone of treatment for the schizophrenias. Social help, with living and work problems are of vital importance as is help for other members of the family. Neglect of these important areas is as harmful as neglect of the proper use of antipsychotic drugs.

The following chapters, each dealing with separate areas of the psychopharmacology of these important drugs, should add to the reader's understanding of these commonly used drugs.

Section II

BASIC RESEARCH

Burrows/Norman/Davies (eds) Antipsychotics

Chapter 2

Neuroendocrine effects of antipsychotic drugs

R. SWAMI NATHAN

Department of Psychiatry, University of Pittsburgh, Western Psychiatric Institute and Clinic, Pittsburgh, PA 15213, U.S.A.

and

DANIEL P. VAN KAMMEN

Department of Psychiatry, University of Pittsburgh, and Psychiatry Service, VA Medical Center, Highland Drive, Pittsburgh, PA 15206, U.S.A.

INTRODUCTION

The endocrine manifestations of dopaminergic drugs have long been recognized. Dopamine exerts a tonic inhibitory control over prolactin (PRL) secretion. When this inhibitory control is decreased, PRL secretion increases. The dopamine receptor blockade has been implicated both in the antipsychotic effects and in raising PRL levels. This hyperprolactinemic state can result in clinically recognizable conditions such as galactorrhea or amenorrhea in some patients. Other hormones, presumably under partial dopaminergic control, are growth hormone (GH), luteinizing hormone (LH) and follicle-stimulating hormone (FSH). Understanding the interactions between the biochemical mechanisms, the endocrine systems and the clinical and side effects of antipsychotic (neuroleptic) drugs will lead to better use of these drugs and to improved clinical care. A schematic representation of the dopaminergic pathways is presented in Fig. 1. The tuberoinfundibular pathway is the major DA pathway involved in the hypothalamo-pituitary axis. Although antipsychotic drugs have the

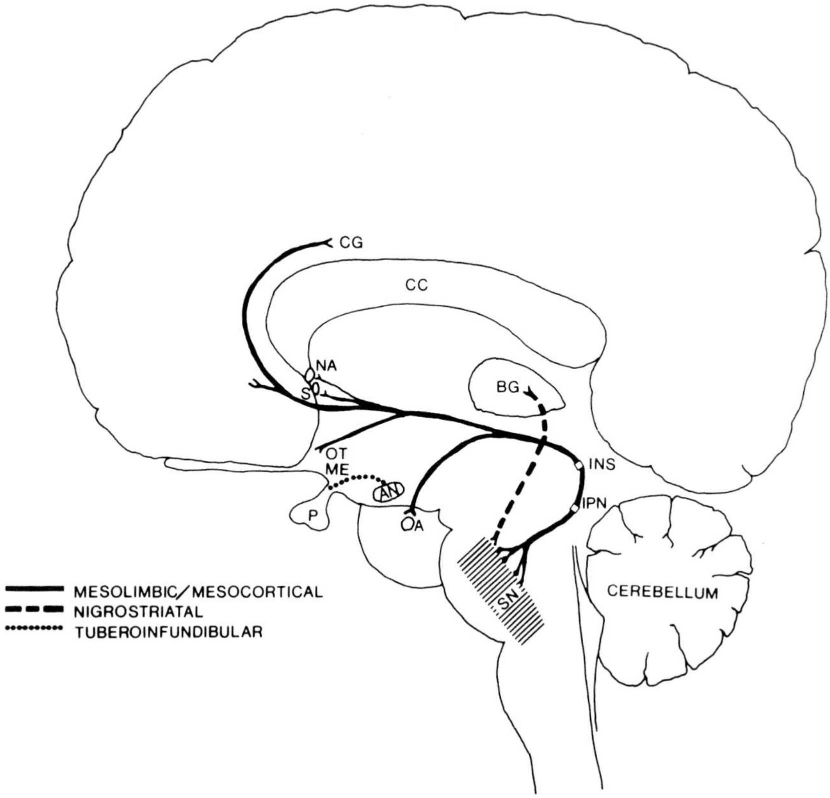

Fig. 1. Schematic representation of dopaminergic pathways. A = amygdaloid; AN = arcuate nucleus; BG = basal ganglia; CC = corpus callosum; CG = cingulate gyrus; INS = interstitial nucleus of stria terminalis; IPN = interpeduncular nucleus; ME = median eminence; NA = nucleus accumbens; OT = olfactory tubercle; P = pituitary; S = septal nucleus; SN = substantia nigra.

TABLE 1

Effect of antipsychotic drugs on hormonal concentrations.

Prolactin	Increased
Growth hormone	No significant change
Cortisol	No significant change
TSH	No significant change
LH	Decreased?
FSH	Decreased?
Testosterone	No significant change
	Decreased

ability to block dopamine receptors, or like reserpine to deplete DA stores, many of them affect other neurotransmitter systems (e.g. norepinephrine, acetylcholine) as well. Furthermore, when larger doses of the drug are administered than needed to block DA transmission, other systems could be non-specifically affected. In this chapter we review studies of antipsychotic drugs upon the following hormones: PRL, GH, cortisol, thyrotropin, gonadotropins and testosterone. A summary of the effects of antipsychotic drugs on hormonal concentrations is presented in Table 1.

PROLACTIN

Frantz and Kleinberg reported in 1970 that chlorpromazine stimulates PRL in man. Since then several studies have confirmed that different classes of dopamine blocking drugs do stimulate PRL release in humans. They include phenothiazines, butyrophenones, diphenylbutylpiperidines, thioxanthenes, dihydroindolones, and dibenzoxazepines. Recently, other drugs that have been added to this list are sulpiride, from the (substituted benzamides) ortopramide group, metoclopramide, a procaineamide derivative and domperidone. There are some exceptions such as clozapine which is an effective antipsychotic that does not significantly induce PRL release. It is believed that clozapine has preferential effect on the mesolimbic dopaminergic system with very little action on the tuberoinfundibular dopaminergic system. On the other hand, metoclopramide stimulates PRL but seems to have antipsychotic effects only at higher doses. Domperidone has been reported to be a peripheral dopamine antagonist which does not cross the blood-brain barrier. However, it does reach the median eminence and the pituitary, stimulating PRL release.

It has reliably been shown that even small amounts of neuroleptics, chlorpromazine 25 mg or haloperidol 0.25 mg, administered parenterally can produce a consistent increase in PRL levels (Rubin et al., 1976a; Langer et al., 1977b, 1979; Gruen et al., 1978b; Rubin and Hays, 1979). There is also a dose-related increase in morning serum PRL levels until the equivalent of 600 – 800 mg of chlorpromazine per day is achieved (Meltzer et al., 1978). Busch et al. (1979) have administered chlorpromazine 25 mg i.m. to drug-free schizophrenic patients and Rubin and Forster (1980) gave haloperidol 0.5 mg i.m. to 18 normal volunteers and 0.5 mg i.v. to 7 volunteers and found that 3 hour monitoring of plasma PRL levels reflect an adequate sampling time. Langer et al. (1977b) reported that doses below 0.25 mg of haloperidol did not consistently release PRL and doses above 1.5 mg of haloperidol (or dose equivalence of another neuroleptic) did not consistently elevate peak PRL responses further. However, several investigators have shown that a further increase in the treatment baseline PRL could be induced by a subsequent challenge dose of a neuroleptic drug (Meltzer, 1980; Kolakowska et al., 1981a, b) or other stimuli (Nathan et al., 1981).

During neuroleptic treatment of up to 12 months, plasma PRL levels remain elevated (DeRivera et al., 1976; Meltzer and Fang, 1976; Meltzer et al., 1978; Gruen et al., 1978a). However, there is some controversy regarding the PRL levels in patients treated with neuroleptics more chronically. DeRivera et al. (1976) reported that acute administration of neuroleptics (2 – 4 weeks) resulted in significantly higher PRL levels than did chronic therapy (5 years or more) with similar daily doses in both the young and older women. They also observed that seven out of 26 of the chronically treated women had normal PRL values, suggesting some degree of adaptation to neuroleptic-induced PRL rise. Zander et al. (1981) observed that CSF and plasma PRL concentrations in 13 schizophrenic patients decreased from high normal range during chronic treatment to lower levels 30 days after drug withdrawal. Beumont et al. (1974a) found PRL levels to be within the normal range in five patients on chronic neuroleptic treatment. Wilson et al. (1975) reported elevated mean PRL levels in chronically (8 years) treated female patients compared to a control population. Naber et al. (1979) reported an absence of increased PRL levels in all 23 male and 29 out of 35 female patients treated with neuroleptics for 13 $\pm$ 4 years, suggesting a tolerance of the tuberoinfundibular (PRL) system. However, Chouinard et al. (1981) found the expected higher PRL levels in patients treated with neuroleptics for several years (median 16 years), supporting a lack of tolerance to long-term neuroleptic treatment in the tuberoinfundibular (PRL) system. It appears that tolerance of the tuberoinfundibular dopamine system with regard to PRL release does not occur at least for several years. Several studies examining the short-term effects of antipsychotic drugs on PRL levels support this view (Gruen et al., 1978a; Siris et al., 1978; Nathan et al., 1981). Three days after discontinuation of antipsychotic drugs, PRL levels decline to normal range in the majority of patients (Meltzer and Fang, 1976).

Factors influencing the PRL response to neuroleptics

Several factors influence the PRL response to neuroleptics.

Estrogens. It is known that woman have higher basal PRL levels than men. Women during their reproductive years respond with enhanced PRL secretion after neuroleptic administration. This is true during both acute and chronic neuroleptic treatment. Higher estrogen levels in women have been suggested to contribute to this enhanced neuroleptic-induced PRL response (Buckman et al., 1976). Exogenous estrogen administration has been shown to potentiate phenothiazine-induced PRL secretion (Buckman and Peake, 1973). In a preliminary report, Nathan et al. (1983a) found that basal PRL levels and PRL response to acute and 6 weeks of penfluridol treatment were consistently higher in female patients compared to male schizophrenic patients. It is of interest to note that the plasma penfluridol levels were lower (although corresponding PRL levels were higher) in female patients compared to male patients.

Anticholinergic drugs. The centrally acting anticholinergic drug, benztropine mesylate has been reported to enhance the PRL response to intramuscular haloperidol in man (Lal and Nair, 1979). Subsequently, Halbreich et al. (1980) observed a delay in the PRL response to intramuscular haloperidol after intramuscular benztropine mesylate. We administered 0.5 mg of benztropine intravenously followed by 0.5 mg of haloperidol intravenously in six healthy young men and observed that benztropine significantly potentiates the PRL response to haloperidol (Nathan et al., 1982a). In collaboration with Perel, we further observed that the plasma haloperidol levels were also increased after benztropine in these subjects (Table 2). In this study, the absorption variables for both the drugs were eliminated because of the choice of intravenous administration. Our data seem to explain the findings of Calil et al. (1979) and Sachar et al. (1975). Calil et al. (1979) found much higher levels of plasma thioridazine than chlorpromazine following chronic administration of both drugs. Sachar et al. (1975) reported that the increase in serum PRL levels produced by 50 mg of thioridazine orally was larger and more rapid than that produced by the same dose of chlorpromazine in the same subjects. It is possible that the administration of thioridazine which has stronger anticholinergic properties may result in higher plasma thioridazine and PRL concentrations compared to chlorpromazine with weaker anticholinergic effects. These data are also consistent with those of Kolakowska et al. (1976), DeRivera et al. (1976) and Martin-du Pan et al. (1979).

Chronobiological effect. Antipsychotic drugs are generally administered in multiple doses or as a single dose at night to schizophrenic patients. Using a chronobiological approach we have already shown that the PRL responses to PRL-releasing stimuli such as insulin-induced hypoglycemia (Nathan et al., 1979) and thyrotropin-stimulating hormone (TSH) (Nathan et al., 1982b) are significantly greater when they are administered in the evening. We observed (Fig. 2) that the PRL response

TABLE 2

Plasma haloperidol concentrations in five healthy men after haloperidol (0.5 mg i.v.) and after benztropine (0.5 mg i.v.) followed by haloperidol (0.5 mg i.v.). These studies were done at 9 a.m. on different days.

Subjects	Plasma haloperidol concentration (ng/ml) (area under the curve)	
	After haloperidol	After benztropine and haloperidol
1	205.8	460.2
2	267.6	1908.0
3	233.4	412.2
4	466.8	1128.0
5	144.0	1032.0

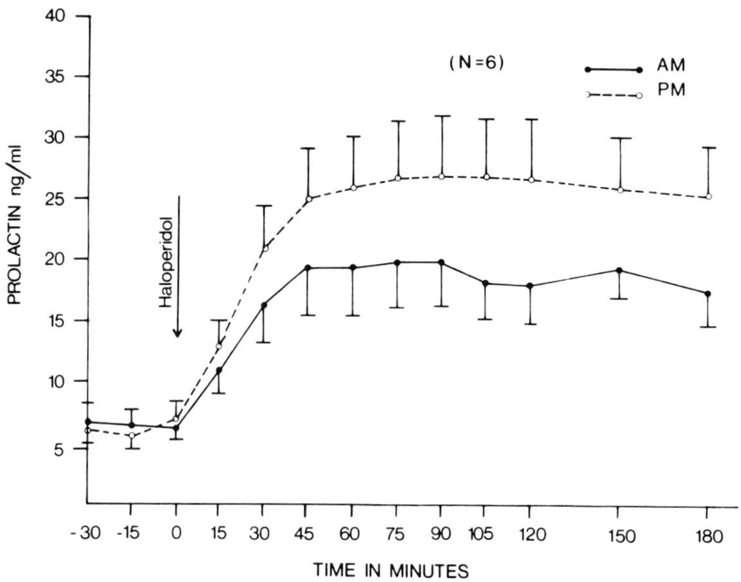

Fig. 2. Diurnal prolactin responses to haloperidol.

to 0.5 mg of intravenous haloperidol was larger in the evening than in the morning in six young healthy men (Nathan et al., 1983b).

Application of PRL releasing effects of neuroleptics

Some of the dopamine receptor blocking antipsychotic drugs are currently employed in clinical endocrinology to test the pituitary PRL reserve, to investigate the hypothalamo-pituitary axis or to explore the dopaminergic involvement in certain conditions including schizophrenia. The hypothesized hyper-dopaminergic activity in schizophrenic patients could be reflected in the basal PRL levels. However, in a majority of studies basal PRL levels were found to be within normal limits in drug-free schizophrenic patients. However, Brambilla et al. (1979) reported that basal PRL levels were markedly decreased in six chronic schizophrenic patients who had been recently withdrawn from antipsychotic drugs. Johnstone et al. (1977) and Kleinman et al. (1982) reported an inverse correlation between PRL concentrations and positive psychotic symptoms. It is of interest to note that Kleinman et al. (1982) found this inverse relationship only in schizophrenic patients with normal cerebral ventricular brain ratio but not in patients with enlarged cerebral ventricles. PRL responses to acute neuroleptic administration were also not significantly different between schizophrenic patients and normal subjects (Gruen et al., 1978b).

Further studies are directed at finding the relationship between PRL levels and improvements in psychotic symptoms in schizophrenic patients. Langer et al.

(1977a) reported a strongly significant correlation between PRL-releasing and antipsychotic potencies of seven neuroleptic drugs at low doses. Meltzer et al. (1978) found a significant correlation between a decrease in psychoses and an increase in PRL during the first 2 weeks of neuroleptic treatment. This correlation between changes in psychoses and in PRL at different time points of neuroleptic treatment has also been observed by several investigators. Ohman and Axelsson (1978) reported significant correlations within subjects over time between their PRL responses and their therapeutic responses to thioridazine. Siris et al. (1978) reported that in a small group of male and female schizophrenic patients there was a decrease in psychoses and an increase in PRL correlated after 4 weeks of pimozide treatment. However, this correlation was not found by other investigators (Langer et al., 1978; Gruen et al., 1978a) and could not be replicated by Siris et al. (1978). Sedvall (1979) and Bowers et al. (1982) have shown that PRL levels in plasma correlate well with CSF PRL levels. Sedvall (1979) reported a significant correlation between treatment outcome and the PRL elevations in both plasma and CSF in patients treated with chlorpromazine but not with other antipsychotic drugs.

The potential use of PRL measurements as a reflection of plasma neuroleptic concentration has been proposed. However, in patients on chronic neuroleptic treatment, plasma PRL levels have not been consistently useful as an index of plasma drug levels. Periodic PRL measurement in patients has also been suggested as a means of detecting non-compliance in drug-taking.

There is some evidence in schizophrenic patients receiving chronic neuroleptic treatment that the basal PRL levels give an indication of their relapse potential. Brown and Laughren (1981) and Laughren et al. (1979) reported that patients who had lowest PRL levels after withdrawal from maintenance treatment showed a greater degree of clinical deterioration.

GROWTH HORMONE (GH)

Benjamin et al. (1969) and Sherman et al. (1971) reported an inhibition of GH levels during neuroleptic administration but later reports by Beumont et al. (1972) Brambilla et al. (1975) Saldanha et al. (1972) and Nathan et al. (1981) did not indicate significant effects on GH levels. Chronic administration of chlorpromazine has been reported to have no effect on GH levels (Beg et al., 1979). More recent studies utilizing more selective dopamine blocking drugs like pimozide (Collu et al., 1975) and penfluridol (Nathan et al., 1981) have reported an absence of any significant effect on GH levels.

CORTISOL

Antipsychotic drugs have been shown, more consistently, not to induce any significant effect on the basal plasma cortisol levels (Franzen, 1971; Sachar, 1975; Nathan et al., 1981). Elevated urinary free cortisol decreased into normal range with pimozide (de Fraite and van Kammen, unpublished data 1979).

THYROID HORMONES

Significant changes in thyroid function have not been noted during neuroleptic drug treatment. Collu et al. (1975) reported a significant decrease in TSH levels in five subjects during pimozide (4 mg) treatment for 4 days. However, Naber et al. (1980a) found no significant change in thyroxin, triiodothyroxin and TSH during acute neuroleptic treatment in nine acute schizophrenic patients and in thyroxin, thyroxin-binding globulin and TSH in 22 chronic schizophrenic patients. Rinieris et al. (1980) reported that T4 and FTI were significantly lower in 24 of 41 schizophrenic patients treated with neuroleptics for 6 years. Wode-Helgodt et al. (1977) found no effect of 4 weeks treatment with chlorpromazine on cerebrospinal fluid or plasma levels of TSH. In summary, there is no convincing evidence to suggest any significant clinical change in thyroid function during antipsychotic drug treatment.

Thyrotropin-releasing hormone (TRH) tests have been performed in schizophrenic patients treated with antipsychotic drugs (Naber et al., 1980b, c; Braddock and Blake, 1981). These studies indicate that TSH, LH and PRL responses to TRH are not markedly impaired by chronic neuroleptic treatment.

GONADOTROPINS

The reported effects of antipsychotic drugs on gonadotropins are mixed. After acute or short-term antipsychotic drug treatment, basal LH levels may be unchanged (Rubin et al., 1976a, b; Cotes et al., 1978) increased (Brambilla et al., 1975) or decreased (Collu et al., 1975; Siris et al., 1980). Chronic neuroleptic treatment produced no significant change in basal LH levels (Beumont et al., 1974a; Naber et al., 1980b). Using a relatively specific dopamine receptor blocker, pimozide, Siris et al. (1980) have shown in nine patients a decrease in LH levels, consistent with the reports of Collu et al. (1975). Conceivably the increasing PRL levels may have stimulated DA turnover, which is compatible with the observations that DA and DA agonists lower LH levels (Leblanc et al., 1976; Lachelin et al., 1977). However, Siris et al. observed that despite the apparent decline in gonadal hormones during pimozide treatment, the circulating concentrations of gonadotropins were within normal range. It is interesting to note that LH values were significantly lower in patients treated chronically with thioridazine compared to those treated with other neuroleptics (Brown et al., 1981).

Similar to LH, FSH levels after neuroleptic administration have been shown to be unchanged (Rubin et al., 1976a, b; Cotes et al., 1978), increased (Brambilla et al., 1975) or decreased (Collu et al., 1975; Siris et al., 1980). Wode-Helgodt et al. (1977) found no effect of 4 weeks of treatment with chlorpromazine on CSF or plasma levels of FSH and LH.

TESTOSTERONE (T)

There are conflicting reports regarding the effect of antipsychotic drugs on T levels. Beumont et al. (1974b) reported low or normal plasma T concentrations that increased after the withdrawal of phenothiazines. Brambilla et al. (1975) observed after haloperidol treatment, a return to normal values of basically reduced T. Rubin et al. (1976b) observed increased T levels in volunteers after acute haloperidol administration. Serum T levels similar to LH were reported to be lower after thioridazine (Brown et al., 1981). Other investigators (Arato et al., 1979; Martin-du Pan et al., 1979; Siris et al., 1980) did not find any significant effect of antipsychotic drug treatment on T levels. Since the effect of dopamine blocking drugs on T may not be a direct one, investigators have tried to define the relationship between T and PRL levels during antipsychotic drug administration. Rubin et al. (1976b) have shown in normal volunteers that PRL may act as a mild, acute stimulus to T secretion, but Nathan et al. (1980), Martin-du Pan et al. (1979) and Arato et al. (1979) did not find any significant relationship between PRL and T in schizophrenic patients on antipsychotic drugs.

The major direct stimulus for the secretion of T from Leydig's cells is LH. LH is secreted by the anterior pituitary under the influence of hypothalamic gonadotropin-releasing hormone and the feedback inhibition exerted by T. PRL appears to reduce endogenous responsiveness to LH and to reduce conversion of T to its active metabolite dihydrotestosterone. This regulating role of PRL seems to be of considerable clinical significance (Franks et al., 1978). In addition, PRL may act as a mild, acute stimulus to T in normal adult men (Rubin et al., 1978). As will be described later in this chapter, these possible interactions between PRL, LH and T may play a role in the development of sexual disorders resulting from antipsychotic treatment.

CLINICAL NEUROENDOCRINE EFFECTS OF ANTIPSYCHOTIC DRUG TREATMENT

Thus, the major and consistent effect of antipsychotic drug treatment appears to be the induction of a hyperprolactinemic state. This hyperprolactinemic condition could, at least in part, explain many of the reported endocrine side effects. The more commonly recognized effects include galactorrhea, menstrual disorders and sexual disturbances (Table 3).

Galactorrhea has long been known as a common side effect of antipsychotic drug treatment. Robinson (1957) found the incidence of galactorrhea to be 10%; Plante and Roy (1967) 57%; Apostolakis et al. (1972) 50%; Rives and Rosier (1959) nearly 50%. Drug-related galactorrhea usually occurs within the first year of antipsychotic medication use.

Menstrual disorders, especially amenorrhea resulting from antipsychotic drug

TABLE 3

Clinical neuroendocrine effects of antipsychotic drug treatment.

1. Galactorrhea
2. Menstrual irregularities – amenorrhea
3. Sexual dysfunctions
   - impotence
   - erectile difficulties
   - ejaculatory difficulties
   - decreased libido
   - decreased semen volume and sperm count
   - absence of orgasm
4. Although suspected, increase in the incidence of human breast cancer has not been established

treatment has been described in many patients. Ghadirian et al. (1982) reported 91% of 29 female patients experienced menstrual irregularities. Beumont et al. (1974a) reported that in amenorrheic patients, basal levels of LH were variable, midcycle peaks were absent, and values of estrogen and progesterone were within the range found normally during the follicular phase of the menstrual cycle. They have shown in two of those patients that these effects were due to the drugs, by the resumption of menstruation and of normal cyclical hormonal changes on withdrawal of medication.

Antipsychotic drugs have been implicated in the production of sexual dysfunction. Kotin et al. (1976) reported an increased incidence of impotence, erectile difficulties, decreased libido and ejaculatory difficulties in patients treated with thioridazine compared to other neuroleptics. Blair and Simpson (1966) reported a decrease in the semen volume and in the sperm count of men treated with neuroleptics. Occurrence of higher incidence of ejaculatory difficulties caused by thioridazine has been observed by several investigators (Blair and Simpson, 1966; Kotin et al., 1976). These authors have also described drug-related decreased libido, erectile impotence and interference with orgasm. Ghadirian et al. (1982) reported 54% of 26 male schizophrenic patients and 30% of 29 female patients experienced moderate to moderately severe sexual dysfunction including orgasmic difficulties during antipsychotic drug treatment.

Antipsychotic drugs may cause sexual dysfunction at several levels: at the CNS level with sedation and parkinsonian effects, at the peripheral level blocking cholinergic and alpha adrenergic receptors or indirectly at the hormonal level increasing PRL levels (Horowitz and Goble, 1979; Nestoros et al., 1980; Ghadirian et al., 1982).

Elevated PRL level increases the incidence of spontaneously occurring mammary tumors in mice and increases the growth of established carcinogen-induced mammary tumors in rats. These observations have raised serious concerns regarding the relationship between antipsychotic drug-induced hyperprolactinemia and carcinoma of the breast in humans. Schyve et al. (1978) extensively reviewed this issue including epidemiological evidence and concluded that at this time there is no unequivocal evidence to support the view that prolonged use of antipsychotic drugs might increase the incidence of breast cancer. In a more recent study, Goode et al. (1981) reviewed the cases of breast cancer in 1969 – 1978 among the female population of a large psychiatric hospital and compared the incidence and prevalence rates of this group to expected rates. They too concluded that the rates of breast cancer among those psychiatric patients were no higher despite their use of antipsychotic drugs.

CONCLUSIONS

The major endocrinological effect of neuroleptics appears to be the rise in PRL levels. Several of the clinical endocrine effects are secondary to this rise in PRL. The sexual dysfunctions observed with neuroleptic treatment may be related to the prolactin increase, to decreased autonomic arousal, to possibly decreased gonadotropin function or to alpha receptor blockade. There is no definitive evidence linking increased incidence of breast cancer to neuroleptic treatment. Anticholinergic agents may lead to increased prolactin response during neuroleptic treatment. Tolerance to the rise in PRL does not occur during short-term neuroleptic administration but may occur late in treatment. Growth hormone and cortisol release and thyroid function do not appear to be significantly affected by neuroleptics. Even though the antipsychotic drugs are potent pharmacological agents, the long-term endocrinological effects are rather small with no evidence of major permanent changes in endocrine function.

REFERENCES

Apostolakis, M., Kapetanakis, S., Lazos, G. and Madena-Pyrgaki, A. (1972) Plasma prolactin activity in patients with galactorrhoea after treatment with psychotropic drugs. In: G. E. W. Wolstenholme and A. Knight (Eds), Lactogenic Hormones. Churchill Livingston, London and Edinburgh, pp. 349 – 354.

Arato, M., Erdos, A. and Polgar, M. (1979) Endocrinological changes in patients with sexual dysfunction under long-term neuroleptic treatment. Pharmacopsychiatrie 12, 426 – 431.

Beg, A. A., Varma, V. K. and Dash, R. J. (1979) The effect of chlorpromazine on human growth hormone. Am. J. Psychiatry 136, 914 – 917.

Benjamin, F., Casper D. J. and Kolodny, H. S. (1969) Immunoreactive human growth hormone in conditions associated with galactorrhea. Obstet. Gynecol. 34, 34 – 39.

Beumont, P. J. V., Harris, G. W., Carr, P. J., Friesen H. G., Kolakowska, T., MacKinnon, P. C. B., Mandelbrote, B. M. and Wiles, D. (1972) Some endocrine effects of phenothiazines: a preliminary report. J. Psychosom. Res. 16, 297 – 304.

Beumont, P. J. V., Gelder, M. G., Friesen, H. G., Harris, G. W., MacKinnon, P. C. B., Mandelbrote,

B. M. and Wiles, D. H. (1974a) The effects of phenothiazines on endocrine function. I. Patients with inappropriate lactation and amenorrhoea. Br. J. Psychiatry 124, 413 – 419.

Beumont, P. J. V., Corker, C. S., Friesen, H. G., Kolakowska, T., Mandelbrote, B. M., Marshall, J., Murray, M. A. F. and Wiles, D. H. (1974b) The effects of phenothiazines on endocrine function. II. Effects in men and post-menopausal women. Br. J. Psychiatry 124, 420 – 430.

Blair, J. H. and Simpson, G. M. (1966) Effect of antipsychotic drugs on reproductive function. Dis. Nerv. Syst. 27, 645 – 647.

Bowers, Jr., M. B., Meltzer, H. Y. and Heniger, G. R. (1982) Correlation of plasma and CSF prolactin with CSF GABA during neuroleptic treatment. Life Sci. 31, 59 – 65.

Braddock, L. E. and Blake, I. M. (1981) The TRH test. Br. J. Psychiatry 139, 404 – 407.

Brambilla, F., Guerrini, A., Guastalla, A., Rovere, C. and Riggi, F. (1975) Neuroendocrine effects of haloperidol therapy in chronic schizophrenia. Psychoneuroendocrinologia 44, 17 – 22.

Brambilla, F., Bellodi, L., Negri, F., Smeraldi, E. and Malagoli, G. (1979) Dopamine receptor sensitivity in the hypothalamus of chronic schizophrenics after haloperidol therapy growth hormone and prolactin response to stimuli. Psychoneuroendocrinology 4, 329 – 339.

Brown, W. A. and Laughren, T. P. (1981) Low serum prolactin and early relapse following neuroleptic withdrawal. Am. J. Psychiatry 138, 237 – 239.

Brown, W. A., Laughren, T. P. and Williams, B. (1981) Differential effects of neuroleptic agents on the pituitary-gonadal axis in men. Arch. Gen. Psychiatry 38, 1270 – 1272.

Buckman, M. T. and Peake, G. T. (1973) Estrogen potentiation of phenothiazine-induced prolactin secretion in man. J. Clin. Endocrinol. Metab. 37, 977 – 980.

Buckman, M. T., Peake, G. T. and Srivastava, L. S. (1976) Endogenous estrogen modulates phenothiazine stimulated prolactin secretion. J. Clin. Endocrinol. Metab. 43, 901 – 906.

Busch, D. A., Fang, V. S. and Meltzer, H. Y. (1979) Serum prolactin levels following intramuscular chlorpromazine. two- and three-hour response as predictors of six-hour response. Psychiatry Res. 1, 153 – 159.

Calil, H. M., Avery, D. H. and Hollister, L. E. (1979) Serum levels of neuroleptics measured by dopamine radio receptor-assay and some clinical observations. Psychiatry Res. 1, 39 – 44.

Chouinard, G., Annable, L., Jones, B. D. and Collu, R. (1981) Lack of tolerance to long-term neuroleptic treatment in dopamine tuberoinfundibular system. Acta Psychiat. Scand. 64, 353 – 362.

Collu, R., Jequier, J. C., Leboeuf, G., Letarte, J. and Ducharme, J. R. (1975) Endocrine effects of pimozide, a specific dopaminergic blocker. J. Clin. Endocrinol. Metab. 44, 981 – 984.

Cotes, P. M., Crow, T. J., Johnstone, E. C., Bartlett, W. and Bourne, R. C. (1978) Neuroendocrine changes in acute schizophrenia as a function of clinical state and neuroleptic medication. Psychol. Med. 8, 657 – 665.

DeRivera, J. L., Lal, S., Ettigi, P., Hontela, S., Muller, H. F. and Friesen, H. G. (1976) Effect of acute and chronic neuroleptic therapy on serum prolactin levels in men and women of different age groups. Clin. Endocrinol. 5, 273 – 282.

Franks, S., Jacobs, H. S., Martin, N. and Nabarro, J. D. N. (1978) Hyperprolactinemia and impotence. Clin. Endocrinol. 8, 277 – 287.

Frantz, A. G. and Kleinberg, D. L. (1970) Prolactin: evidence that it is separate from growth hormone in human blood. Science 170, 745 – 747.

Franzen, G. (1971) Serum cortisol in chronic schizophrenia. Acta Psychiatr. Scand. 47, 150 – 162.

Ghadirian, A. M., Chouinard, G. and Annable, L. (1982) Sexual dysfunction and plasma prolactin levels in neuroleptic-treated schizophrenic outpatients. J. Nerv. Ment. Dis. 170, 463 – 467.

Goode, D. J., Corbett, W. T., Schey, H. M., Suh, S. H., Woodie, B., Morris, D. L. and Morrisey, L. (1981) Breast cancer in hospitalized psychiatric patients. Am. J. Psychiatry 138, 804 – 806.

Gruen, P. H., Sachar, E. J., Altman, N., Langer, G., Tabrizi, M. A. and Halpern, F. S. (1978a) Relation of plasma prolactin to clinical response in schizophrenic patients. Arch. Gen. Psychiatry 35, 1222 – 1227.

Gruen, P. H., Sachar, E. J., Langer, G., Altman, N., Leifer, M., Frantz, A. and Halpern, F. S. (1978b) Prolactin response to neuroleptics in normal and schizophrenic subjects. Arch. Gen. Psychiatry 35, 108 – 116.

Halbreich, U., Sachar, E. J., Nathan, R. S., Asnis, G. M. and Halpern, F. S. (1980) The effect of benztropine methylate on the prolactin response to haloperidol. Psychopharmacology 72, 61 – 65.

Horowitz, J. D. and Goble, A. J. (1979) Drugs and impaired male sexual function. Drugs 18, 206 – 217.

Johnstone, E. C., Crow, T. J. and Mashiter, K. (1977) Anterior pituitary hormone secretion in chronic schizophrenia – an approach to neurohumoral mechanisms. Psychol. Med. 7, 223 – 228.

Kleinman, J. E., Weinberger, D. R., Rogol, A. D., Bigelow, L. B., Klein, S. T., Gillin, J. C. and Wyatt, R. J. (1982) Plasma prolactin concentrations and psychopathology in chronic schizophrenia. Arch. Gen. Psychiatry 35, 655 – 657.

Kolakowska, T., Wiles, D. H., Gelder, M. G. and McNeilly, A. S. (1976) Clinical significance of plasma chlorpromazine levels. II. Plasma levels of the drug, some of its metabolites and prolactin in patients receiving long term phenothiazine treatment. Psychopharmacology 49, 101 – 107.

Kolakowska, T., Braddock, L., Wiles, D., Franklin, M. and Gelder, M. (1981a) Neuroendocrine tests during treatment with neuroleptic drugs. I. Plasma prolactin response to haloperidol challenge. Br. J. Psychiatry 139, 400 – 412.

Kolakowska, T., Fraser, S., Franklin, M. and Knox, J. (1981b) Neuroendocrine tests during treatment with neuroleptic drugs. I. Plasma prolactin response to chlorpromazine challenge. Psychopharmacology 72, 283 – 285.

Kotin, J., Wilbert, D. E., Verburg, D. and Soldinger, S. M. (1976) Thioridazine and sexual dysfunction. Am. J. Psychiatry 133, 82 – 85.

Lachelin, G. C. L., Leblanc, H. and Yen, S. S. C. (1977) The inhibitory effect of dopamine agonist on LH release in women. J. Clin. Endocrinol. and Metabolism 44, 728 – 732.

Lal, S. and Nair, N. P. V. (1979) Growth hormone and prolactin responses in neuropsychiatric research. In: E. Muller and A. Agnoli (Eds), Neuroendocrine Correlates in Neurology and Psychiatry. Elsevier/North-Holland Biomedical Press, Amsterdam, pp. 179 – 194.

Langer, G., Sachar, E. J. and Gruen, P. H. (1977a) Human prolactin responses to neuroleptic drugs correlate with antischizophrenic potency. Nature (London) 226, 639 – 640.

Langer, G., Sachar, E. J., Halpern, F. S., Gruen, B. H. and Solomon, M. (1977b) The prolactin response to neuroleptic drugs. A test of dopaminergic blockade: neuroendocrine studies in normal men. J. Clin. Endocrinol. Metab. 45, 996 – 1002.

Langer, G., Sachar, E. S. and Gruen, P. H. (1978) Prolactin response to neuroleptic drugs in normal and schizophrenic subjects. Psychopharmacol. Bull. 14, 8 – 9.

Langer, G., Sachar, E. J., Nathan, R. S., Tabrizi, M. A., Perel, J. M. and Halpern, F. S. (1979) Dopaminergic factors in human prolactin regulation: a pituitary model for the study of a neuroendocrine system in man. Psychopharmacology 65, 161 – 164.

Laughren, T. P., Brown, W. A. and Williams, B. W. (1979) Serum prolactin and clinical state during neuroleptic treatment and withdrawal. Am. J. Psychiatry 136, 108 – 110.

Leblanc, H., Lachelin, G. C. L., Abu-Fadil, S. and Yen, S. S. C. (1976) Effects of dopamine infusion on pituitary hormone secretion in humans. J. Clin. Endocrinol. Metab. 43, 668 – 674.

Martin-du Pan, R., Baumann, P., Magrini, G. and Felber, J. P. (1979) Neuroendocrine effects of chronic neuroleptic therapy in male psychiatric patients. Psychoneuroendocrinology 3, 245 – 252.

Meltzer, H. Y. (1980) Effect of psychotropic drugs on neuroendocrine function. Psychiatr. Clin. North Am. 3, 277 – 298.

Meltzer, H. Y. and Fang, V. S. (1976) The effect of neuroleptics on serum prolactin in schizophrenic patients. Arch. Gen. Psychiatry 33, 279 – 286.

Meltzer, H. Y., Goode, D. J. and Fang, V. S. (1978) The effect of psychotropic drugs on endocrine function. I. Neuroleptics, precursors and agonists. In: M. A. Lipton, A. D. Mascio and K. F. Killam

(Eds), Psychopharmacology: A Generation of Progress. Raven Press, New York, pp. 509–529.

Naber, D., Fischer, H. and Ackenheil, M. (1979) Effect of long-term neuroleptic treatment on dopamine tuberoinfundibular system: development of tolerance? Commun. Psychopharmacol. 3, 59–65.

Naber, D., Steinböck, H. and Greil, W. (1980a) Effects of short- and long-term neuroleptic treatment on thyroid function. Prog. Neuropsychopharmacol. 4, 199–206.

Naber, D., Ackenheil, M. and Laakmann, G. (1980b) Basal and stimulated levels of prolactin, TSH, and LH in serum of chronic schizophrenic patients long-term treated with neuroleptics: relations to psychopathology. Adv. Biochem. Psychopharmacol. 24, 419–423.

Naber, D., Ackenheil, M., Laakman, G., Fischer, H. and von Werder, K. (1980c) Basal and stimulated levels of PRL, TSH and LH in serum of chronic schizophrenic patients, long-term treated with neuroleptics. Pharmacopsychiatry 13, 325–330.

Nathan, R. S., Sachar, E. J., Langer, G., Tabrizi, M. A. and Halpern, F. S. (1979) Diurnal variation in the response of plasma PRL, cortisol and GH to insulin-induced hypoglycemia in normal men. J. Clin. Endocrinol. Metab. 49, 231–235.

Nathan, R. S., Asnis, G. M., Dyrenfurth, I., Halpern, F. S., Halbreich, U, Ostrow, L. C. and Sachar, E. J. (1980) Plasma prolactin and testosterone during penfluridol treatment. Lancet ii, 94.

Nathan, R. S., Sachar, E. J., Ostrow, L., Asnis, G. M., Halbreich, U. and Halpern, F. S. (1981) Failure of dopaminergic blockade to affect prolactin, growth hormone, and cortisol responses to insulin-induced hypoglycemia in schizophrenics. J. Clin. Endocrinol. Metab. 52, 807–809.

Nathan, R. S., Perel, J. M., McCarthy, T. and Jarrett, D. (1982a) Factors potentiating the prolactin responses to neuroleptics. APA Meeting, 1982. New Research Abstracts, NR10, Toronto, Canada, May 15–21, 1982.

Nathan, R. S., Sachar, E. J., Tabrizi, M. A., Asnis, G. M., Halbreich, U. and Halpern, F. S. (1982b) Diurnal hormonal responses to thyrotropin-releasing hormone in normal men. Psychoneuroendocrinology 7, 235–238.

Nathan, R. S., Sachar, E. J., Ostrow, L., Asnis, G. M., Halbreich, U., Halpern, F. S., Renzi, N. L. and Slotnick, V. (1983a) Sex related differences in the prolactin responses to dopamine blockade, to insulin hypoglycemia and in the plasma penfluridol level in schizophrenic patients. Psychopharmacology 80, 46–49.

Nathan, R. S., Perel, J. M., McCarthy, T. and Jarrett, D. B. (1983b) Diurnal pattern in the prolactin responses to haloperidol in man. In: G. Tolis, C. Stefanis, T. Mountokalakis and F. Labrie (Eds), Prolactin and Prolactinomas. Raven Press, New York, pp. 143–149.

Nestoros, J. N., Lehmann, H. E. and Ban, T. A. (1980) Neuroleptic drugs and sexual functions in schizophrenia. In: T. A. Ban (Ed.), Modern Problems in Pharmacopsychiatry, Vol. 15. Karger, Basel, pp. 111–130.

Ohman, R., and Axelsson, R. (1978) The relationship between prolactin response and antipsychotic effect of thioridazine in psychiatric patients. Eur. J. Clin. Pharmacol. 14, 111–116.

Plante, N. and Roy, P. (1967) Galactorrhoea and neuroleptics. Laval Med. 38, 103–107.

Rinieris, P., Christodoulou, G. N., Souvatzoglou, A., Koutras, D. A. and Stefanis, C. (1980) Free-thyroxine index in schizophrenic patients before and after neuroleptic treatment. Neuropsychobiology 6, 29–33.

Rives, O. P. and Rosier, Y. (1959) The frequent occurrence of galactorrhoea during prolonged treatment with phenothiazines. Entretiens Franco-allemands de Therapeutique Psychiatrique, pp. 177–178, Lyon.

Robinson, B. (1957) Breast changes in the male and female with chlorpromazine or reserpine therapy. Med. J. Aust. 44, 239–241.

Rubin, R. T. and Hays, S. E. (1979) Variability of prolactin response to intravenous and intramuscular haloperidol in normal adult men. Psychopharmacology 61, 17–24.

Rubin, R. T. and Forster, B. (1980) Haloperidol stimulation of prolactin secretion: how many blood samples are needed to define the hormone response? Commun. Psychopharmacol. 4, 41 – 47.

Rubin, R. T., Poland, R. E., O'Connor, D., Gouin, P. R. and Tower, B. B. (1976a) Selective neuroendocrine effects of low-dose haloperidol in normal adult men. Psychopharmacology 47, 135 – 140.

Rubin, R. T., Poland, R. E. and Tower, B. B. (1976b) Prolactin-related testosterone secretion in normal adult men. J. Clin. Endocrinol. Metab. 42, 112 – 116.

Rubin, R. T., Poland, R. E., Sobil, I., Tower, B. B. and Odell, W. D. (1978) Effects of prolactin and prolactin plus luteinizing hormone on plasma testosterone levels in normal adult men. J. Clin. Endocrinol. Metab. 47, 447 – 452.

Sachar, E. J. (1975) Twenty-four hour cortisol secretory patterns in depressed and manic patients. In: W. H. Gispen, T. J. B. van Wimersma Greidanus, B. Bohus and D. de Wied (Eds), Progress in Brain Research: Hormones, Homeostasis and the Brain, Vol. 42. Elsevier, Amsterdam, pp. 81 – 91.

Sachar, E. J., Gruen, P. H., Karasu, T. B., Altman, N. and Frantz, A. G. (1975) Thioridazine stimulates prolactin secretion in man. Arch. Gen. Psychiatry 32, 885 – 886.

Saldanha, V. F., Havard, C. W. H, Bird, R. and Gardner, R. (1972) The effect of chlorpromazine on pituitary function. Clin. Endocrinol. 1, 173 – 180.

Schyve P. M., Smithline, F. and Meltzer, H. Y. (1978) Neuroleptic-induced prolactin level elevation and breast cancer. Arch. Gen. Psychiatry 35, 1291 – 1301.

Sedvall, G. (1979) Neuroendocrine correlates in schizophrenia. In: E. E. Muller and A. Agnoli (Eds), Neuroendocrine Correlates in Neurology and Psychiatry. Elsevier Biomedical Press, Amsterdam, pp. 195 – 209.

Sherman, L., Kim, S., Benjamin, F. and Kolodny, H. D. (1971) Effect of chlorpromazine on serum growth-hormone concentration in man. N. Engl. J. Med. 284, 72 – 74.

Siris, S. G., van Kammen, D. P. and DeFraites, E. G. (1978) Serum prolactin and antipsychotic responses to pimozide in schizophrenia. Psychopharmacol. Bull. 14, 11 – 14.

Siris, S. G., Siris, E. S., van Kammen, D. P., Docherty, J. P., Alexander, P. E. and Bunney, Jr., W. E. (1980) Effects of dopamine blockade on gonadotropins and testosterone in man. Am. J. Psychiatry 137, 211 – 215.

Wilson, R. G., Hamilton, J. R., Boyd, W. D., Forrest, A. P. M., Cole, E. N., Boyns, A. R. and Griffiths, K. (1975) The effect of long-term phenothiazine therapy on plasma prolactin. Br. J. Psychiatry 127, 71 – 74.

Wode-Helgodt, B., Eneroth, P., Fyro, B., Gullberg, B. and Sedvall, G. (1977) Effect of chlorpromazine treatment on prolactin levels in cerebrospinal fluid and plasma of psychotic patients. Acta Psychiatr. Scand. 56, 280 – 293.

Zander, K. J., Fischer, B., Zimmer, R. and Ackenheil, M. (1981) Long-term neuroleptic treatment of chronic schizophrenic patients: clinical and biochemical effects of withdrawal. Psychopharmacology 73, 43 – 47.

Burrows/Norman/Davies (eds) Antipsychotics

Chapter 3

Antipsychotic actions of the endorphins

JAN M. VAN REE, WIM M.A. VERHOEVEN*

and

DAVID DE WIED

*Rudolf Magnus Institute for Pharmacology, Medical Faculty, University of Utrecht, Vondellaan 6, 3521 GD Utrecht, and *Department of Psychiatry, Medical Faculty, University of Utrecht, Nic. Beetsstraat 24, 3511 HG Utrecht, The Netherlands*

NEUROPEPTIDE CONCEPT

The pituitary gland secretes a number of hormones, which control a variety of endocrine processes in the body. These hormones are peptide molecules, consisting of a chain of amino acids. The sequence of the different amino acids determines the information encoded in the peptide molecule. This principle is comparable with features of our language. The amino acids are the letters of the alphabet, which as such have little significance for communication. But placing the letters in a certain sequence, we can make words with a specific meaning and apply them in our communication. Similarly, the pituitary hormones serve as building stones of the endocrine communication network. They carry specific information from the pituitary to different organs in the body.

During recent decades evidence has accumulated that pituitary hormones in addition to their classical endocrine actions, affect distinct central nervous system (CNS) functions as well (De Wied, 1969; De Wied, 1977; Van Ree et al., 1978a). In particular, animal behavioural test procedures have been employed to demonstrate the

intrinsic effects of peptide molecules on CNS processes. It has subsequently been shown that pituitary hormones and a variety of other peptides are present in the brain. Interestingly, it was observed that fragments of pituitary hormones which are practically devoid of the classical endocrine activities of the parent hormones, were as effective as the parent hormones in a number of behavioural tests. Thus, the behavioural and endocrine effects of pituitary hormones are dissociated. This led to the postulate that these hormones act as precursor molecules from which behaviourally active fragments may be enzymatically generated. These fragments have been designated as neuropeptides (De Wied et al., 1974). Analogous to the peripheral function of pituitary hormones, the neuropeptide systems can be regarded as the endocrine communication network of the brain. They carry a lot of specific information, encoded in the peptide structure, from one place to another. The control of neuropeptides over brain functions has led to several postulates assigning disturbances in these peptide systems to various psychopathological disorders and disturbed behaviour. This chapter will summarize the present information about the possible relationship between endogenous opioids and related peptides, and schizophrenic psychoses.

OUTLINE OF THE ENDORPHIN SYSTEM

The discovery in the early 1970's of the presence of specific opiate binding sites in brain tissue (Terenius, 1973; Simon et al., 1973; Pert and Snyder, 1973) was soon followed by isolation of endogenous substances in brain extracts or cerebrospinal fluid (CSF), that compete for opiate receptor binding or mimic the effects of morphine on isolated tissue preparations (Terenius and Wahlström, 1975; Pasternak et al., 1975; Hughes, 1975). The first identified endogenous substances with morphine-like actions – endorphins – are pentapeptides called enkephalins (Hughes et al., 1975). Subsequent research has revealed that a number of opioid peptides are present in the brain. They seem to belong to three major families, arising from three distinct systems (Table 1). Firstly, the pro-enkephalin system, yielding enkephalins, which is located peripherally (e.g. in the adrenal cortex) and in widely distributed short neuronal pathways in the brain (Watson et al., 1979; Noda et al., 1982). Secondly, the pro-opiomelanocortin system, yielding α-, β- and γ-endorphins, which is located predominantly in the pituitary, but also in a neuronal pathway in the brain. From the basal hypothalamus (nucleus arcuatus) this system spreads to several structures of the limbic system and to the brain stem (Nakanishi et al., 1979; Watson et al., 1979). Thirdly, the pro-dynorphin system, yielding dynorphins, which is located in the hypothalamic-hypophyseal neuronal system, but also in other parts of the brain, such as the hippocampus (Watson et al., 1981; Kakidani et al., 1982). Some evidence is available that the opioid peptides belonging to a certain family can activate a specific subclass of opioid receptors (Table 1; Wood, 1982). Enkephalins may activate the δ-receptors, while β-endorphin and dynorphins may

TABLE 1

Endorphins and opiate receptors.

	Pro-opiomelanocortin (245 aa)		Pro-enkephalin (239 aa)		Pro-dynorphin (236 aa)	
Endorphins	α-endorphin	(16 aa)	(Met)-enkephalin	(5 aa)	dynorphin	(8 aa)
	γ-endorphin	(17 aa)	(Leu)-enkephalin	(5 aa)	β-neo-endorphin	(9 aa)
	β-endorphin	(31 aa)	heptapeptide	(7 aa)	α-neo-endorphin	(10 aa)
			octapeptide	(8 aa)	dynorphin	(17 aa)
					'new' big dynorphin	(29 aa)
Structure	Tyr-Gly-Gly-Phe-Met . . .		Tyr-Gly-Gly-Phe-Met (Leu) . . .		Tyr-Gly-Gly-Phe-Leu . . .	
Prototype	β-endorphin		Met/Leu-enkephalin		dynorphin	
Opiate receptor	$\mu(\delta)$		$\delta(\mu)$		κ	

aa = amino acids.

activate μ- and κ-receptors respectively. However, the relationship between these subclasses of the opioid receptors and the physiological roles of the different opioid peptides have so far not been clearly elucidated.

In the three systems a big precursor molecule of about 230–240 amino acids is formed, which is subsequently further processed to smaller fragments. For example, pro-opiomelanocortin is a 31K molecule which is the precursor molecule of adrenocorticotrophic hormone (ACTH) and β-lipotropin (β-LPH). The latter is the precursor molecule of β-endorphin. Proteolytic processing of β-endorphin yields α- and γ-endorphin and smaller fragments (Burbach et al., 1980). All these subsequently formed neuropeptides have specific information for brain mechanisms. Enzymatic processing can evoke specific information enclosed in the peptide molecule, or select a certain information out of others. For example, β-lipotropin (89 amino acids) lacks morphine-like activity, but its C-terminal part β-endorphin (31 amino acids) exerts morphinomimetic effects. The N-terminal fragment of β-endorphin, γ-endorphin (17 amino acids) has both opiate-like and neuroleptic-like actions, but in the C-terminal fragment of γ-endorphin, des-Tyr^1-γ-endorphin (16 amino acids) only the neuroleptic-like effects are conserved. Since these principles may be operative in all brain neuropeptide systems, it is evident that the endocrine communication network of the brain is complex, but enables a precise and integrative control over brain functions.

ENDORPHINS AND SCHIZOPHRENIA

Soon after the discovery of endorphins, they were implicated in chronic pain and various psychopathological disorders such as psychosis, depression, mania and addiction. Interest has been focussed mainly on psychosis, particularly of the schizophrenic type. Three lines of research were followed: endorphin excess, endorphin deficiency and disturbances in β-endorphin fragmentation.

Endorphin excess

Animal data

Injection of β-endorphin into the cerebrospinal fluid leads to a variety of behavioural changes which are also observed after administration of morphine. Thus, β-endorphin induces antinociception, hypothermia, hormonal changes, excessive grooming and at higher dose levels profound immobilization and muscular rigidity (Van Ree et al., 1976; Gispen et al., 1976; Bloom et al., 1976; Holaday et al., 1978). Most, if not all, of these effects are blocked by the opiate antagonists naloxone and naltrexone. β-Endorphin also shows common actions with morphine-like drugs after repeated administration, e.g. development of tolerance and physical dependence and induction of experimental addiction (Van Ree et al., 1976; Wei and Loh, 1976; Van Ree et al., 1979). Other endorphins like α- and γ-endorphin, enkephalins and dynorphins can produce most of these behavioural effects but less markedly. This may be due to a more rapid biotransformation of the shorter endorphins in vivo. The animal data showing that β-endorphin caused a naloxone-reversible postural rigidity, which may be reminiscent of the catatonic posture sometimes seen in schizophrenic psychosis, have been interpreted as supporting evidence for the postulate that an endorphin excess is involved in the symptomatology of schizophrenic patients (Bloom et al., 1976; Segal et al., 1977).

Endorphins in blood and CSF

Mixed opiate agonists and antagonists, such as cyclazocine and pentazocine, unlike pure opiate agonists and antagonists, can produce psychotomimetic effects, e.g. hallucinations and delusions, that are frequently observed in schizophrenic psychosis. This stimulated Terenius and coworkers to measure endorphin levels in CSF of schizophrenic patients. Two fractions with endorphin-like material could be distinguished using a receptor assay method. Later studies revealed several opioid peptides to be present in these fractions, e.g. fraction I contains dynorphin 1 – 8 and fraction II the hexapeptide (Met)-enkephalin-Lys (Nyberg et al., 1983). An increased concentration of endorphin-like material, especially of fraction I, was found in a number of acute schizophrenic patients, while only a few chronic schizophrenics had an enhanced level. Treatment with neuroleptics significantly lowered the fraction I level in acute schizophrenics (Terenius et al., 1976; Lindström et al., 1978; Rimón et al., 1980).

β-Endorphin levels were determined in blood and CSF using the radioimmunoassay technique. Blood levels of β-endorphin-like immunoreactivity in schizophrenic patients were not different from those in control subjects, although increased and decreased levels have also been reported (Emrich et al., 1979; Ross et al., 1979; Brambilla et al., 1981; Nagel et al., 1982). An enhanced level of β-endorphin in CSF has been observed in patients with acute schizophrenic psychoses, but others found no clear changes in CSF β-endorphin-like immunoreactivity, either in acute or in chronic schizophrenia (Domschke et al., 1979; Emrich et al., 1979; Naber et al., 1981). Also, no marked differences in the level of β-endorphin in selected areas of post-mortem brains from schizophrenic patients and in those of control patients were observed (Lightman et al., 1979). Thus, at present there is some evidence for an increase in endorphin-like material in CSF in a number of schizophrenic patients, although this material may not be β-endorphin.

Clinical trials with opioid antagonists

To evaluate the endorphin excess hypothesis, clinical studies were performed with the opioid antagonists naloxone and naltrexone. The idea was that if an excess of endorphin activity contributes to psychotic symptomatology, then opioid receptor blockade should cause improvement. The initial report on this subject was encouraging, in that a single intravenous injection with a low dose of naloxone resulted in a transient reduction of psychotic symptoms, in particular auditory hallucinations in a number of schizophrenic patients (Gunne et al., 1977). This stimulated a number of trials with opioid antagonists, including two WHO collaborative projects. Summarizing the presently available data, there is circumstantial evidence that blockade of opiate receptors following a single administration of opioid antagonists is associated with a decrease of symptomatology in a naloxone-sensitive subgroup of patients suffering from schizophrenic psychosis (Verhoeven et al., 1981a; Pickar et al., 1982). In particular, auditory hallucinations and symptoms belonging to the paranoid-suspiciousness subscale of the Brief Psychiatric Rating Scale (BPRS) (hostility, suspiciousness, unco-operativeness) appeared to be sensitive to naloxone treatment. Approximately 30% of the patients responded to treatment. Trials with repeated injections with naloxone are currently under way, but the outcome of the first studies is not impressive (Verhoeven et al., 1984a; Naber and Leibl, 1983). Thus, endorphins may be implicated in certain but not all psychotic symptoms of schizophrenic patients.

Haemodialysis of patients
It has been reported that weekly haemodialysis of some schizophrenic patients resulted in substantial improvement of psychotic symptomatology (Wagemaker and Cade, 1977). It was proposed that this procedure eliminates from the blood an abnormal endorphin or other substances sustaining the illness. Subsequently, a high level of (Leu^5)-β-endorphin was found in dialysates of some, but not all schizophrenic patients (Palmour et al., 1978). So far, at least 200 schizophrenic patients have been dialysed using open- and double-blind designs (for ref. see Van Ree and De Wied, 1981). Although 25 – 40% of the patients improved more or less upon haemodialysis in the open studies, this response was not replicable under double-blind conditions (Wagemaker et al., 1983; Vanherweghem et al., 1983). Moreover, the enhanced level of (Leu^5)-β-endorphin in blood or dialysates of schizophrenic patients could not be confirmed (for ref. see Van Ree and De Wied, 1981). Thus, although haemodialysis may be useful for treating certain schizophrenic patients, its routine application as a treatment for schizophrenics is inappropriate and the background of its possible beneficial effect is as yet unknown.

Endorphin deficiency

Animal data
The opposite hypothesis to endorphin excess, is the assumption that psychosis may be related to endorphin deficiency in the brain. Injection of β-endorphin into the periaqueductal grey matter of the brain stem of rats induces postural rigidity (Jacquet and Marks, 1976). This rigidity was interpreted as being similar to the symptoms of catalepsy produced by neuroleptic drugs. Consequently, it was postulated that β-endorphin may be an endogenous antipsychotic compound.

Clinical trials with β-endorphin

β-Endorphin was intravenously injected in some schizophrenic patients using an open design (Kline et al., 1977; Lehmann et al., 1979). It was reported that initially cognitive difficulties were worsened, difficulty in conceptualizing was increased and mood was elevated. Thereafter a long-term progressive reduction of psychotic symptomatology was observed starting 1 – 3 days after injection and lasting up to 10 days. Subsequently, four double-blind studies were performed in which a total of 29 schizophrenic patients received an intravenous injection or infusion with β-endorphin (Berger et al., 1980; Gerner et al., 1980; Pethö et al., 1981; Pickar et al., 1981). Although the influence of β-endorphin appeared to be marginal, a tendency to worsening was found shortly after injection (1 – 4 hours), whereas a slight, but not clinically obvious improvement was noticed in the 5-day period following treatment. In view of the reported beneficial after effects, it may be of interest to study the effect of repeated injections with β-endorphin. Interestingly, β-endorphin induced some antidepressant and mood-elevating effects in patients suffering from different types of depressive syndromes.

Clinical trials with FK 33-824

Enkephalins are rapidly broken down in the body. However, synthetic analogues have been synthesized which are less susceptible to degradation enzymes, e.g. FK 33-824 (Roemer et al., 1977). This potent peptide shares many of the biological properties of β-endorphin and has been used in three studies (2 open, 1 single blind) including 17 schizophrenic patients (Jørgensen et al., 1979; Nedopil and Rüther, 1979; Krebs and Roubicek, 1979). The peptide was administered for 2 – 8 days. Nine patients improved upon treatment, in that psychotic symptoms decreased for several days, but the peptide induced some morphine-like side effects shortly after injection.

In conclusion, the data collected so far with β-endorphin and FK 33-824 are inconclusive and do not favour the postulate that schizophrenia is due to an endorphin deficiency, at least with respect to the opiate-like effects of these peptides.

Disturbances in β-endorphin fragmentation

Animal studies

Towards the hypothesis. Besides morphinomimetic activity, β-endorphin (βE) and some of its fragments (e.g. α-endorphin (βE 1 – 16)) exert behavioural effects in rats which are apparently not mediated by opiate receptor systems. Thus, α- and β-endorphin delay extinction of pole jumping avoidance behaviour, an effect which persists in the presence of naltrexone (De Wied et al., 1978a). Interestingly, γ-endorphin (βE 1 – 17), which is only one amino acid longer than α-endorphin (Fig. 1) facilitated extinction of pole jumping avoidance behaviour (De Wied et al., 1978b). This effect is also not mediated by opiate receptor systems, since removal of the N-terminal amino acid tyrosine, which is essential for opiate-like activity, yields the peptide des-Tyr[1]-γ-endorphin (DTγE, βE 2 – 17), which is even more potent than γ-endorphin in facilitating extinction of active avoidance behaviour. Since it is well known that neuroleptic drugs decrease acquisition and facilitate extinction of conditioned avoidance behaviour, further studies were designed to compare DTγE with haloperidol, using a variety of behavioural test procedures (pole jumping avoidance behaviour, passive avoidance behaviour, electrical brain self-stimulation, the so-called grasping response) (De Wied et al., 1978b; Kovács and De Wied, 1978; Dorsa et al., 1979; Van Ree et al., 1980a; Van Ree and Otte, 1980). The effects of DTγE are in several aspects comparable to those of haloperidol, although the peptide, unlike haloperidol, causes less sedation and reduction of locomotor activity and does not show affinity to neuroleptic brain binding sites in vitro (Van Ree et al., 1978b). In view of this, it was postulated that DTγE or a closely related peptide may be an endogenous neuropeptide with neuroleptic-like activity and consequently may be implicated in the pathogenesis of schizophrenic psychoses (De Wied, 1978).

α-Endorphin and its non-opiate fragment des-Tyr[1]-α-endorphin, induce an opposite effect in a number of behavioural test procedures as compared to γ-endorphin and DTγE. The effects of the α-type endorphins show in some aspects similarities with those of psychostimulant drugs like amphetamine (De Wied, 1978;

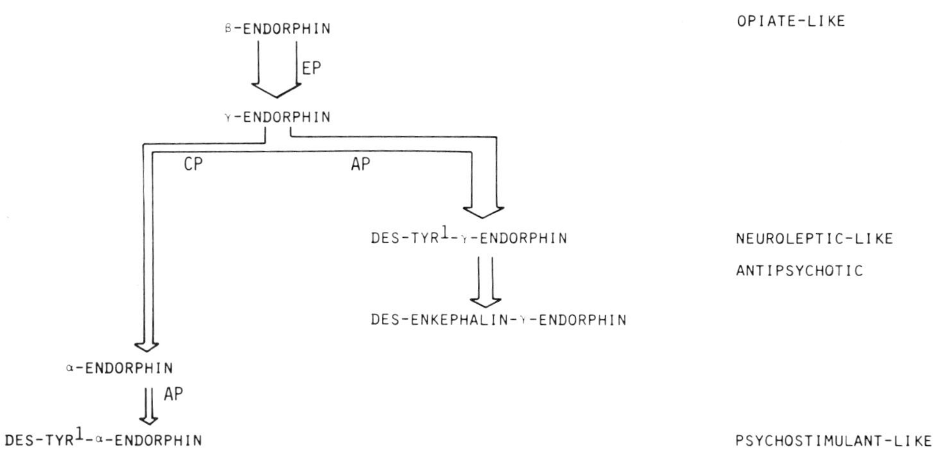

Fig. 1. CNS Effects of β-endorphin and related peptides, formed from β-endorphin by SPM associated peptidases. β-Endorphin (βE) contains 31 amino acids. γ-Endorphin = βE 1 – 17; α-endorphin = βE 1 – 16; des-Tyr[1]-α-endorphin = DTαE, βE 2 – 16; des-Tyr[1]-γ-endorphin = DTγE, βE 2 – 17; des-enkephalin-γ-endorphin = DEγE, βE 6 – 17. EP = Endopeptidase activity; AP = aminopeptidase activity; CP = carboxypeptidase activity. α-, β- and γ-Endorphins possess opiate activity; the most potent peptide in this respect being β-endorphin. α-Endorphin and DTαE have behavioural effects which are in some aspects similar to those induced by psychostimulant drugs, while DTγE and DEγE exert effects in rats and humans, which are in several aspects comparable to neuroleptic drugs.

Van Ree et al., 1980a). This observation extended the original hypothesis, since it is well known that psychostimulant drugs can induce psychoses and exaggerate psychotic symptoms of schizophrenic patients. Thus, the balance between α- and γ-type endorphins may be disturbed in schizophrenia, leading to a relative deficiency of γ-type endorphins or a relative excess of α-type endorphins (Fig. 1; De Wied, 1978).

γ-Type endorphins and brain dopamine. The dopamine (DA) hypothesis of schizophrenia, which in its simple format states that DA-ergic hyperactivity in the brain plays a key role in the pathogenesis of schizophrenia, stems from the coincidence of the psychosis-inducing and DA-ergic activity-enhancing effects of amphetamine and of the anti-psychotic and the DA-ergic blocking action of most neuroleptic drugs in current use. Thus, the interaction between γ-type endorphins and brain DA-ergic systems was studied in detail. Administration of DTγE to rats resulted in an increased DA disappearance in some restricted brain areas, while α-endorphin led to a decreased DA disappearance in these and other brain nuclei in rats pretreated with a catecholamine synthesis inhibitor (Versteeg et al., 1979, 1982). Haloperidol induced similar effects to DTγE, but the influence of this drug was more widespread (Versteeg, unpublished data). In a series of experiments the interaction between γ-type endorphins and the directly (apomorphine) or indirectly (amphetamine) acting DA-mimetics was investigated. These drugs are commonly used to detect anti-psychotic and neuroleptic actions of new compounds. Low doses of apomorphine, injected either systemically or into the nucleus accumbens result in hypoactivity, while systemic treatment with high doses of apomorphine and amphetamine induce hyperactivity and stereotypy, which responses are likely mediated by DA-ergic systems in the nucleus accumbens and nucleus caudatus respectively (Van Ree and Wolterink, 1981; Van Ree et al., 1982a, b, 1984; Van Ree, 1982). The effect of low doses of apomorphine may result from stimulation of self-inhibiting DA receptor systems (presynaptic DA receptors and/or DA autoreceptors), which are involved in feedback regulation, while the effect of high doses presumably stems from stimulation of postsynaptically located DA receptors. DTγE and DEγE (desenkephalin-γ-endorphin, βE 6 – 17), the shortest sequence with neuroleptic-like action (De Wied et al., 1980), did not interfere with the behavioural effects elicited by high doses of apomorphine or amphetamine. However, these peptides dose-dependently antagonized the hypoactivity induced by low doses of apomorphine injected either systemically or into the nucleus accumbens (Van Ree et al., 1982a, b). This effect of γ-type endorphins was mimicked by injecting low doses of the classical neuroleptic haloperidol and the atypical neuroleptic sulpiride (Van Ree et al., 1982b; Serra et al., 1983). The neuroleptic drugs, particularly the classical ones however, antagonize in addition the effect of high doses of apomorphine i.e. hyperactivity and stereotypy (Table 2). Thus, γ-endorphins may interfere with DA receptor systems in the nucleus accumbens, presumably located

TABLE 2

The influence of antipsychotic compounds on the behavioural changes elicited by injection of apomorphine into the nucleus accumbens and the nucleus caudatus of rats.

Apomorphine	Nucleus accumbens		Nucleus caudatus
	low doses	high doses	high doses
Classic neuroleptics	– –	– –	– –
Atypical neuroleptics	– –	–	–
γ-Type endorphins (DTγE, DEγE)	– –	0	0

Low and high doses of apomorphine injected into the nucleus accumbens induce hypolocomotion and hyperlocomotion, respectively. High doses of apomorphine injected into the nucleus caudatus induce stereotyped sniffing. 0 = No effect; – = inhibition (– moderate potency, – – marked potency).

presynaptically and sensitive to low doses of both DA agonists and antagonists. This is in line with other studies showing that the nucleus accumbens is sensitive to γ-type endorphins (Gispen et al., 1980; Van Ree and Otte, 1980; Kovács et al., 1982) and with the suggestion that particularly the mesolimbic DA system with terminals in the nucleus accumbens is hyperactive in schizophrenia (Crow, 1982). In fact, it seems that the action of neuroleptics in the nucleus accumbens is related to their antipsychotic effects and that the actions of the drugs in the nucleus caudatus are more related to their side effects (Parkinsonism, tardive dyskinesia).

γ-Type endorphin may be involved in regulating γ-type endorphin sensitive DA receptor systems in the nucleus accumbens. Indeed, animals treated subchronically with DEγE are more sensitive to the effects of low doses of apomorphine (Van Ree et al., 1982a, b). Moreover, chronic intra-accumbal treatment with DEγE results in a decrease in activity, whereas identical treatment with γ-endorphin antiserum leads to hyperactivity, which outlasts the treatment with the antiserum (Van Ree et al., 1982d). Treatment with the antiserum may inactivate the physiologically available γ-endorphin fragments, and thus result in a chronic deficiency of these peptides. Thus, γ-type endorphins may modulate the setpoint for feedback regulation in neurons equipped with γ-type endorphin sensitive DA receptor systems. According to the hypothesis that psychosis of the schizophrenic type is due to a relative deficiency of γ-type endorphins, the setpoint for feedback regulation in these DA neurons of the mesolimbic DA system may be lower in schizophrenics than in control subjects. This would result in a sustained increase in DA activity. Treatment of such patients with γ-type endorphins may restore the disturbed DA feedback systems to its physiological equilibrium and consequently decrease symptoms. This postulate may somehow link the γ-type endorphin hypothesis with the dopamine hypothesis of schizophrenia (Van Ree and De Wied, 1982).

Clinical trials with γ-type endorphins. Outline of the studies: The postulate that DTγE or a closely related neuropeptide may be implicated in schizophrenia, stimulated research into the purported antipsychotic action of γ-type endorphins. So far, we have completed a number of clinical trials, including a total of 43 patients treated with DTγE and 21 patients with DEγE (Verhoeven et al., 1979, 1981b, 1982, 1984b and unpublished data of four patients). The patients were classified nosologically as suffering from schizophrenia or schizo-affective psychosis. This diagnosis was based on the Research Diagnostic Criteria (RDC, Spitzer et al., 1978), the DSM-III diagnostic criteria for schizophrenia (DSM-III, 1980), the Present State Examination criteria (PSE, Wing et al., 1975) and the course of illness (Van Praag, 1976). All patients showed positive psychotic symptoms such as delusions and/or hallucinations, were more of less resistant to neuroleptic treatment and most of the patients had relapsed several times despite maintenance therapy with conventional neuroleptic drugs. DTγE was used in four studies (one open ($n = 6$) and three double-blind, cross-over trials ($n = 8$, 10 and 18, respectively)) and administered intramuscularly (i.m.) at a dose of 1 mg/day for 8 to 14 days. DEγE was used in a double-blind, placebo-controlled trial ($n = 19$); 13 patients received 3 mg DEγE/day i.m. for 10 days. This trial was preceded by a pilot study in which four patients were treated single blind with DEγE. Neuroleptic treatment was maintained (one DTγE trial and the DEγE trial) or discontinued one week (1st DTγE trial) or at least 3 weeks (2nd DTγE trials) before the start of the experimental period. Scoring of the symptoms was performed using among others the BPRS. The response to DTγE and DEγE was assessed by calculating the difference between the total BPRS score of each patient before the trial (baseline) and that at the end of γ-type endorphin treatment and in the period of 2 weeks after treatment. The response of each patient was expressed as percentage of the baseline score and the maximal response was used for dividing the patients among four groups: 1) < 20% improvement (no response); 2) 20 – 50% improvement (slight response); 3) 50 – 80% improvement (moderate response); 4) > 80% improvement (marked response).

Clinical effects: None of the six patients treated with placebo responded to treatment, neither did any of the patients, whose treatment started with placebo. Of the 64 patients, 13 did not respond, 19 patients showed a slight response, 16 patients displayed a moderate response and 16 patients showed a marked response to γ-type endorphins (Table 3). A more than 50% maximal response to treatment was taken as indicating improvement of clinical significance. Thus, in half of the patients a clinically obvious therapeutic effect was observed during or just after treatment with γ-type endorphins. When patients responded to treatment, the effect usually started at 3 – 7 days of active treatment. No marked differences among the specific symptoms of these patients were observed, either in degree of improvement shown or in the time course of improvement. In fact, both positive and negative psychotic symptoms similarily decreased during active treatment (Fig. 2). Plasma levels of growth hormone and cortisol were not changed by γ-type endorphin treatment, neither did

TABLE 3

Maximal decrease (in %) of symptoms according to the BPRS score at the end or during 2 weeks after des-Tyr[1]-γ-endorphin (DTγE) or des-enkephalin-γ-endorphin (DEγE) treatment of patients suffering from different types of schizophrenic psychoses.

	Diagnosis	*n*	Response % BPRS				Mean ± S.E.M.
			< 20	20 – 50	50 – 80	> 80	
DTγE	Hebephrenic type	9	–	1	4	4	68.3 ± 8.8
	Paranoid type	18	–	5	6	7	64.4 ± 5.7
	Catatonic type	3	–	3	–	–	39.3 ± 5.5
	Undifferentiated type	3	1	2	–	–	22.3 ± 9.7
	Residual type	4	4	–	–	–	11.3 ± 4.5
	Schizo-affective manic type	1	–	–	–	1	94.0
	Schizo-affective depressed type	5	5	–	–	–	13.4 ± 3.1
	All diagnoses	43	10	11	10	12	50.3 ± 4.7
DEγE	Hebephrenic type	1	–	–	–	1	100.0
	Catatonic type	5	1	3	1	–	40.8 ± 5.9
	Paranoid type	14	2	4	5	3	55.5 ± 6.6
	Schizo-affective depressed type	1	–	1	–	–	37.0
	All diagnoses	21	3	8	6	4	53.3 ± 5.3

CSF levels of homovanillic acid (HVA), methoxy-hydroxy-phenyl-glycol (MHPG) and 5-hydroxyindole-acetic acid (5-HIAA). Interestingly, plasma prolactin levels were decreased during DTγE treatment, which contrasts with the increasing effect after neuroleptics, but is in line with animal experiments, showing that under certain conditions γ-type endorphins inhibit the release of prolactin (Lamberts et al., 1982). Thus, the influence of γ-type endorphins on plasma levels of hormones and CSF levels of monoamine metabolites is quite different from that of classical and atypical neuroleptics, because neuroleptic drugs markedly change a number of these parameters. This may be related to the more selective action of γ-type endorphins.

Others also have studied the effects of DTγE in patients. In eight trials, DTγE was administered to a total of 83 schizophrenic patients (Bourgeois et al., 1980; Emrich et al., 1980; Casey et al., 1981; Fink et al., 1981; Manchanda and Hirsch, 1981; Tamminga et al., 1981; Meltzer et al., 1982; Volavka et al., personal communication). In general, the response to peptide treatment was less marked than in our studies; 24 patients responded to treatment. This diminished response may be related to the characteristics of the selected patients, in that more patients suffering

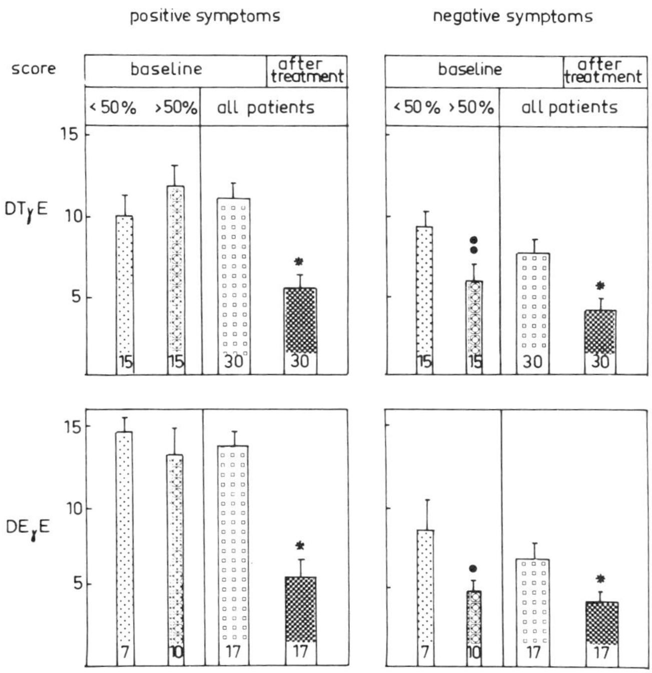

Fig. 2. Positive and negative psychotic symptoms derived from the BPRS scoring before and after treatment with γ-type endorphins. Presented are baseline BPRS scoring of all patients, the baseline scoring of the patients whose maximal response to treatment was less (<) or more (>) than 50% and the BPRS scoring on the day of maximal response (after treatment). Positive symptoms: conceptual disorganization, grandiosity, suspiciousness, hallucinatory behaviour, unusual thought content. Negative symptoms: emotional withdrawal, motor retardation, blunted affect. Maximal score of individual items is 6; data are expressed as mean scores of positive and negative symptoms; vertical bars indicate S.E.M.; number of patients is depicted in the columns. DTγE = des-Tyr[1]-γ-endorphin; DEγE = des-enkephalin-γ-endorphin; ●, different from the scoring of the patients who responded less than 50% (●, $p = 0.07$; ●●, $p = 0.01$, Student's t-test); *, different from baseline scoring ($p < 0.001$, Student's paired t-test).

from chronic schizophrenia were included in the other studies. Such patients seem to be less sensitive to treatment with γ-type endorphins than those suffering from sub-acute schizophrenia (see below).

Long-term effect of γ-type endorphins: Eleven of the 64 patients treated with γ-type endorphins for one or two consecutive treatment periods, remained free of psychotic symptoms for at least 6 months (Van Ree et al., 1982c; Verhoeven, 1983). It appeared that in these patients the degree of treatment with neuroleptics after the experimental treatment was significantly lower as compared to that in the period before γ-type endorphin treatment. The time interval between two psychotic episodes was extended after peptide treatment. Moreover, a significant improvement was observed in social functioning, in that a higher percentage of the patients functioned at their pre-morbid level without complaints and with a job in normal society (before treatment: 1 patient; after treatment: 6 patients), while a lower percentage of the patients functioned at an inadequate level, socially inactive with major psychosocial disturbances (before treatment: 7 patients; after treatment: none). Typing the lymphocytes of the patients with a long-lasting response for antigens of the HLA system, the major histocompatibility complex in the body, revealed a higher occurrence of HLA-B15-antigen as compared to that found in the other patients (De Jongh et al., 1982). Maybe a subpopulation of schizophrenic patients exists, with a marked and long-lasting response to treatment with γ-type endorphins and which is characterized by a certain HLA typology, suggesting the involvement of genetic factors.

Characterization of patients responding to γ-type endorphins: Since the response of the patients varied between no response at all to complete remission of psychotic symptoms, we have looked in more detail at the symptomatology and course of illness and the history of the patients so as to find whether the degree of response to γ-type endorphins co-varied with these characteristics of the individual patients (Van Ree et al., 1980b, 1981, 1982c; Verhoeven, 1983).

– *Diagnostic subtypes:* Patients suffering from hebephrenic (disorganized) and paranoid types of schizophrenia responded best (Table 3). Less response was found in patients with a catatonic type of schizophrenia. Patients with undifferentiated or residual type of schizophrenia hardly responded. Interestingly, patients suffering from schizo-affective psychosis depressed type did not respond to γ-type endorphins, while in the patient with a schizo-affective psychosis manic type, a marked response was observed.

– *PSE syndrome profile:* According to the CATEGO analysis, most patients belonged to the class of schizophrenic psychosis (S^+) and subclass nuclear schizophrenia (NS^+). It appeared that patients with a response of less than 50% showed significantly more symptoms belonging to the syndromes of Slowness, Catatonic syndrome and Residual syndrome. Thus, motor symptoms such as retardation and catatonic symptoms seem especially to have a negative influence on the response to treatment with γ-type endorphins.

– *Positive versus negative symptoms:* The positive symptoms (conceptual disorganization, grandiosity, suspiciousness, hallucinatory behaviour and unusual thought content) and the negative symptoms (emotional withdrawal, motor retardation and blunted effect) of the baseline BPRS scoring were added for each individual subject. It was found that the intensity of the negative symptoms was more severe in the patients with a response of less than 50% to γ-type endorphin treatment as compared to the other patients (Fig. 2). No differences were found between the two response groups with respect to the positive symptoms.

– *Other characteristics:* The age of the patients, the duration of the disease and the duration of neuroleptic treatment did not covary with the response to γ-type endorphin treatment. The duration of the last psychotic episode however was negatively correlated with the patient's response. The same was observed with the dose of neuroleptics the patient received during the last 6 weeks before the start of the trials. Thus, a long duration of the recent psychotic episode and treatment with high doses of neuroleptics may lead to a reduced responsiveness to γ-type endorphin treatment.

Summarizing, the data suggest that a subgroup of schizophrenic patients is preferentially sensitive to treatment with γ-type endorphins. The patients of this subgroup are characterized by the occurrence of relatively less negative psychotic symptoms, a relatively short duration of the last psychotic episode and previous treatment with low doses of neuroleptic drugs. Thus, patients responding to γ-type endorphins may belong to the type I schizophrenic syndrome as proposed by Crow (1982) (characterized by relatively less negative symptoms and susceptible to neuroleptic treatment) rather than to type II (characterized by relatively more negative symptoms, poor prognosis, and less susceptible to neuroleptic treatment). Distinct pathological processes may underlie this subclassification, i.e. hyperactivity of dopaminergic systems especially in the nucleus accumbens (type I) and perhaps an encephalitis-like process (type II). This accords with the animal data showing that γ-type endorphins may control certain dopaminergic systems in the nucleus accumbens (Van Ree and De Wied, 1982).

CONCLUDING REMARKS

The discovery of opioid peptides in the pituitary and brain has led to several postulates implicating these peptides in schizophrenia. The available data do not support the hypothesis that a deficiency of endorphins is operative in schizophrenia. It is more likely that at least in some patients the activity of the endorphin system is stimulated. Animal and human data suggest that disturbances in β-endorphin homeostasis, resulting in a relative deficiency of the non-opiate γ-type endorphins, is involved in schizophrenia. However, it remains to be shown that such disturbances exist in the brain of schizophrenics. Moreover, it should be kept in mind that other peptide systems, e.g. cholecystokinin-octapeptide, may be implicated in this psychopathological disorder too (Moroji et al., 1982; Nair et al., 1983; Van Ree et al., 1983). Nevertheless, the antipsychotic action of γ-type endorphins as observed in a number of patients supports the view that schizophrenic and other psychopathologic symptoms may be due to disturbances in the endocrine communication network of the brain.

REFERENCES

Berger, Ph. A., Watson, S. J., Akil, H., Elliott, G. R., Rubin, R. T., Pfefferbaum, A., Davis, K. L.,

Barchas, J. D. and Li, C. H. (1980) β-Endorphin and schizophrenia. Arch. Gen. Psychiatry 37, 635 – 640.

Bloom, F., Segal, D., Ling, N. and Guillemin, R. (1976) Endorphins: profound behavioral effects in rats suggest new etiological factors in mental illness. Science 194, 630 – 632.

Bourgeois, M., Laforge, E., Muyard, J., Blayac, J. and Lemoine, J. (1980) Endorphins et schizophrénies. Ann. Med. Psychol. 138, 1112 – 1119.

Brambilla, F., Genazzani, A. R., Facchinetti, F., Parrini, D., Petraglia, F., Sacchetti, E., Scarone, S., Guastalla, A. and D'Antona, N. (1981) β-Endorphin and β-lipotropin plasma levels in chronic schizophrenia, primary affective disorders and secondary affective disorders. Psychoneuroendocrinology 6, 321 – 330.

Burbach, J. P. H., Loeber, J. G., Verhoef, J., Wiegant, V. M., De Kloet, E. R. and De Wied, D. (1980) Selective conversion of β-endorphin into peptides related to γ- and α-endorphin. Nature (London) 283, 96 – 97.

Casey, D. E., Korsgaard, S., Gerlach, J., Jørgensen, A. and Simmelsgaard, H. (1981) Effect of Des-Tyrosine-γ-endorphin in tardive dyskinesia. Arch. Gen. Psychiatry 38, 158 – 160.

Crow, T. J. (1982) Two syndromes in schizophrenia? Trends Neurosci. 5, 351 – 354.

De Jongh, B. M., Verhoeven, W. M. A., Van Ree, J. M., De Wied, D. and Van Rood, J. J. (1982) HLA, and the response to treatment with γ-type endorphins in schizophrenia. J. Immunogenet. 9, 381 – 388.

De Wied, D. (1969) Effects of peptide hormones on behavior. In: W. F. Ganong and L. Martini (Eds), Frontiers in Neuroendocrinology. Oxford University Press, New York, pp. 97 – 140.

De Wied, D. (1977) Peptides and behaviour. Life Sci. 20, 195 – 204.

De Wied, D. (1978) Psychopathology as a neuropeptide dysfunction. In: J. M. Van Ree and L. Terenius (Eds), Characteristics and Function of Opioids. Elsevier/North-Holland Biomed. Press, Amsterdam, pp. 113 – 122.

De Wied, D., Van Wimersma Greidanus, Tj. B. and Bohus, B. (1974) Pituitary peptides and behavior: influence on motivational, learning and memory processes. In: Excerpta Medica International Congress Series No. 359, Proc. IX Congress Collegium Int. Neuropsychopharmacol., Excerpta Medica, Amsterdam, pp. 653 – 658.

De Wied, D., Bohus, B., Van Ree, J. M. and Urban, I. (1978a) Behavioral and electrophysiological effects of peptides related to lipotropin (β-LPH). J. Pharmacol. Exp. Ther. 204, 570 – 580.

De Wied, D., Kovács, G. L., Bohus, B., Van Ree, J. M. and Greven, H. M. (1978b) Neuroleptic activity of the neuropeptide β-LPH_{62-77} ([des-Tyr^1]-γ-endorphin; DTγE). Eur. J. Pharmacol. 49, 427 – 436.

De Wied, D., Van Ree, J. M. and Greven, H. M. (1980) Neuroleptic-like activity of peptides related to (des-tyr^1)-γ-endorphin: structure activity studies. Life Sci. 26, 1575 – 1579.

Domschke, W., Dickschas, A. and Mitznegg, P. (1979) CSF β-endorphin in schizophrenia. Lancet i, 1024.

Dorsa, D. M., Van Ree, J. M. and De Wied, D. (1979) Effects of [Des-Tyr^1]-γ-endorphin and α-endorphin on substantia nigra self-stimulation. Pharmacol. Biochem. Behav. 10, 899 – 905.

DSM-III. (1980) Diagnostic and Statistical Manual of Mental Disorders. The American Psychiatric Association.

Emrich, H. M., Höllt, V., Kissling, W., Fischler, M., Laspe, H., Heinemann, H., Von Zerssen, D. and Herz, A. (1979) β-Endorphin-like immunoreactivity in cerebrospinal fluid and plasma of patients with schizophrenia and other neuropsychiatric disorders. Pharmakopsychiatrie 12, 269 – 276.

Emrich, H. M., Zaudig, M., Kissling, W., Dirlich, G., Von Zerssen, D. and Herz, A. (1980) Des-Tyrosyl-γ-endorphin in schizophrenia: a double-blind trial in 13 patients. Pharmakopsychiatrie 13, 290 – 298.

Fink, M., Papakostas, Y., Lee, J., Meehan, Th. and Johnson, L. (1981) Clinical trials with des-tyr-gamma-endorphin (GK-78). In: C. Perris, G. Struwe and B. Jansson (Eds), Biological Psychiatry. Elsevier/North-Holland Biomed. Press, Amsterdam, pp. 398 – 401.

Gerner, R. H., Catlin, D. H., Gorelick, D. A., Hui, K. K. and Li, C. H. (1980) β-Endorphin: intravenous infusion causes behavioural change in psychiatric inpatients. Arch. Gen. Psychiatry 37, 642 – 647.

Gispen, W. H., Wiegant, V. M., Bradbury, A. F., Hulme, E. C., Smyth, D. G., Snell, C. R. and De Wied, D. (1976) Induction of excessive grooming in the rat by fragments of lipotropin. Nature (London) 264, 794 – 795.

Gispen, W. H., Ormond, D., Ten Haaf, J. and De Wied, D. (1980) Modulation of ACTH-induced grooming by (des-Tyr[1])-γ-endorphin and haloperidol. Eur. J. Pharmacol. 63, 203 – 207.

Gunne, L.-M., Lindstrom, L. and Terenius, L. (1977) Naloxone-induced reversal of schizophrenic hallucinations. J. Neural Transm. 40, 13 – 19.

Holaday, J. W., Loh, H. H. and Li, C. H. (1978) Unique behavioral effects of β-endorphin and their relationship to thermoregulation and hypothalamic function. Life Sci. 22, 1525 – 1536.

Hughes, J. (1975) Isolation of an endogenous compound from the brain with pharmacological properties similar to morphine. Brain Res. 88, 295 – 308.

Hughes, J., Smith, T. W., Kosterlitz, H. W., Fothergill, L. A., Morgan, B. A. and Morris, H. R. (1975) Identification of two related pentapeptides from the brain with potent opiate agonist activity. Nature (London) 258, 577 – 579.

Jacquet, Y. F. and Marks, N. (1976) The C-fragment of β-lipotropin: an endogenous neuroleptic or antipsychotogen? Science 194, 632 – 635.

Jørgensen, A., Fog, R. and Veilis, B. (1979) Synthetic enkephalin analogue in treatment of schizophrenia. Lancet i, 935.

Kakidani, H., Furutani, Y., Takahashi, H., Noda, M., Morimoto, Y., Hirose, T., Asai, M., Inayama, S., Nakanishi, S. and Numa, S. (1982) Cloning and sequence analysis of cDNA for porcine β-neo-endorphin/dynorphin precursor. Nature (London) 298, 245 – 249.

Kline, N. S., Li, C. H., Lehmann, H. E., Lajtha, A., Laski, E. and Cooper, Th. (1977) β-Endorphin-induced changes in schizophrenic and depressed patients. Arch. Gen. Psychiatry 34, 1111 – 1113.

Kovács, G. L. and De Wied, D. (1978) Effects of amphetamine and haloperidol on avoidance behavior and exploratory activity. Eur. J. Pharmacol. 53, 103 – 107.

Kovács, G. L., Telegdy, G. and de Wied, D. (1982) Selective attenuation of passive avoidance behaviour by micro-injection of β-$LPH_{62\text{-}77}$ and β-$LPH_{66\text{-}77}$ into the nucleus accumbens in rats. Neuropharmacology 21, 451 – 454.

Krebs, E. and Roubicek, J. (1979) EEG and clinical profile of a synthetic analogue of methionine-enkephalin – FK 33-824. Pharmakopsychiatrie 12, 86 – 93.

Lamberts, S. W. J., De Quijda, M., Van Ree, J. M. and De Wied, D. (1982) Non-opiate β-endorphin fragments and dopamine. V. γ-Type endorphins and prolactin secretion in rats. Neuropharmacology 21, 1129 – 1135.

Lehmann, N. P., Nair, N. P. V. and Kline, N. S. (1979) β-Endorphin and naloxone in psychiatric patients: clinical and biological effects. Am. J. Psychiatry 136, 762 – 766.

Lightman, S. L., Spokes, E. G., Sagnella, G. A., Gordon, D. and Bird, E. D. (1979) Distribution of β-endorphin in normal and schizophrenic human brains. Eur. J. Clin. Invest. 9, 377 – 379.

Lindström, L. H., Widerlöv, E., Gunne, L.-M., Wahlström, A. and Terenius, L. (1978) Endorphins in human cerebrospinal fluid: clinical correlations to some psychotic states. Acta Psychiatr. Scand. 57, 153 – 164.

Manchanda, R. and Hirsch, S. R. (1981) (Des-Tyr[1])-γ-endorphin in the treatment of schizophrenia. Psychol. Med. 11, 401 – 404.

Meltzer, H. Y., Busch, D. A., Tricou, B. J. and Robertson, A. (1982) Effect of (Des-Tyr)-gamma-endorphin in schizophrenia. Psychiatry Res. 6, 313 – 326.

Moroji, T., Watanabe, N., Aoki, N. and Itoh, S. (1982) Antipsychotic effects of ceruletide (caerulein) on chronic schizophrenia. Arch. Gen. Psychiatry 39, 485.

Naber, D. and Leibl, K. (1983) Repeated high dosage naloxone treatment without therapeutic efficacy in schizophrenic patients. Pharmakopsychiatrie 16, 43 – 45.

Naber, D., Pickar, D., Rost, R., Van Kammen, D., Waters, R. N., Ballenger, J. C., Goodwin, F. K. and Bunney, W. E. (1981) Endogenous opioid activity and β-endorphin immunoreactivity in CSF of psychiatric patients and normal volunteers. Am. J. Psychiatry 138, 1457 – 1462.

Nagel, S., Tegeler, J. and Goertz, B. (1982) Serum-Konzentration des β-Endorphins bei schizophrenen und depressiven Erkrankungen. Nervenarzt 63, 659 – 663.

Nair, N. P. V., Bloom, D. M., Nestoros, J. N. and Schwartz, G. (1983) Therapeutic efficacy of cholecystokinin in neuroleptic-resistant schizophrenic subjects. Psychopharmacol. Bull. 19, 134 – 136.

Nakanishi, S., Inoue, A., Kita, T., Nakamura, M., Chang, A. C. Y., Cohen, S. N. and Numa, S. (1979) Nucleotide sequence of cloned cDNA for bovine corticotropin-β-lipotropin precursor. Nature (London) 278, 423 – 427.

Nedopil, N. and Rüther, E. (1979) Effects of the synthetic analogue of methionine enkephalin FK 33-824 on psychotic symptoms. Pharmakopsychiatrie 12, 277 – 280.

Noda, M., Furutani, Y., Takahashi, H., Toyosato, M., Hirose, T., Inayama, S., Nakanishi, S. and Numa, S. (1982) Cloning and sequence analysis of cDNA for bovine adrenal preproenkephalin. Nature (London) 295, 202 – 206.

Nyberg, F., Wahlström, A., Sjölund, B. and Terenius, L. (1983) Characterization of electrophoretically separable endorphins in human CSF. Brain Res. 259, 267 – 274.

Palmour, R. M., Ervin, F. R., Wagemaker, H. and Cade, R. (1978) Characterization of a peptide from the serum of psychotic patients. In: E. Usdin, W. E. Bunney, Jr. and N. S. Kline (Eds), Endorphins in Mental Health Research. Macmillan and Co., New York, pp. 581 – 593.

Pasternak, G. W., Goodman, R. and Snyder, S. H. (1975) An endogenous morphine-like factor in mammalian brain. Life Sci. 16, 1765 – 1769.

Pert, C. B. and Snyder, S. H. (1973) Properties of opiate-receptor binding in rat brain. Proc. Natl. Acad. Sci. USA 70, 2243 – 2247.

Pethö, B., Gräf, L., Karczag, I., Bitter, I., Tolna, J., Baraczka, K. and Li, C. H. (1981) β-Endorphin and schizophrenia. Lancet i, 212 – 213.

Pickar, D., Davis, G. C., Schulz, S. Ch., Extein, I., Wagner, R., Naber, D., Gold, Ph. W., Van Kammen, D. P., Goodwin, F. K., Wyatt, R. J., Li, C. H. and Bunney, Jr., W. E. (1981) Behavioral and biological effects of acute β-endorphin injection in schizophrenic and depressed patients. Am. J. Psychiatry 138, 160 – 166.

Pickar, D., Vartanian, F., Bunney, Jr., W. E., Maier, H. P., Gastpar, M. T., Prakash, R., Sethi, B. B., Lideman, R., Belyaev, B. S., Tsutsulkovakaja, M. V. A., Jungkunż, G., Nedopil, N., Verhoeven, W. and Van Praag, H. (1982) Short-term naloxone administration in schizophrenic and manic patients. Arch. Gen. Psychiatry 39, 313 – 319.

Rimón, R., Terenius, L. and Kampman, R. (1980) Cerebrospinal fluid endorphins in schizophrenia. Acta Psychiatr. Scand. 61, 395 – 403.

Roemer, D., Buescher, H. H., Hill, R. C., Pless, J., Bauer, W., Cardinaux, F., Closse, A., Hauser, D. and Huguenin, R. (1977) A synthetic enkephalin analogue with prolonged parenteral and oral analgesic activity. Nature (London) 268, 547 – 549.

Ross, M., Berger, P. A. and Coldstein, A. (1979) Plasma β-endorphin immunoreactivity in schizophrenia. Science 205, 1163 – 1164.

Segal, D. S., Browne, R. G., Bloom, F., Ling, N. and Guillemin, R. (1977) β-Endorphin: endogenous opiate or neuroleptic? Science 198, 411 – 414.

Serra, G., Van Ree, J. M. and De Wied, D. (1983) Influence of classical and atypical neuroleptics on apomorphine-induced behavioral changes and on extinction of a conditioned avoidance response. J. Pharm. Pharmacol. 35, 255 – 257.

Simon, E. J., Hiller, J. M. and Edelman, I. (1973) Stereospecific binding of the potent narcotic analgesic [^{3}H]etorphine to rat brain homogenate. Proc. Natl. Acad. Sci. USA 70, 1947 – 1949.

Spitzer, R. L., Endicott, J. and Robins, E. (1978) Research diagnostic criteria. Arch. Gen. Psychiatry 35, 773 – 782.

Tamminga, C. A., Tighe, P. J., Chase, Th. N., DeFraites, E. G. and Schaffer, M. H. (1981) Des-Tyrosine-γ-endorphin administration in chronic schizophrenics. Arch. Gen. Psychiatry 38, 167 – 168.

Terenius, L. (1973) Characteristics of the 'receptor' for narcotic analgesics in synaptic plasma membrane fraction from rat brain. Acta Pharmacol. Toxicol. 33, 377 – 384.

Terenius, L. and Wahlström, A. (1975) Morphine-like ligang for opiate receptors in human CSF. Life Sci. 16, 1759 – 1764.

Terenius, L., Wahlström, A., Lindström, L. and Widerlöv, E. (1976) Increased CSF levels of endorphins in chronic psychosis. Neurosci. Lett. 3, 157 – 162.

Vanherweghem, J.-L., Linkowski, P. and Mendlewicz, J. (1983) Hemodialysis in schizophrenics. Arch. Gen. Psychiatry 40, 211 – 214.

Van Praag, H. M. (1976) About the impossible concept of schizophrenia. Compr. Psychiatry 17, 481 – 497.

Van Ree, J. M. (1982) Non-opiate β-endorphin fragments and dopamine. II. β-endorphin 2 – 9 enhances apomorphine-induced stereotypy following subcutaneous and intrastriatal injection. Neuropharmacology 21, 1103 – 1109.

Van Ree, J. M. and De Wied, D. (1981) Endorphins in schizophrenia. Neuropharmacology 20, 1271 – 1277.

Van Ree, J. M. and De Wied, D. (1982) Neuroleptic-like profile of γ-type endorphins as related to schizophrenia. Trends Pharmacol. Sci. 3, 358 – 361.

Van Ree, J. M. and Otte, A. P. (1980) Effects of (Des-Tyr[1])-γ-endorphin and α-endorphin as compared to haloperidol and amphetamine on nucleus accumbens self-stimulation. Neuropharmacology 19, 429 – 434.

Van Ree, J. M. and Wolterink, G. (1981) Injection of low doses of apomorphine into the nucleus accumbens of rats reduces locomotor activity. Eur. J. Pharmacol. 72, 107 – 111.

Van Ree, J. M., De Wied, D., Bradbury, A. F., Hulme, E. C., Smyth, D. G. and Snell, C. R. (1976) Induction of tolerance to the analgesic action of lipotropin C-fragment. Nature (London) 264, 792 – 794.

Van Ree, J. M., Bohus, B., Versteeg, D. H. G. and De Wied, D. (1978a) Neurohypophyseal principles and memory processes. Biochem. Pharmacol. 27, 1793 – 1800.

Van Ree, J. M., Witter, A and Leysen, J. E. (1978b) Interaction of des-tyrosine-γ-endorphin (DTγE, β-LPH_{62-77}) with neuroleptic binding sites in various areas of rat brain. Eur. J. Pharmacol. 52, 411 – 413.

Van Ree, J. M., Smyth, D. G. and Colpaert, F. (1979) Dependence creating properties of lipotropin C-fragment (β-endorphin): evidence for its internal control of behavior. Life Sci. 24, 495 – 502.

Van Ree, J. M., Bohus, B. and De Wied, D. (1980a) Similarity between behavioral effects of Des-Tyrosine-γ-endorphin and haloperidol and of α-endorphin and amphetamine. In: E. Leong Way (Ed.), Endogenous and Exogenous Opiate Agonists and Antagonists. Pergamon Press, New York, pp. 459 – 462.

Van Ree, J. M., De Wied, D., Verhoeven, W. M. A. and Van Praag, H. M. (1980b) Antipsychotic effect of γ-type endorphins in schizophrenia. Lancet ii, 1363 – 1364.

Van Ree, J. M., Verhoeven, W. M. A., Van Praag, H. M. and De Wied, D. (1981) Neuroleptic-like and antipsychotic effects of γ-type endorphins. In: H. M. Emrich (Ed.), Modern Problems of Pharmacopsychiatry, Vol. 17: The Role of Endorphins and Neuropsychiatry. Karger, Basel, pp. 226 – 278.

Van Ree, J. M., Innemee, H., Louwerens, J. W., Kahn, R. S. and De Wied, D. (1982a) Non-opiate β-endorphin fragments and dopamine. I. The neuroleptic-like γ-endorphin fragments interfere with behavioural effects elicited by small doses of apomorphine. Neuropharmacology 21, 1095 – 1101.

Van Ree, J. M., Caffé, A. M. and Wolterink, G. (1982b) Non-opiate β-endorphin fragments and dopamine. III. γ-Type endorphins and various neuroleptics counteract the hypoactivity elicited by injection of apomorphine into the nucleus accumbens. Neuropharmacology 21, 1111 – 1117.

Van Ree, J. M., Verhoeven, W. M. A., De Wied, D. and Van Praag, H. M. (1982c) The use of the synthetic peptides γ-type endorphins in mentally ill patients. Ann. N. Y. Acad. Sci. 398, 478 – 495.

Van Ree, J. M., Wolterink, G., Fekete, M. and De Wied, D. (1982d) Non-opiate β-endorphin fragments and dopamine. IV. γ-Type endorphins may control dopaminergic systems in the nucleus accumbens. Neuropharmacology 21, 1119 – 1127.

Van Ree, J. M., Gaffori, O. and De Wied, D. (1983) Behavioral profile of CCK-8 related peptides in rats resembles that of antipsychotic agents. Eur. J. Pharmacol. 93, 63 – 78.

Van Ree, J. M., Gaffori, O. and Király, I. (1984) γ-Endorphin and N^{α}-acetyl-γ-endorphin interfere with distinct dopaminergic systems in the nucleus accumbens via opioid and non-opioid mechanisms. Life Sci. 34, 1317 – 1324.

Verhoeven, W. M. A. (1983) Endogenous Opioids and γ-Type Endorphins in Schizophrenia. Thesis, Utrecht.

Verhoeven, W. M. A., Van Praag, H. M., Van Ree, J. M. and De Wied, D. (1979) Improvement of schizophrenic patients by treatment with [Des-Tyr^1]-γ-endorphin (DTγE). Arch. Gen. Psychiatry 36, 294 – 298.

Verhoeven, W. M. A., Van Praag, H. M. and De Jong, J. T. V. M. (1981a) Use of naloxone in schizophrenic psychoses and manic syndromes. Neuropsychobiology 7, 159 – 168.

Verhoeven, W. M. A., Westenberg, H. G. M., Gerritsen, A. W., Van Praag, H. M., Thijssen, J. H. H., Schwarz, F., Van Ree, J. M. and De Wied, D. (1981b) (Des-$tyrosine^1$)-γ-endorphin in schizophrenia: clinical, biochemical and hormonal aspects. Psychiatry Res. 5, 293 – 309.

Verhoeven, W. M. A., Van Ree, J. M., Heezius-Van Bentum, A., De Wied, D. and Van Praag, H. M. (1982) Antipsychotic properties of (des-enkephalin)-γ-endorphin (DEγE; β-LPH 66-77) in schizophrenic patients. Arch. Gen. Psychiatry 39, 648 – 654.

Verhoeven, W. M. A., Van Praag, H. M. and Van Ree, J. M. (1984a) Repeated naloxone administration in schizophrenia. Psychiatry Res. 12, 297 – 312.

Verhoeven, W. M. A., Van Ree, J. M., Westenberg, H. G. M., Krul, J. M., Brouwer, G. J., Thijssen, J. H. H., De Wied, D., Van Praag, H. M., Ceulemans, D. L. S. and Kahn, R. S. (1984b) Clinical, biochemical and hormonal aspects of treatment with des-Tyr^1-γ-endorphin in schizophrenia. Psychiatry Res. 11, 329 – 346.

Versteeg, D. H. G., De Kloet, E. R. and De Wied, D. (1979) Effects of α-endorphin, β-endorphin and (Des-Tyr^1)-γ-endorphin on α-MPT-induced catecholamine disappearance in discrete regions of the rat brain. Brain Res. 179, 85 – 93.

Versteeg, D. H. G., Kovács, G. L., Bohus, B., De Kloet, E. R. and De Wied, D. (1982) Effect of Des-Tyr^1-γ-endorphin and Des-Tyr^1-α-endorphin on α-MPT-induced catecholamine disappearance in rat brain nuclei: a dose-response study. Brain Res. 231, 343 – 351.

Wagemaker, H. and Cade, R. (1977) The use of hemodialysis in chronic schizophrenia. Am. J. Psychiatry 134, 684 – 685.

Wagemaker, H., Rogers, J. L. and Cade, R. (1983) The experimental use of hemodialysis in a double-blind study of 24 chronic schizophrenics. Psychopharmacol. Bull. 19, 33 – 36.

Watson, S. J., Akil, H., Berger, Ph. A. and Barchas, J. D. (1979) Some observations on the opiate peptides and schizophrenia. Arch. Gen. Psychiatry 36, 35 – 41.

Watson, S. J., Akil, H., Ghazarossian, V. E. and Goldstein, A. (1981) Dynorphin immunocytochemical localization in brain and peripheral nervous system: preliminary studies. Proc. Natl. Acad. Sci. USA 78, 1260 – 1263.

Wei, E. and Loh, H. (1976) Psysical dependence on opiate-like peptides. Science 193, 1262 – 1263.

Wing, J. K., Cooper. J. E. and Sartorius, N. (1975) The Measurement and Classification of Psychiatric Symptoms. Cambridge University Press, London.

Wood, P. L. (1982) Multiple opiate receptors: support for unique mu, delta and kappa sites. Neuropharmacology 21, 487 – 497.

Burrows/Norman/Davies (eds) Antipsychotics

Chapter 4

Prediction of response to antipsychotic drugs

THEODORE VAN PUTTEN[1,2], PHILIP R.A. MAY[2]
and
STEPHEN R. MARDER[1,2]

[1]*Veterans Administration Medical Center, West Los Angeles, Brentwood Division, CA 90073, and* [2]*Department of Psychiatry and Biobehavioural Sciences, University of California at Los Angeles, CA, U.S.A.*

INTRODUCTION

The odds are in favor of a prediction that any schizophrenic will improve if given medication. Nevertheless, a substantial number do just as well without it and some get worse or develop adverse effects. Regrettably, controlled research on prediction of response has been meager (May and Goldberg, 1977), and our present state of knowledge is not impressive, epitomized by Hollister's (personal communication, 1976) observation that drug treatment is unlikely to make a patient play the violin if he has never played before.

It must, of course, be conceded that we are not totally ignorant in the matter of prognosis. A few predictors are obvious. Chronic illness is likely to remain chronic; acute reactions usually get better; and patients with a poor premorbid history or a 'process' disorder are unlikely to attain a high level of adjustment. Also, if a patient has been treated previously with drugs, his prior response may be a good guide to future treatment.

The question is whether over and above crude statements of the obvious, one can predict whether drug treatment is likely to be of advantage to a particular person.

Having failed in 7 years of painstaking research to develop methods that predict the outcome for a specific patient from pretreatment information, the investigators came to the unhappy conclusion that they may have been trying to predict from the wrong set of variables and that one might learn something relevant about the eventual clinical response by studying the immediate response to the drug itself (May et al., 1976, 1978, 1981a, b).

EARLY CLINICAL CHANGE AS A PREDICTOR

It makes intuitive sense to attempt to predict outcome from the patient's early response to drug treatment. To this end, we gave an initial test dose of antipsychotic drug and additional doses at 24 and 36 hours to newly admitted patients suffering from a functional psychosis with definite schizophrenic features but not from significant physical disease, drug addiction, or alcoholism. Clinical response was measured at 48 hours and at the end of 28 days of subsequent treatment with a controlled standardized course of drug therapy.

As described elsewhere (May et al., 1976) the diagnosis was substantiated by using four different sets of diagnostic criteria. (DSM-III was not in use when these studies were performed.) Our objective was to select patients for whom treatment with antipsychotic drugs was clearly indicated, an issue that we suspect may be of greater concern to the clinician than achieving complete certainty about a diagnosis of schizophrenia. Although there is no substantive evidence that drug response is predicted better by any particular set of diagnostic criteria, whether stringent or relaxed, the majority of these patients met the criteria for DSM-III schizophrenic disorder; the remainder met criteria for schizophreniform, schizoaffective or atypical (psychosis) disorder.

With chlorpromazine (CPZ) the initial dose was 2.2 mg/kg; the same dose was repeated at 24 hours, and 4.4 mg/kg was given at 36 hours (just before bedtime). After this, a fixed daily dose of 6.6 mg/kg was given at bedtime, for 28 days. With thiothixene (THX) the test dose was 0.22 mg/kg. The same dose was repeated at 24 hours and 0.44 mg/kg was given daily at bedtime, for 28 days.

Clinical status was rated by the treating psychiatrist at baseline, at 48 hours, and at 28 days on the Brief Psychiatric Rating Scale (BPRS) (total score and 4 factors; Overall and Gorham, 1962); and by nursing staff on the MACC scale (total score and 4 sub-scales; Ellsworth, 1957). The raters at post-treatment were blind to the earlier values.

Table 1 shows consistent correlations between 48-hour change and the eventual amount of improvement for both drugs. With the exception of three correlations in the THX patients [BPRS anxious-depression (N.S.), BPRS total score (N.S), and BPRS thought disorder ($p < 0.05$)], all other correlations were significant at the 0.001 level. The BPRS plots of the THX patients showed one extreme outlier; deleting this one case strengthened the BPRS correlations.

TABLE 1

Correlations (*r*) of early change (at 48 hours) with eventual improvement (at 28 days) for thiothixene (THX) and chlorpromazine (CPZ). (Number of cases in parentheses.)

		THX	THX (outlier removed)	CPZ
BPRS	thought disorder	0.365 (37)	0.425 (37)	0.631 (33)
	anxious depression	0.208	0.276	0.669
	paranoia	0.567	0.650	0.537
	withdrawal	0.365	0.339	0.513
	total score	0.305	0.410	0.669
MACC	mobility	0.577 (39)		0.597 (29)
	mobility	0.642		0.558
	affect	0.650		0.511
	cooperation	0.612		0.507
	communication	0.635		0.573

With THX, a separate analysis compared the correlations for cases where the diagnosis of schizophrenia was confident ('certain') with those for whom it was less certain or questionable ('uncertain'). The correlations were comparable. We conclude that there was no demonstrable difference in prediction of drug response between the certain and the questionable cases.

We do not wish to enter too deeply into the controversy that surrounds the various diagnostic systems that purport to establish a 'valid' diagnosis of schizophrenia. The findings of our study, however, seem to confirm the wisdom of Overall and Hollister's (1979 a, b) view that there are practical and scientific disadvantages to defining concepts too narrowly. In our study, stringency of diagnosis had little or no bearing on predictability of response or non-response to drug; indeed if anything our data support the view that a broader diagnosis may be more useful. Our findings apply, however, only to prediction of immediate short-term outcome on drug treatment; not to prediction of long-range outcome. For this later task chronicity-laden criteria such as those of the St. Louis group [Feighner et al. (1972) and Bland and Orne (1979)] may be more appropriate.

In general, these findings indicate that early change is a respectable predictor of eventual improvement. Neborsky and Janowsky (1981) similarly found that improvement in general psychopathology one hour after receiving an injection of haloperidol correlated significantly ($r = 0.516, p < 0.02$) with a decrease in the total BPRS after 7 days of treatment. In addition, they found that improvement in the BPRS thinking disorder, excitement, and hostility-suspiciousness subscales measured 4 and 24 hours after the haloperidol injection(s) correlated significantly ($r = 0.495 - 0.791, p < 0.05 - 0.01$) with a decrease in the BPRS total score after 7 days of haloperidol treatment.

To the clinician, this will come as no surprise. He, however, will want to know what is in store for those who are the same or worse after 48 hours of drug treatment. With THX, 7 were unimproved after 48 hours of treatment: of these 7, 1 became even worse after further treatment; 4 remained the same; 1 improved slightly; and 1 (the extreme outlier) was much improved. With CPZ, only one of the five patients who were rated worse on the BPRS thought disorder scale after 48 hours went on to a very good outcome.

Although our findings are subject to the usual caveats about preliminary findings from a relatively small number of patients, the consistency and magnitude of the correlations are impressive. It is easy in clinical practice to monitor 48-hour improvement, and we, therefore, suggest that this simple prognostic indicator be given further clinical trial.

SUBJECTIVE RESPONSE AS A PREDICTOR

Early on, while studying EEG and other psychophysiologic measures, we noticed that some patients unexpectedly became extremely dysphoric several hours after the test dose. Some of these dysphoric responders became panicked and distinctly more psychotic; several started to speak of suicide and death. 'Syntonic' responders, by contrast, perceived the medication effect as helpful and agreeable. Aside from the clinical necessity of managing dysphoric responses, the question was what – if anything – did subjective response after a test dose augur?

The nature of subjective response

Syntonic responders, already at 4 hours after a test dose of THX (0.22 mg/kg), CPZ (2.2 mg/kg), or haloperidol (5 mg), tended to describe an improvement in thought disorder or mood. Some examples are: 'It's easier to concentrate on one thought', 'I don't feel threatened anymore', 'It brings my mind into focus', or 'I can cope with the voices better'. Dysphoric responders, on the other hand, experienced the drug effect quite differently. Some examples are: 'It makes everything slower', 'takes me away from my normal frame of mind', 'slows my thinking', 'makes me panic', 'makes me confused', 'I am calmer without the medication', 'my whole body feels like it is in a physical prison', 'suppresses me from having ideas', 'makes me think jittery'.

Frequency of dysphoric response

We found that with test doses of CPZ, THX and haloperidol, some 25% of patients experience a distinct dysphoric response (Van Putten et al., 1984).

Implications of subjective response

Clinical sense suggests that a syntonic response should augur favorably. This is so. We found that patients with a syntonic response to a test dose of CPZ (2.2 mg/kg), THX (0.22 mg/kg), or haloperidol (5 mg) did well; compliance was good and, at least with chlorpromazine, short-term clinical outcome superior (Van Putten and May, 1978; Van Putten et al., 1981, 1984).

We also found that a dysphoric response, if nothing else, is a powerful predictor of non-compliance. With THX, 16 (25%) of 65 patients had a dysphoric response to the first dose. Of these 16, 10 (63%) would not continue with medication past 14 days, no matter how much we reasoned or cajoled. (Only 11% of the syntonic responders refused continued drug treatment; chi square = 15.4, $p < 0.001$.). With haloperidol, in a different sample, similar percentages emerge: 9 of 40 (23%) patients had a dysphoric response to the first dose; of the 9 dysphoric responders 6 (67%) could not be persuaded to continue with treatment. [Of the 30 syntonic responders only 6 (20%) did not continue with treatment; the chi square, however, is not significant]. In the sense that non-compliance can be equated with a poor outcome, an initial dysphoric response is predictive of it.

Can patients with an initial dysphoric response go onto a good outcome? Of the 35% of patients with a dysphoric response who continued with treatment for another 28 days, some did have a good clinical response – often at very low doses (say 2 – 5 mg of haloperidol) and with antiparkinson drugs. (The antiparkinson drugs are required because, in our experience, dysphoric responses are nearly always fueled by extrapyramidal side effects, particularly akathisia; Van Putten et al., 1981.)

DEPRESSIVE HEREDITY AS A PREDICTOR

Galdi et al. (1981) studied drug response in two large samples (total $n = 251$) of schizophrenic inpatients treated with a variety of neuroleptics. In both samples, schizophrenics with depressed relatives experienced more depression and anxiety as measured by the BPRS. Hogarty et al. (1979) similarly found depressive heredity in neuroleptic-treated outpatients who relapsed with depressive symptoms. In our own work, also, schizophrenic patients with depressive heredity, although they improved in terms of psychotic symptoms, also developed more depressive symptoms than schizophrenic patients without depressive heredity.

PERFORMANCE TESTS AS A PREDICTOR

Since there is the consensus that schizophrenics suffer attentional dysfunction, we reasoned that a measure of attention (or any performance test for that matter) might be a useful predictor of drug response. Accordingly, a number of such performance tests were incorporated into the test-dose procedure.

The results were negative. Neither baseline performance nor early change in such performance measures as the Continuous Performance Test (reportedly a rather sensitive measures of schizophrenic deficit; Kornetsky, 1972), tapping speed, movie comprehension (Goldstein et al., 1966), Word Association Test or Digit Symbol Substitution Test were useful as predictors of symptomatic improvement (May et al., 1981b).

VENTRICULAR SIZE AS A PREDICTOR

Schizophrenic patients with enlarged ventricles as determined by CT scans may have a poor response to neuroleptic treatment. Weinberger et al. (1980) compared 10 chronic schizophrenic patients with enlarged cerebral ventricles with 10 similar patients with normal ventricles. The groups were closely matched for age, age at onset of illness, years of hospitalization and illness, drug dosage and plasma neuroleptic concentration. Response was significantly worse in those with enlarged ventricles.

It now seems established that some schizophrenics have ventricular enlargement, even at the onset of their illness (Weinberger et al., 1982; Luchins, 1982). It is, however, too early to tell whether ventricular size is a meaningful biologic sign with therapeutic and prognostic significance.

PHARMACOKINETIC DATA AS A PREDICTOR

Prediction of steady-state plasma levels from a 24-hour (or earlier) sample after a single dose has been demonstrated for some tricyclic antidepressants and lithium (Cooper et al., 1981). Such a procedure 'appears to present an exciting and substantial advance in the applications of pharmacokinetics to the clinical setting' (Slattery et al., 1980). Assuming a useful therapeutic range for antipsychotic drugs exists, a similar procedure, particularly one utilizing saliva levels, would be clinically useful.

Yesavage et al. (1982) found a correlation of 0.51 ($p < 0.005$) between a plasma THX level 2.5 hours after a 20 mg dose and improvement in the total BPRS after one week of treatment with a fixed dose of THX.

In our laboratory, saliva levels of CPZ at 2 hours correlated significantly ($p < 0.05$) with 3 of the improvement criteria (BPRS paranoid, $r = 0.58$; MACC total score, $r = 0.43$; MACC pathological affect, $r = 0.67$), and 4-hour saliva levels correlated significantly with 3 improvement criteria (BPRS paranoid, $r = 0.63$; MACC total score, $r = 0.47$; MACC pathological affect, $r = 0.61$).

CPZ plasma levels at 24 hours correlated significantly with improvement by 2 criteria (BPRS thought disorder, $r = 0.55$; BPRS withdrawal-retardation, $r = 0.71$) – so did saliva levels (BPRS thought disorder, $r = 0.55$; BPRS paranoid, r

= 0.61) (May et al., 1981a). Trimming off outliers did not materially alter these relationships.

Subject to caveats that the number of cases is modest and that interpretation of the significance of substantial numbers of correlations must necessarily be cautious, our findings suggest that saliva levels or 24-hour plasma levels after a test dose of CPZ can help to forecast whether a patient is likely to improve on the given drug.

CONCLUSION

The most promising approach to prediction of response in the individual patient lies in that patient's earliest responses to antipsychotic medication. So far, the most practical predictors of outcome appear to be early clinical change and the subjective response after the first or the first several dose(s). A dysphoric response means that the patient will likely stop the medication; if he continues to take it, early clinical change seems to be the most powerful predictor. Plasma (or saliva) levels may be promising; but they are cumbersome and expensive and the correlations – few as they are – are smaller than the correlations with such a simple measure as early clinical change.

The above measures need substantiation. Further, they may only be useful for the early identification of potentially good and poor responders to drug treatment. They may be more powerful in predicting the speed and amount of early drug-induced restitution than in predicting the ultimate level attained, since this latter depends heavily on ancillary psychological and social therapies for which drugs can only set the stage.

ACKNOWLEDGEMENT

This work was supported by the Veterans Administration Medical Research Service.

REFERENCES

Bland, R. C. and Orne, H. (1979) Schizophrenia: diagnostic criteria and outcome. Br. J. Psychiatry 134, 34 – 81.

Cooper, T. B., Bark N. and Simpson, G. M. (1981) Prediction of steady state plasma and saliva levels of desmethylimipramine using a single dose, single time point procedure. Psychopharmacology 74, 115 – 121.

Ellsworth, R. B. (1957) The MACC Behavioral Adjustment Scale. Western Psychol. Services, Santa Monica, CA.

Feighner, J. P., Robins, E., Guze, S. B., Woodruff, R. A., Winokur, G. and Munoz, R. (1972) Diagnostic criteria for use in psychiatric research. Arch. Gen. Psychiatry 26, 57 – 63.

Galdi, J., Rieder, R. O., Silber, D. and Bonato, R. R. (1981) Genetic factors in the response to neuroleptics in schizophrenia: a psychopharmacogenetic study. Psychol. Med. 11, 713 – 728.

Goldstein, M. J., Acker, C. W., Crockett, J. T. and Riddle, J. J. (1966) Psychophysiological reactions to films by chronic schizophrenics. I. Effects of drug states. J. Abnorm. Psychol. 71, 335 – 344.

Hogarty, G. E., Schooler, N. R., Ulrich, R., Mussare, F., Ferro, P. and Herron, E. (1979) Fluphenazine and social therapy in the aftercare of schizophrenic patients: relapse analyses of a two-year controlled study of fluphenazine decanoate and fluphenazine hydrochloride. Arch. Gen. Psychiatry 36, 1283 – 1294.

Kornetsky, C. (1972) The use of a simple test of attention as a measure of drug effects in schizophrenic patients. Psychopharmacologia 24, 99 – 106.

Luchins, D. J. (1982) Computed tomography in schizophrenia. Arch. Gen. Psychiatry 349, 859 – 860.

May, P. R. A. and Goldberg, S. C. (1977) Prediction of schizophrenic patients' response to pharmacotherapy. In: M. A. Lipton, A. DiMascio and K. F. Killam (Eds), Psychopharmacology: A Generation of Progress. Raven Press, New York, pp. 1139 – 1153.

May, P. R. A., Van Putten, T., Yale, C., Potepan, P., Jenden, D. J., Fairchild, M. D. and Dixon, W. J. (1976) Predicting individual responses to drug treatment in schizophrenia. A test dose model. J. Nerv. Ment. Dis. 162, 177 – 184.

May, P. R. A., Van Putten, T., Jenden, D. J. and Cho A. K. (1978) Test dose response in schizophrenia: chlorpromazine blood and saliva levels. Arch. Gen. Psychiatry 35, 1091 – 1097.

May, P. R. A., Van Putten, T. and Yale, C. (1980) Predicting the outcome of antipsychotic drug treatment from early response. Am. J. Psychiatry 137, 1088 – 1089.

May, P. R. A., Van Putten, T., Jenden, D. J., Yale, C. and Dixon, W. J. (1981a) Chlorpromazine in blood and saliva levels and the outcome of treatment in schizophrenic patients. Arch. Gen. Psychiatry 38, 202 – 207.

May, P. R. A., Van Putten, T., Jenden, D. J., Yale, C., Dixon, W. J. and Goldstein, M. J. (1981b) Individual differences in psychological response to a test dose of antipsychotic drug and their relationship to blood and saliva levels and treatment outcome. Compr. Psychiatry 22, 147 – 152.

Neborsky, R. J. and Janowsky, D. S. (1981) Early treatment response and predicting outcome. Am. J. Psychiatry 138, 538.

Overall, J. E. and Gorham, D. R. (1962) The brief psychiatric rating scale. Psychol. Rep. 10, 799 – 812.

Overall, J. E. and Hollister, L. E. (1979a) Comparative evaluation of research criteria for schizophrenia. Arch. Gen. Psychiatry 36, 1198 – 1205.

Overall, J. E. and Hollister, L. E. (1979b) Research Diagnostic Criteria. Arch. Gen. Psychiatry 36, 1381 – 1382.

Slattery, J. T., Gibaldi, M. and Koup, J. R. (1980) Prediction of maintenance dose required to attain a desired drug concentration at steady-state from a single determination of concentration after an initial dose. Clin. Pharmacokinet. 5, 377 – 385.

Van Putten, T. and May, P. R. A. (1978) Subjective response as a predictor of outcome in pharmacotherapy: the consumer has a point. Arch. Gen. Psychiatry 35, 477 – 480.

Van Putten, T., May, P. R. A., Marder, S. R. and Wittman, L. A. (1981) Subjective response to antipsychotic drugs. Arch. Gen. Psychiatry 38, 187 – 190.

Van Putten, T., May, P. R. A. and Marder, S. R. (1984) Response to antipsychotic medication: the doctor's and the consumer's view. Am. J. Psychiatry (in press).

Weinberger, D. R., Bigelow, L. B., Kleinman, J. E., Klein, S. T., Rosenblatt, J. E. and Wyatt, R. J. (1980) Cerebral ventricular enlargement in chronic schizophrenia. Arch. Gen. Psychiatry 37, 11 – 13.

Weinberger, D. R., DeLisi, L. E. and Perman, G. P. (1982) Computed tomography in schizophreniform disorder and other acute psychiatric disorders. Arch. Gen. Psychiatry 39, 778 – 783.

Yesavage, J. A., Becker, J., Werner, P. D., Mills, M. J., Holman, C. A. and Cohn, R. (1982) Serum level monitoring of thiothixene in schizophrenia: acute single-dose levels at fixed doses. Am. J. Psychiatry 139, 174 – 178.

Section III

PLASMA LEVEL MEASUREMENT, PHARMACOKINETICS AND CLINICAL RESPONSE

Burrows/Norman/Davies (eds) Antipsychotics

Chapter 5

Antipsychotics: Plasma levels and clinical response

JOHN M. DAVIS, JAVAID I. JAVAID, PHILIP G. JANICAK

and

MARCELLE A. MOSTERT

Illinois State Psychiatric Institute, Chicago, Illinois, U.S.A.

INTRODUCTION

The obvious purpose of drug treatment is to achieve adequate clinical response with minimum toxicity. In order for a drug to be effective, an optimal amount of the drug must be delivered to the site of action in the body. A large body of evidence indicates that patients treated with the same dose of a drug achieve markedly different concentrations in the blood due to large variations in pharmacokinetic behavior in different individuals. Therefore, monitoring blood levels, rather than standard doses of drugs, may provide a better indication of therapeutic failures and side effects of drug treatment.

The measurement of lithium and some antidepressants (notably, nortriptyline) in plasma has proved clinically useful for adjusting the dosage to experimentally determined therapeutic concentrations. Although antipsychotic drugs were introduced for the treatment of schizophrenia some 30 years ago, the required limits for therapeutic or toxic concentrations in blood have not been well established for most of the antipsychotic drugs. The scarcity of information with regard to therapeutic and toxic concentrations of antipsychotic drugs in blood has been due in part to the lack of specific and sensitive methods for measuring low therapeutic levels of these drugs. In recent years, however, there has been much emphasis on the development of such methods, and at present a variety of analytical methods have become available. To date, however, there have been only a few methodologically valid studies on plasma levels of antipsychotic drugs and clinical efficacy. In this chapter, we will discuss the conceptual basis for the plasma level/clinical efficacy relationship and the requirements for methodologically valid studies and also review the literature of controlled investigations on plasma level-clinical efficacy relationships.

THEORETICAL BASIS FOR PLASMA LEVEL/CLINICAL RESPONSE STUDIES

The basic assumption that underlies plasma level/clinical response relationship studies is that pharmacogenetic and environmental factors vary the quantity of a drug that reaches the receptor site in different individuals and that there is a relationship between drug concentration in blood and the site of action. There is an optimum concentration of drug at which maximum pharmacologic response will occur. Thus, at low concentration there will be no response, followed by an increased response with increasing drug concentrations. After the maximum pharmacologic response is achieved, a further increase in drug concentration will not increase the response. Thus the plot of drug levels vs. clinical response will be the typical sigmoid dose-response curve (Davis et al., 1978). This is graphically shown in Fig. 1. The left part of the theoretical curve shows the relative lack of clinical response at low plasma levels. After a certain drug concentration, as the plasma levels of the drug increase, there is a proportional increase in clinical response (linear part of the curve). Once enough drug reaches the receptor sites to elicit maximum response, further increase in plasma levels does not affect clinical response. At higher concentrations, various toxic effects of the drug may become more prominent and there may also be a relationship between plasma levels and various side effects of the drug (Fig. 1, middle panel). Thus a composite plot of total clinical benefits and side effects of the drug vs. plasma levels will result in an inverted U-shaped relationship which will indicate an optimum range or 'therapeutic window' of plasma levels for maximum beneficial response. This is shown in Fig. 1 (bottom panel).

For most of the drugs, the upper end of the therapeutic window will represent toxicity. However, some drugs may, in fact, lose their clinical effectiveness as a result of their action on different receptors at higher concentrations. A drug which has neither serious toxic effects nor loss of beneficial effects at higher concentrations would not display the descending portion of the therapeutic window. The plasma level/clinical response relationship in this case will be sigmoidal or linear. The ability to measure drug concentrations in plasma helps to empirically determine the nature of relationship between plasma levels and clinical response or a given side effect.

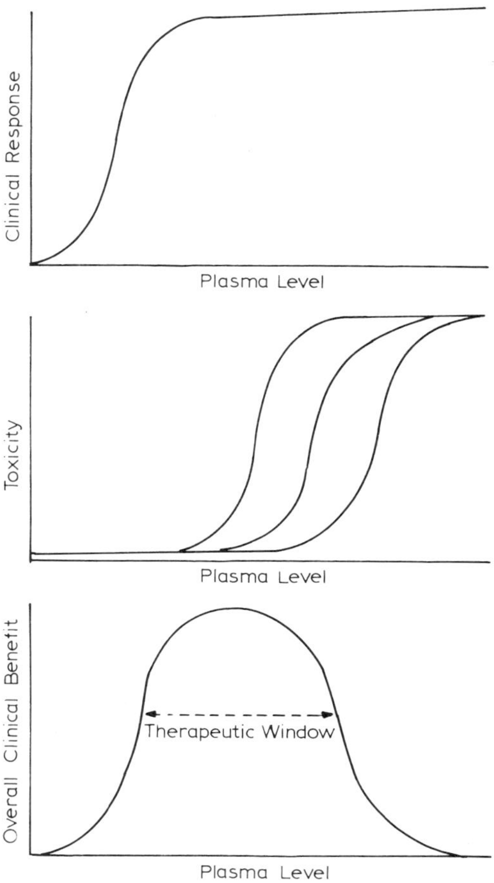

Fig. 1. Theoretical concept of therapeutic window in drug plasma-level/clinical-response relationship.

WHEN IS PLASMA LEVEL MONITORING USEFUL?

If a drug produces immediate pharmacologic effects, then the monitoring of plasma levels may not be clinically very useful. For example, an anesthesiologist can directly monitor the clinical stages of anesthesia. In this case, plasma levels will not be very useful because the clinician can adjust the dosage of the anesthetic by simply monitoring the clinical effects. On the other hand, if there is a long interval between clinical response and drug treatment, a number of weeks are required to adjust the dosage on the basis of clinical response. In this situation, if the plasma concentrations required for clinical response are known, dosage can be adjusted based on blood levels. Plasma levels are also useful when there are large interindividual differences in plasma levels and clinical response in patients with the same clinical diagnoses and treated with the same doses of the drug.

In psychiatry, the introduction of antipsychotic drugs in the early 1950's has made possible fundamental changes in patient management. However, it takes several weeks of drug treatment before the psychiatrist can make a decision on dose adjustment based on clinical outcome. Essentially, the clinician treats each patient with what is regarded as a reasonable dose. After several weeks of treatment, if there is no clinical response the clinician increases the dose until either the patient shows clinical improvement or undesirable side effects. Since large interindividual variations in plasma levels of antipsychotic drugs are now well established, the knowledge of therapeutic ranges of plasma levels of these drugs could provide scientific guidelines to clinicians for dosage adjustment in different patients.

HISTORY OF PLASMA-LEVEL STUDIES IN PSYCHIATRY

The history of plasma levels in psychiatry dates to World-War II, when the pharmacologist Shannon (later head of NIH) was trying to develop synthetic antimalarial drugs as substitutes for quinine. Fundamental knowledge about the clinical pharmacology of many drugs used in internal medicine was developed by B. B. Brodie, a student of Shannon's. Brodie's student, Julius Axelrode (later to win the Nobel Prize), became interested in the metabolism of amphetamine and discovered the liver microsomal enzymes that metabolize amphetamine. Subsequent work indicated that these liver microsomal enzymes metabolize a great variety of drugs including antipsychotics and tricyclic antidepressants. Stephen Curry, another student of Brodie's, developed the first method for measuring chlorpromazine in plasma from patients (Curry, 1968). Davis, Janowsky, and Marshall (students of Curry's) determined correlations between antipsychotic drug plasma levels and clinical effects in man (Curry and Marshall, 1968; Curry et al., 1970a, b). Since then, a large number of laboratories have developed different methods for measuring various antipsychotic drugs and have shown large interindividual differences in plasma levels of these drugs (Hobbs et al., 1974; Alfredsson et al., 1976; Gottschalk et al., 1978; Franklin et al., 1978; Simpson et al., 1978; Papadopoulos et al., 1980; Javaid et al., 1981, 1982; Yesavage et al., 1981; see also Burrows and Norman, 1981 for reviews).

Although, at present, there is a large number of studies that generally find an inverted U-shaped relationship between plasma levels of different antipsychotic drugs and clinical response, many of these studies have methodological problems (see below). The monitoring of plasma levels of antipsychotic drugs is still at an experimental stage.

METHODOLOGICAL REQUIREMENTS FOR VALID STUDIES

Requirement of fixed dosage

Since most investigations claiming to relate clinical efficacy to plasma levels have used flexible doses, it is important to analyze the influence of varying the dose on clinical response. In a flexible dose design, when patients do not show a good clinical response the clinician increases the dose, thereby increasing the plasma level. In those patients who show side effects, the clinician will decrease the dose, thus lowering the plasma level. Because clinicians adjust dosage on the basis of clinical effects and toxicity, this will have secondary effects on plasma levels. This will alter the relationship between clinical response and plasma levels. To illustrate this, consider two examples of patients with poor clinical response. In the first, suppose that the poor response is due to a low plasma level. When the clinician increases the dose, the plasma level will also rise. Thus, the lower end of the therapeutic window will be obscured. In the second, suppose the patient has an adequate plasma level but would be unresponsive to the drug at any dose. When the dose is increased, the plasma level will also rise, biasing the upper end of the therapeutic window. Thus, a flexible-dose strategy will, by design, confound the relationship of plasma level and clinical efficacy. Flexible-dose studies are, therefore, of no use for interpreting plasma level/clinical response relationships. Indeed, the only valid design to meaningfully define the upper end of the therapeutic window is to use a constant dose and observe that patients who have very high plasma levels do not do well. This can be further substantiated if, after lowering the dose in a randomly chosen subsample, thereby lowering the plasma level, the patient does better in comparison to patients with high levels whose dose was not lowered.

In valid plasma level studies, a fixed-dose design should be used. It can be a single fixed dose or it can have patients randomly assigned to several different fixed doses, perhaps a low fixed and a high fixed dose, to investigate the low and the high end of the therapeutic window.

Need for floridly-ill patients

Some patients will not improve with neuroleptics because they are not floridly ill. Their reason for hospitalization may be deterioration in their social situation; their degree of psychosis during hospitalization is about the same as before hospitalization. Such patients who are admitted without a relapse in their disease, i.e. with only their residual psychopathology, are not an adequate population for therapeutic trials. In a therapeutic trial, it is necessary to have patients who have florid illness and, therefore, have the capacity to demonstrate a substantial degree of therapeutic improvement. To be valid, plasma level/clinical response relationship studies should exclude schizophrenics who have only residual symptoms. In suitable floridly-ill patients, improvement with antipsychotics should be measured over a time course of 2 or 3 weeks.

Need responsive patients

Placebo responders will recover regardless of plasma level, and some patients will not respond to neuroleptics at any dose. In such cases, one would anticipate no correlation between plasma levels and therapeutic response.

Necessity to measure drug-induced improvements

It is important to distinguish rate of improvement from maximum possible improvement. Some schizophrenics will improve to a point of complete remission of symptoms. Many other patients, however, will still have residual symptoms even after adequate drug treatment and substantial improvement. In our opinion, the degree of residual symptoms indicates the patient's maximum capacity to improve. We therefore do not expect a correlation between plasma levels and maximum improvement possible as this likely reflects the underlying psychopathology.

In assessing the relationship between clinical response and plasma level in chronic patients, it is important to measure rate of drug-induced improvement, as distinct from capacity to improve. Taking patients off drugs for several weeks is not necessarily an adequate clinical procedure. There is a substantial body of data to show that patients relapse very slowly after the discontinuance of antipsychotic drugs. A drug-free interval of one year perhaps would be necessary to ensure that 80% or so of the patient population would have relapsed in that period of time.

LITERATURE REVIEW

The studies by Curry and co-workers (Curry et al., 1968, 1970a, b; Curry and Marshall, 1968) were the first investigations of antipsychotic plasma levels. These studies noted that there were marked individual differences in plasma levels of chlorpromazine among patients on comparable doses of the drug. A wide range of almost 20-fold (approximately 25 – 500 ng/ml) in plasma levels was seen in patients on fairly standard clinical doses. Several patients who had very low levels of chlorpromazine failed to show either side effects or clinical response. One patient with a high chlorpromazine plasma level showed excessive sedation. The patient demonstrated a clinical response when the dose was lowered and plasma level decreased. These exploratory open studies must be verified by properly controlled studies.

Controlled studies of chlorpromazine

There have been very few methodologically appropriate investigations of the relationship between antipsychotic drug-plasma levels and clinical efficacy. Sakalis et al. (1972) treated a small number of schizophrenics and manics with 300 mg of chlorpromazine daily. However, the study is complicated by the fact that the original sample deliberately included nonfloridly-ill patients (because patients amenable to psychophysiological studies were chosen). Lader (1976) subsequently extended the study to include a larger group of new patients, many of whom were floridly ill. However, the 300 mg dose used is probably lower than the ED_{50} dose of chlorpromazine (the average dose necessary to produce 50% of maximal improvement). Therefore, although some patients may have had plasma levels below the therapeutic window, it is unlikely that any patient would have had plasma levels above the therapeutic window. This dose would be useful to define the lower end of the therapeutic window, and at this dose, a linear relationship between plasma level and clinical efficacy would be anticipated. Patients with low plasma levels would be expected to show poor clinical response; patients with slightly higher levels would be expected to show good clinical response. A recent report of results on the first 32 patients indicates the investigators found a correlation of −0.32 between clinical efficacy and plasma levels, which is of borderline significance ($p = 0.04$, one-tailed).

Wode-Helgodt and co-workers (1977, 1978, 1981) did a methodologically excellent study on patients who were treated with randomly assigned fixed-doses of either 200, 400, or 600 mg of chlorpromazine per day. A 200 or 400 mg fixed-dose schedule would be considered low; 600 mg would be a moderate dose. Studying 15 male schizophrenics, the investigators found a positive correlation ($r = 0.82$, $p < 0.01$) between improvement and prolactin elevation at 4 weeks. There was a similar correlation between plasma levels and clinical response. Van Putten et al. (1981) and May et al. (1981) studied schizophrenic patients treated with fixed doses of chlorpromazine (6.6 mg/kg per day) for 28 days. They did not find any correlation between drug-plasma level and prolactin level or clinical outcome.

Chlorpromazine theoretically can be metabolized to 168 different metabolites, many of which may be active. If clinical effects are produced to a fair extent by metabolites, and if a chemical assay measures only the unchanged chlorpromazine, and if the amount of metabolite is not highly correlated with the amount of unchanged drug, then the presence of active metabolites may obscure the correlation between chlorpromazine-plasma levels and therapeutic efficacy. In other words, if clinical improvement is produced by active metabolites, then plasma levels of unchanged drug would not be expected to correlate highly with improvement because the improvement is being produced by something other than the unchanged drug. This may complicate the interpretation of the chlorpromazine studies.

Other antipsychotics

Because the presence of unmeasured chlorpromazine metabolites may complicate

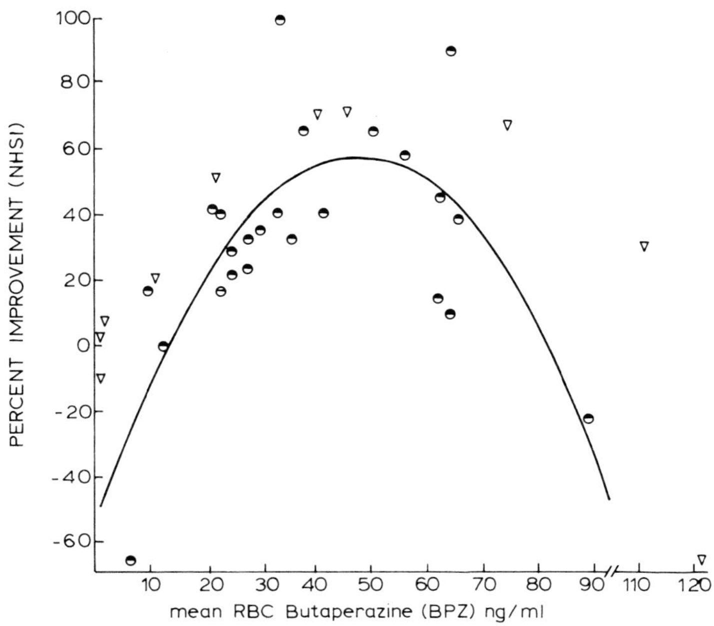

Fig. 2. Therapeutic response as a function of butaperazine concentrations. △, Plasma level; ○, red blood cell level.

the interpretation of plasma level efficacy studies (Manian et al., 1965, 1971), it may be desirable to use antipsychotic drugs without active metabolites to work out plasma level and therapeutic efficacy relationships. The metabolism of many antipsychotic drugs has not been worked out, so it is difficult to be certain which drugs do or do not have active metabolites. For this reason, Simpson et al. (1973) and Cooper et al. (1975) have suggested that butaperazine may be a particularly fruitful drug to investigate.

Our group studied the relationship between plasma levels and clinical response in schizophrenic patients treated with constant maintenance doses of butaperazine (Garver et al., 1977; Smith et al., 1979; Casper et al., 1980) and found that there was an inverted U-shaped relationship between RBC levels and clinical response. Optimum clinical response was obtained when levels were between 25 and 65 ng of butaperazine per milliliter RBC. These results are shown in Fig. 2. We have also found an inverted U-shaped relationship between fluphenazine concentrations in plasma and clinical response in 29 schizophrenic patients treated with fixed doses of fluphenazine (Dysken et al., 1981). In this study (Fig. 3), both an upper and lower end of therapeutic concentration are suggested by three nonresponders whose plasma levels were above 2.8 ng/ml and by two nonresponders and one partial responder whose plasma levels were below 0.3 ng/ml.

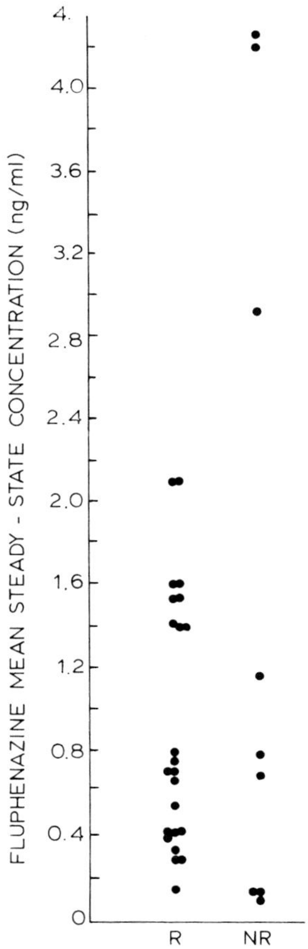

Fig. 3. Plasma levels of fluphenazine in responders (R) and non-responders (NR) to the antipsychotic effects of the drug administered at a fixed dosage. $n = 29$.

Smith et al. (1982) reported that in 26 hospitalized schizophrenic patients treated with fixed doses of haloperidol, there was an inverted U-shaped relationship between blood levels and clinical response. They reported that patients with steady-state RBC haloperidol levels in the range of 2.4 – 5.4 ng/ml showed greater response than those with lower or higher levels. In their study, a similar, although nonsignificant, curvilinear relationship between plasma haloperidol levels and clinical response was found. We have similarly found a curvilinear relationship between haloperidol plasma levels and clinical response in schizophrenic patients treated with fixed doses of haloperidol (unpublished results).

Cotes et al. (1978) treated patients with fixed doses of flupenthixol and reported a correlation 0.56 between prolactin levels and total symptom changes ($p < 0.05$).

USE OF FREE DRUG LEVELS

All blood level studies in the literature have reported total (bound + free) drug concentrations in blood. It is the concentration of free drug which is in equilibrium with tissue-drug levels; at present, however, the quantification of free drug is technically very difficult. Drugs must cross the blood-brain barrier to reach central receptor sites. Thus the factors which affect pharmacokinetics will determine the amount of drug at the receptor site. If some of the mechanisms involved in the drugs' distribution across the RBC membrane mimic those mechanisms governing the passage of drug through the blood-brain barrier, then drug levels within RBC (or RBC/plasma ratio) may provide information that total plasma levels alone cannot. In fact, Manian et al. (1974) have shown similarities between RBC and rat-brain synaptosomes-chlorpromazine levels. If the assumption is valid, then RBCs may be a preferred tissue for measurement.

As pointed out earlier, our group administered butaperazine on a constant dose schedule to acutely symptomatic schizophrenic patients while measuring plasma and RBC levels. Although both plasma and RBC levels and response were best characterized by an inverted U-shaped curve, the relationship of RBC levels to response was more striking (see Fig. 2). Smith et al. (1979) have reported similar results with haloperidol. These findings support the hypothesis that RBC levels of antipsychotic drugs correlate better with clinical response and side effects than do plasma levels.

BLOOD LEVELS IN CHRONIC SCHIZOPHRENIC PATIENTS

Ideally, concentration of drug should be measured at the receptor site. Since CSF level may reflect free levels in plasma, it is relevant to note that Alfredsson et al. (1976) found plasma-chlorpromazine levels to be highly correlated to CSF-chlorpromazine levels ($r = 0.91$).

Although most hospitalized schizophrenics will respond in some measure to neuroleptic treatment and then return home, there are occasional patients who demonstrate no response to drugs whatsoever and need to be hospitalized continuously on a lifetime basis. A possible explanation of their chronicity may be that some of these chronic patients are fast metabolizers and fail to respond to drugs. Our research group (Smith et al., 1979) studied such a chronic population and found that both their plasma and red cell levels were substantially below those seen in the acute population. In Fig. 4 (right column), we have presented as a bar graph the plasma and red cell level of our acute patients, including both relatively good and relatively poor responders. The left column of the graph represents the mean response of the very unresponsive, chronic group. Also studied was a similar group of very unresponsive patients in an acute setting, many of whom had absolutely no clinical response to antipsychotic drugs; many were, indeed, considered for transfer

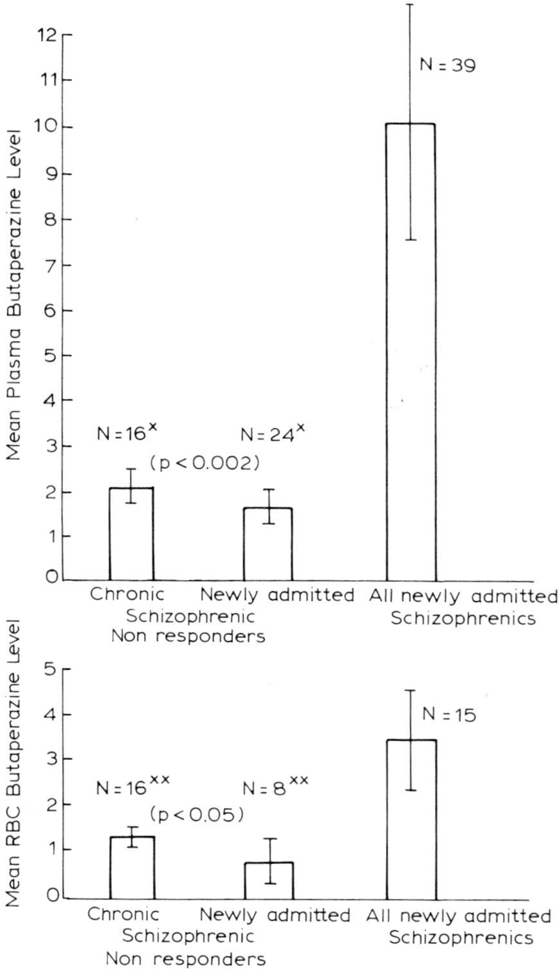

Fig. 4. Mean levels of butaperazine in chronic non-responders, and in newly admitted non-responders and responders. Plasma levels (above) and red blood cell levels (below).

to a long-term facility. In essence, this was the same population as the chronic nonresponders, but identified in an acute setting. These patients also showed extremely low plasma and red cell levels (see middle column of Fig. 4). A fair number of these nonresponders ultimately did respond, however, after administration of higher-than-normal doses of fluphenazine enanthate or decanoate. Since chlorpromazine undergoes first-pass metabolism, an intramuscular formulation may bypass this first-pass effect and thus reach a therapeutically adequate plasma level.

CONCLUSION

There is a substantial number of studies that show large differences in plasma levels among patients treated with the same doses of antipsychotic drugs. Furthermore, there is some evidence to suggest that these plasma or red cell levels of antipsychotic drugs do correlate with clinical response. This provides one rationale why a clinician should adjust the dose to clinical response based on blood levels of the drug. Although these data are fairly consistent, we do not feel that there are enough methodologically valid studies to demonstrate just exactly what the therapeutic window is for different antipsychotic drugs. The therapeutic window must be worked out for each drug separately. Thus a substantial body of information is required before even a rough approximation of the therapeutic window can be determined. We feel the use of antipsychotic plasma levels is experimental at this point.

For plasma levels to be clinically useful, they must be more precisely defined. Not only must valid data define a therapeutic window's existence, but it is also necessary for laboratories to agree on its exact limits. Unlike a plasma sodium, which is either low, normal, or high, drug plasma levels differ widely among individuals due to differences in rate of liver metabolism. Therefore, the clinician must adjust each patient's dosage individually to achieve maximum benefit with minimal side effects. Accurately determined plasma levels can occasionally aid in dose adjustment when the literature provides sufficient data to make sense of the value obtained. We believe the best way to understand plasma levels is not through arbitrarily selected numbers defining the upper or lower limits of the therapeutic window, but by placing a given plasma level in the context of the published data from methodologically valid studies.

REFERENCES

Alfredsson, G., Wode-Helgodt, B. and Sedvall, G. (1976) A mass fragmentographic method for the determination of chlorpromazine and two of its active metabolites in human plasma and CSF. Psychopharmacology 48, 123 – 131.

Burrows, G. D. and Norman, T. R. (Eds) (1980) Psychotropic Drugs – Plasma Concentration and Clinical Response. Marcel Dekker, Inc., New York.

Casper, R., Garver, D. L., Dekirmenjian, H., Chang, S. and Davis, J. M. (1980) Phenothiazine levels in plasma and red blood cells. Arch. Gen. Psychiatry 37, 301 – 305.

Cooper, T. B., Simpson, G. M., Haher, E. J. and Bergner, P. E. (1975) Butaperazine pharmacokinetics. Arch. Gen. Psychiatry 37, 903 – 905.

Cotes, P. M., Crow, T. J., Johnstone, E. C., Bartlett, W. and Bourne, R. C. (1978) Neuroendocrine changes in acute schizophrenia as a function of clinical state and neuroleptic medication. Psychol. Med. 8, 657 – 665.

Curry, S. H. (1968) Determination of nanogram quantities of chlorpromazine and some of its metabolites in plasma using gas-liquid chromatography with an electron-capture detector. Anal. Chem. 40, 1251 – 1256.

Curry, S. H. and Marshall, J. H. L. (1968) Plasma levels of chlorpromazine and some of its relatively non-polar metabolites in psychiatric patients. Life Sci. 7, 9 – 17.

Curry, S. H., Marshall, J. H. L., Davis, J. M. and Janowsky, D. S. (1970a) Factors affecting chlorpromazine plasma levels in psychiatric patients. Arch. Gen. Psychiatry 22, 209 – 215.

Curry, S. H., Marshall, J. H. L., Davis, J. M. and Janowsky, D. S. (1970b) Chlorpromazine plasma level and effects. Arch. Gen. Psychiatry 22, 289 – 296.

Davis, J. M., Janowsky, D. S., Sekerke, H., Manier, D. and El-Yousef, M. K. (1974) The pharmacokinetics of butaperazine in serum. In: I. Forrest, C. Carr and E. Usdin (Eds), The Phenothiazines and Structurally Related Drugs. Raven Press, New York, pp. 433 – 443.

Davis, J. M., Ericksen, S. and Dekirmenjian H. (1978) Plasma levels of antipsychotic drugs and clinical response. In: M. A. Lipton A. Dimascio, and K. F. Killam (Eds), Psychopharmacology: A Generation of Progress. Raven Press, New York, pp. 905 – 915.

Dysken, M. W., Javaid, J. I., Chang, S. S., Schaffer, C., Shaid, A. and Davis, J. M. (1981) Fluphenazine pharmacokinetics and therapeutic response. Psychopharmacology 73, 205 – 210.

Franklin, M., Wiles, D. H. and Harvey, D. J. (1978) Sensitive gas chromatographic determination of fluphenazine in human plasma. Clin. Chem. 24, 41 – 44.

Garver, D. L., Dekirmenjian, H., Davis, J. M., Casper, R. and Erickson, S. (1977) Neuroleptic drug levels and therapeutic response: preliminary observations with red blood cell bound butaperazine. Am. J. Psychiatry 134, 304 – 307.

Gottschalk, L. A., Dinovo, E. C. and Nandi, B. R. (1978) The assay of plasma concentration of thioridazine and its metabolites as a function of time. Commun. Psychopharmacol. 2, 475 – 479.

Hobbs, D. C., Welch, W. M., Short, M. J., Moody, W. A. and Van der Velde, C. D. (1974) Pharmacokinetics of thiothixene in man. Clin. Pharmacol. Ther. 16, 473 – 478.

Javaid, J. I., Dekirmenjian, H., Liskevych, U., Lin, R. L. and Davis, J. M. (1981) Fluphenazine determination in human plasma by a sensitive gas chromatographic method using nitrogen detector. J. Chromatogr. Sci. 19, 439 – 443.

Javaid, J. I., Dekirmenjian, H. and Davis, J. M. (1982) GLC analysis of trifluoperazine in human plasma. J. Pharm. Sci. 71, 63 – 66.

Lader, M. H. (1976) Monitoring plasma concentrations of neuroleptics. Pharmacopsychiatry 9, 170 – 177.

Manian, A. A., Efron, D. H. and Goldbert, M. E. (1965) A comparative pharmacological study of a series of monohydroxylated and methoxylated chlorpromazine derivatives. Life Sci. 4, 2425 – 2438.

Manian, A. A., Efron, D. H. and Harris, S. R. (1971) Appearance of monohydroxylated chlorpromazine metabolites in the central nervous system. Life Sci. 10, 679 – 684.

Manian, A. A., Piette, L. H., Holland, D., Grover, T. and Leterrier F. (1974) Red blood cell drug binding as a possible mechanism for tranquilization. In: I. S. Forrest, C. J. Carr and E. Usdin (Eds), Advances in Biochemical Pyschopharmacology. Raven Press, New York, pp. 149 – 161.

May, P. R. A., van Putten, T., Jenden, D. J., Yale, C. and Dixon, W. J. (1981) Chlorpromazine levels and outcome of treatment in schizophrenic patients. Arch. Gen. Psychiatry 38, 202 – 207.

Midha, K. K., Hubbard, J. W., Cooper, J. K., Hawes, E. M., Fournier, S. and Yeung, P. (1981) Radioimmunoassay for trifluoperazine in human plasma. Br. J. Clin. Pharmacol. 12, 189 – 193.

Papdopoulos, A. S., Ghand, T. G., Crammer, J. L. and Lader, S. (1980) A pilot study of plasma thioidazine and metabolites in chronically treated patients. Br. J. Psychiatry 13, 591 – 596.

Sakalis, G., Curry, S. H., Mould, G. P. and Lader, M. H. (1972) Psychologic and clinical effects of chlorpromazine and their relationship to plasma level. Clin. Pharmacol. Ther. 13, 931 – 946.

Simpson, G. M., Lament, R., Cooper, T. B., Lee, J. H. and Bruce, R. B. (1973) The relationship between blood levels of different forms of butaperazine and clinical response. J. Clin. Pharmacol. 13, 288 – 297.

Simpson, G. M., Cooper, T. B., Lee, J. H. and Young, M. A. (1978) Clinical and plasma level characteristics of intramuscular and oral loxapine. Psychopharmacol. 56, 225 – 232.

Smith, R. C., Crayton, J. W., Dekirmenjian, H., Klass, D. and Davis, J. M. (1979) Blood levels of neuroleptic drugs in nonresponding chronic schizophrenic patients. Arch. Gen. Psychiatry 36, 579 – 584.

Smith, R. C., Vroulis, G., Shvartsburd, A., Allen, R., Lewis, N., Schoolar, J. C., Chojnacki, M. and Johnson, R. (1982) RBC and plasma levels of haloperidol and clinical response. Am. J. Psychiatry 139, 1054 – 1056.

Van Putten, T., May, P. R. A., Marder, S. R. and Wittman, L. A. (1981) Subjective response to antipsychotic drugs. Arch. Gen. Psychiatry 38, 187 – 191.

Wode-Helgodt, B. and Alfredsson, G. (1981) Concentrations of chlorpromazine and two of its active metabolites in plasma and cerebrospinal fluid of psychotic patients treated with fixed drug doses. Psychopharmacology 73, 55 – 62.

Wode-Helgodt, B., Eneroth, P., Fyro, B., Gullberg, B. and Sedvall, G. (1977) Effect of chlorpromazine treatment on prolactin levels in cerebrospinal fluid and plasma of psychotic patients. Acta Psychiatr. Scand. 56, 280 – 293.

Wode-Helgodt, B., Borg, S., Fyro, B. and Sedvall, G. (1978) Clinical effects and drug concentrations in plasma and cerebrospinal fluid in psychotic patients treated with fixed doses of chlorpromazine. Acta Psychiatr. Scand. 58, 149 – 173.

Yesavage, J. A., Holman, C. A. and Cohn, R. (1981) Correlation of thiothixene serum levels and age. Psychopharmacol. 74, 170 – 172.

Burrows/Norman/Davies (eds) Antipsychotics

Chapter 6

Plasma level measurement of phenothiazines and butyrophenones

KAY P. MAGUIRE

Department of Psychiatry, University of Melbourne, Australia

and

TREVOR R. NORMAN

Department of Psychiatry, University of Melbourne, Austin Hospital, Australia

INTRODUCTION

A variety of methods have been reported for the measurement of phenothiazines and butyrophenones since the introduction of chlorpromazine (CPZ) in the fifties. It is only recently that methods of sufficient sensitivity and specificity for the analysis of plasma concentrations have been developed. This is largely due to two factors, the first being the numerous active metabolites of drugs such as CPZ and thioridazine, and the second, the very low concentrations achieved following the long-acting depot preparations such as fluphenazine decanoate.

The first suitable method for the determination of plasma CPZ concentrations was developed in 1968 (Curry, 1968). This method utilized gas chromatography with electron-capture detection. Recent developments include gas chromatography with nitrogen-selective detection, gas chromatography-mass fragmentography, radioimmunoassay, radioreceptor assay and high performance liquid chromatography.

The limitations and advantages of these techniques will be reviewed and the appropriate method to select, depending on the required application, discussed. In addition, the requirements of a good assay will be outlined and the above techniques assessed in that light.

REQUIREMENTS OF A GOOD ASSAY

A good assay must meet certain criteria. Definitions of analytical parameters to be considered are as follows: *Precision* (reproducibility) – the closeness of agreement between the results obtained by applying the experimental procedure several times under prescribed conditions. *Accuracy* – the closeness of agreement between the true value and the mean results obtained by applying the experimental procedure a very large number of times. In practice this should involve as many results as possible, the total number being stated. *Limit of detection* – the smallest concentration of substance which can be reported with a specified degree of certainty. *Sensitivity* – the change in measured value resulting from a concentration change of one unit. The assay should be capable of a precision of approximately $\pm$ 5 – 10% (CV) over the total concentration range required. A procedure is considered specific if drug metabolites or endogenous plasma constituents do not interfere. In addition, only drugs which do not interfere in the assay procedure should be administered concomitantly.

Several practicalities should also be considered when assessing assay procedures. These are expense, in terms of initial outlay for equipment and running costs, time required to complete the assays, convenience and ease of performing the procedure.

ANALYTICAL TECHNIQUES

Gas chromatography

Gas chromatography (GC) involves injection of a plasma extract onto the GC column where separation of compounds takes place. Commonly used column stationary phases for the phenothiazines or butyrophenones are the methyl or phenyl silicone phases (OV – 101, OV – 17). Compounds are detected as they elute from the GC column. The most frequently used detectors are the electron-capture (ECD) and the nitrogen-specific detectors (ND). Similar sensitivity (low nanogram range) is achieved with both detectors but the latter appears simpler to use on a routine basis. GC techniques have acceptable accuracy, precision and sensitivity for the measurement of plasma drug concentrations following multiple oral doses and for some single oral doses (e.g. CPZ).

Simultaneous quantitation of parent drug and active metabolites may be possible depending on the drug of interest. Simultaneous analysis of CPZ and some of its metabolites have been carried out (Curry, 1968) but problems were found when thioridazine and metabolites were examined by GC (see section on HPLC, p. 74).

Some published reports using GC-ND showing excellent sensitivity for fluphenazine and trifluoperazine include Javaid et al. (1981, 1982) and Roscoe et al. (1982).

Gas chromatography-mass fragmentography (GC-MF)

GC-MF involves the use of a mass spectrometer as an ion-specific detector for the GC. Simultaneous and continuous monitoring of mass spectral ions representing typical fragments of the compounds to be measured provides for a high degree of selectivity. Combining this with the separative powers of GC has produced one of the most powerful analytical techniques available. However, the high cost of the instrumentation restricts the use of the technique.

An advantage of this procedure is that it can be used for screening of plasma from overdose patients. It is more sensitive than the other GC methods (sub-nanogram range) hence is extremely useful for single dose pharmacokinetic studies, and for monitoring plasma concentrations following the long-acting intramuscular depot preparations such as fluphenazine decanoate.

Several phenothiazine or butyrophenone compounds have been successfully measured using GC-MF, including CPZ and some metabolites (Alfredsson et al., 1976), trifluoperazine (Midha et al., 1982) and fluphenazine (McKay et al., 1983).

Radioimmunoassay (RIA)

The basic principle of radioimmunoassay is that of competitive protein-binding where a radioactive and a non-radioactive compound compete for a fixed number of antibody binding sites. The antibodies are generated by raising antisera in animals. A major problem with this type of assay is that many antisera show substantial cross-reactivity between parent drug and metabolites. Furthermore, the cross-reactivity between drug and metabolites is not identical so that an accurate measurement of total drug and metabolites is not obtained.

RIAs are very sensitive techniques (sub-nanogram range) and have acceptable precision and accuracy. Provided a specific antiserum can be developed, RIAs are excellent techniques for single-dose kinetics. As a screening procedure for checking compliance, RIA is most suitable as the technique is simple, rapid, and requires small volumes of plasma.

Few RIA methods have been published recently but earlier publications include methods for CPZ (Midha et al., 1979), perphenazine (Midha et al., 1981a), fluphenazine (Wiles and Franklin, 1978), and haloperidol (Rubin et al., 1980).

Radioreceptor assay (RRA)

RRAs for antipsychotic drugs are based on the hypothesis that these drugs act by selectively blocking the brain dopamine receptors. The principle of the assay is the in vitro competitive binding of these drugs in plasma with radioactively labelled compounds (e.g. [^{3}H]spiroperidol) that bind selectively to membrane receptors.

The technique measures total pharmacological activity (i.e. parent drug and any metabolites possessing dopamine blocking activity), and results are usually expressed as 'CPZ equivalents'.

Sensitivity is generally in the nanogram range but a lack of precision (CV 20 – 30%) has been reported (Lader, 1980). Non-specific interference by serum constituents has also been reported recently (Mailman et al., 1984) which is a major problem.

Although RRA was initially thought to have great potential for studies correlating clinical response with drug plasma concentrations, recent reviewers have been more critical (Rivera-Calimlim and Hershey, 1984). As a screening procedure, RRA may be useful as it is simple, rapid and requires small volumes of plasma. If high concentrations of pharmacologically active but not psychoactive metabolites are present in any samples then misleading results would ensue.

The first report of the use of RRAs was by Creese and Snyder (1979) and further published assays have been based on this method.

High performance liquid chromatography (HPLC)

HPLC methodology has developed rapidly over the last few years and appears to have several advantages over other techniques. Following extraction of the plasma sample, separation of components can be achieved by either ion-pair partition, adsorption, reversed phase or most recently using radially compressed silica gel columns. Detection modes include fluorimetric, UV absorbance or electrochemical detection (EC).

Radial compression has been shown to offer significant improvements in resolution of thioridazine and four metabolites (Kilts et al., 1982), and other phenothiazines (Curry et al., 1982). The latter study compared two detection systems, finding that the sensitivity achieved with UV was approximately 10 ng/ml and that electrochemical detection lowers this by two orders of magnitude.

Since HPLC is carried out at room temperature, reduction of metabolites to their parent drug (e.g. CPZ-*N*-oxide to CPZ) which occurs during high temperature GC analysis, is not a problem. Sample derivatisation is often necessary with GC assays to improve chromatographic separations but the derivatising reagents can sometimes alter metabolites (e.g. thioridazine 2-sulfoxide was converted to the sulfide when reacted with trifluoroacetic anhydride). This also is not a problem with HPLC as good separation can be achieved without derivatisation.

The two publications referred to above provide detailed information on the application of HPLC to the analysis of phenothiazines. A method for the measurement of haloperidol and reduced haloperidol has been reported by Korpi et al. (1983).

Comparative studies

Some recent studies have compared two or more different analytical procedures for the same drug. Due to its excellent sensitivity and specificity, GC-MF is usually used as the reference method. McKay et al. (1982) compared GC-MF and HPLC-EC for CPZ and found good agreement for 90 samples over the range 0.25 – 10 ng/ml. A GC-ND assay for trifluoperazine showed agreement with a GC-MF assay whereas RIA gave slightly higher values, probably due to metabolic interference (Roscoe et al., 1982).

Comparisons of RRA and either GC or GC-MS have shown reasonable agreement for some drugs but not others. Kurland et al. (1981) found good agreement between RRA and GC-MF for haloperidol suggesting that haloperidol has few active metabolites. Javaid and colleagues' (Javaid et al., 1980) findings were similar for both haloperidol and butaperazine, however, the values obtained by RRA were 7 – 8 times greater than GC-ND for fluphenazine and trifluoperazine. It may be that RRAs are useful for certain drugs but larger comparative studies are required to confirm this.

Although it is good practice to check a newly developed assay with an established assay within laboratories, interlaboratory comparisons are even more desirable. This was attempted earlier for CPZ (Turner et al., 1976) and some assays found lacking. Commercially available quality control samples would be most helpful in ensuring that all laboratories are obtaining comparable results.

PLASMA EXTRACTION

Extraction of parent drug and metabolites from the plasma is necessary prior to analysis by GC or HPLC. RIA or RRA generally can be carried out using unextracted plasma. Extraction procedures for these drugs involve alkalinisation of the plasma and extraction into an organic solvent such as hexane or diethyl ether. This one-step procedure is adequate for some assays. For others such as GC-MF or for HPLC where concentrations are expected to be low, a three-step extraction is necessary to provide clean extracts. Following the first extraction into an organic solvent, a back extraction into acid, and a further extraction into an organic solvent is carried out. A paper by Curry et al. (1982) has suggested the following scheme for HPLC extractions – for parent drug alone use hexane; for metabolites in addition to parent drug use diethyl ether; for difficult problems, whole blood or low concentrations use a three-step procedure with chloroform as the second solvent. Other authors (Roscoe et al., 1982) suggest adding isopropyl alcohol to the extraction solvent to retard adsorption of these drugs onto glass during the extraction. Silanisation of glassware used for extraction is also recommended to overcome this problem (Kilts et al., 1982). Use of high quality solvents is recommended to provide clean extracts.

SAMPLE COLLECTION AND STORAGE

Blood is usually collected into glass or polystyrene tubes containing heparin or EDTA as anticoagulants. Collection of blood into evacuated tubes may be carried out provided that the blood does not contact the stopper. A redistribution of drug between the plasma and red cells is caused by a plasticiser from the stopper (Javaid et al., 1980; Midha et al., 1981b), leading to a lowering of the plasma concentration.

Some early reports were concerned about the stability of frozen plasma samples but recent papers have shown that this is not a problem for most drugs in the short term. Methanolic solutions were stable in the dark at 4°C for at least one month, and plasma standards and samples were stable when frozen for the same time (Curry et al., 1982; Midha et al., 1982). Little data has been published on the effect of storage over a longer timespan except for Javaid et al. (1982), who found that samples without preservatives added were more prone to losses during storage over one year. The suggested preservatives were either sodium metabisulfite or ascorbic acid (0.5 mg/ml). Some authors also recommend that assays be carried out in subdued lighting to minimise decomposition during extraction and analysis.

SUMMARY

The method of choice for the determination of plasma levels of phenothiazines and butyrophenones, depends largely on the concentration of the drug in the plasma, and whether simultaneous measurement of metabolites is also required. For phenothiazines such as CPZ and thioridazine, plasma concentrations above 10 ng/ml would be expected. Either a GC-ND of HPLC-UV would be the method of choice for single dose kinetics requiring only parent drug levels. For clinical response studies requiring metabolites as well, only HPLC would be appropriate.

For fluphenazine and trifluoperazine, where low or sub-nanogram per millilitre concentrations would be expected, GC-MF would be the method of choice for single dose kinetics, or RIA if a specific antiserum was available. For clinical studies involving metabolites, GC-MF, HPLC-EC and possibly GC-ND procedures would be appropriate.

Haloperidol may be estimated using a variety of methods as it does not have any active metabolites (although Korpi et al., 1983 have suggested that reduced haloperidol may be psychoactive). Plasma concentrations in plasma are in the nanogram range, even after the i.m. decanoate, thus RIA, GC-ND, HPLC-EC and possibly RRA could be used for clinical response and pharmacokinetic studies.

For studies where more than one antipsychotic medication is being prescribed, HPLC would be the method of choice (Curry et al., 1982).

REFERENCES

Alfredsson, G., Wode-Helgodt, B. and Sedvall, G. (1976) A mass fragmentographic method for the determination of chlorpromazine and two of its active metabolites in human plasma and CSF. Psychopharmacol. 48, 123–131.

Creese, I. and Snyder, S. H. (1977) A simple and sensitive radioreceptor assay for antischizophrenic drugs in blood. Nature (London) 270, 180–182.

Curry, S. H. (1968) Determination of nanogram quantities of chlorpromazine and some of its metabolites in plasma with an electron capture detector. Anal. Chem. 40, 1251–1255.

Curry, S. H., Brown, E. A., Hu, O. Y-P. and Perrin, J. H. (1982) Liquid chromatographic assay of phenothiazine, thioxanthene and butyrophenone neuroleptics and antihistamines in blood and plasma with conventional and radial compression columns and UV and electrochemical detection. J. Chromatogr. 231, 361–376.

Javaid, J. I., Pandey, G. N., Duslak, B., Hu, H. Y. and Davis, J. M. (1980) Measurement of neuroleptic concentrations by GLC and radioreceptor assay. Commun. Psychopharmacol. 4, 467–475.

Javaid, J. I., Dekirmenjian, H., Liskevych, U., Lin, R-L., and Davis, J. M. (1981) Fluphenazine determination in human plasma by a sensitive gas chromatographic method using nitrogen detector. J. Chromatogr. Sci. 19, 439–443.

Javaid, J. I., Dekirmenjian, H. and Davis, J. M. (1982) GLC analysis of trifluoperazine in human plasma. J. Pharm. Sci. 71, 63–66.

Kilts, C. D., Patrick, K. S., Breese, G. R. and Mailman, R. B. (1982) Simultaneous determination of thioridazine and its S-oxidised and N-demethylated metabolites using high performance liquid chromatography on radially compressed silica. J. Chromatogr. 231, 377–391.

Korpi, E. R., Phelps, B. H., Granger, H., Chang, W-H, Linnoila, M., Meek, J. L. and Wyatt, R. J. (1983) Simultaneous determination of haloperidol and its reduced metabolite in serum and plasma by isocratic liquid chromatography with electrochemical detection. Clin. Chem. 29, 624–628.

Kurland, A. A., Nagaraju, A., Hanlon, T. E., Wilkinson, E. H. and Ng, K. T. (1981) A comparison of dopamine receptor blocking assay with plasma drug levels of haloperidol in schizophrenic patients. J. Clin. Pharmacol. 21, 42–47.

Lader, S. R. (1980) A radioreceptor assay for neuroleptic drugs in plasma. J. Immunoassay. 1, 57–75.

Mailman, R. B., Dehaven, D. L., Halpern, E. A. and Lewis, M. H. (1984) Serum effects confound the neuroleptic radioreceptor assay. Life Sci. 34, 1057–1064.

McKay, G., Hall, K., Cooper, J. K. Hawes, E. M. and Midha, K. K. (1982) Gas chromatographic-mass spectrometric procedure for the quantitation of chlorpromazine in plasma and its comparison with a new high performance liquid chromatographic assay with electrochemical detection. J. Chromatogr. 232, 275–282.

McKay, G., Hall, K., Edom, R. Hawes, E. M. and Midha, K. K. (1983) Subnanogram determination of fluphenazine in human plasma by gas chromatography-mass spectrometry. Biomed. Mass Spectrom. 10, 550–555.

Midha, K. K., Loo, J. C. K., Hubbard, J. W., Rowe, M. L. and McGilveray, I. J. (1979) Radioimmunoassay for chlorpromazine in plasma. Clin. Chem. 25, 166–168.

Midha, K. K., MacKonka, C., Cooper, J. K., Hubbard, J. W. and Yeung P. K. F. (1981a) Radioim-

munoassay for perphenazine in human plasma. Br. J. Clin. Pharmacol. 1, 85 – 88.
Midha, K. K., Cooper, J. K., Lapierre, Y. D. and Hubbard, J. W. (1981b) Fluphenazine, trifluoperazine and perphenazine in vacutainers. Can. Med. Assoc. J. 124, 264 – 265.
Midha, K. K., Roscoe, R. M. H., Hall, K., Hawes, E. M. Cooper, J. K., McKay, G. and Shetty, H. U. (1982) A gas chromatographic-mass spectrometric assay for plasma trifluoperazine concentrations following single doses. Biomed. Mass Spectrom. 9, 186 – 189.
Rivera-Calimlim, L. and Hershey, L. (1984) Neuroleptic concentrations and clinical response. Ann. Rev. Pharmacol. Toxicol. 24, 361 – 386.
Roscoe, R. M. H., Cooper, J. K., Hawes, E. M. and Midha, K. K. (1982) A GLC nitrogen phosphorus detector assay for trifluoperazine in plasma. J. Pharm. Sci. 71, 625 – 627.
Rubin, R. T., Forsman, A., Heykants, J., Ohman, R., Tower, B. and Michiels, M. (1980) Serum haloperidol determinations in psychiatric patients. Arch. Gen. Psychiatry 37, 1069 – 1074.
Turner, W. J., Turano, P. and Badzinski, S. (1976) An attempt to establish quality control in determination of plasma chlorpromazine by a multi-laboratory collaboration. In: L. Gottschalk and S. Merlis (Eds), Pharmacokinetics of Psychoactive Drugs. Spectrum, New York, pp. 33 – 43.
Wiles, D. H. and Franklin, M. (1978) Radioimmunoassay for fluphenazine in human plasma. Br. J. Clin. Pharmacol. 5, 265 – 268.

Burrows/Norman/Davies (eds) Antipsychotics

Chapter 7

Phenothiazines: Metabolism and pharmacokinetics

STEPHEN H. CURRY

Division of Clinical Pharmacokinetics, College of Pharmacy, University of Florida, Gainesville, FL 32610, U.S.A.

INTRODUCTION

Research into the metabolism and pharmacokinetics of drugs is a crucial part of the objective study of the time course of drug action, which in turn should be the basis for the selection of logical sizes of doses and frequency of drug administration. This philosophy became firmly established as the result of the pioneering work of Bernard B. Brodie between 1945 and 1970 (Curry and Brodie, 1967; Brodie, 1968). The phenothiazine drugs were subjected to intensive study in regard to their metabolites in the period 1955 – 1965, and since 1965 there has been considerable interest in their pharmacokinetic properties, while interest in the metabolites has abated somewhat. This chapter is designed to review the established truths of this area of research, and to bring up-to-date information previously reviewed between 1976 and 1981, and published in several other book chapters (Curry, 1976a, b, 1980, 1981a, b).

METABOLISM

Metabolic reactions

The phenothiazines are substrates for a remarkably large number of metabolic reactions. The known initial reactions involved in chlorpromazine metabolism include sulphoxidation (addition of oxygen to the phenothiazine ring sulphur), hydroxylation (substitution of an OH group for protons in the phenothiazine ring), demethylation (removal of CH_3 groups from the tertiary amine group at the end of the side chain, in two stages), and *N*-oxidation (addition of oxygen to the nitrogen of the tertiary amine group). The products of hydroxylation, such as 7-hydroxychlorpromazine, become conjugated with glucuronic acid to form *O*-glucuronides, Additionally, there has long been a suspicion that the side chain can be deaminated, and also that sulphones (disulphoxides) can be formed, although whether or not either of these reactions truly occurs has never been adequately resolved. Another paper reported formation of a new group of glucuronides of tertiary amine drugs, including chlorpromazine, arising by direct coupling of the tertiary amine group and the glucuronic acid residue to give a quaternary amine glucuronide. Another previous paper reported discovery of aminoethylation of the phenothiazine ring (Vierfond et al., 1983).

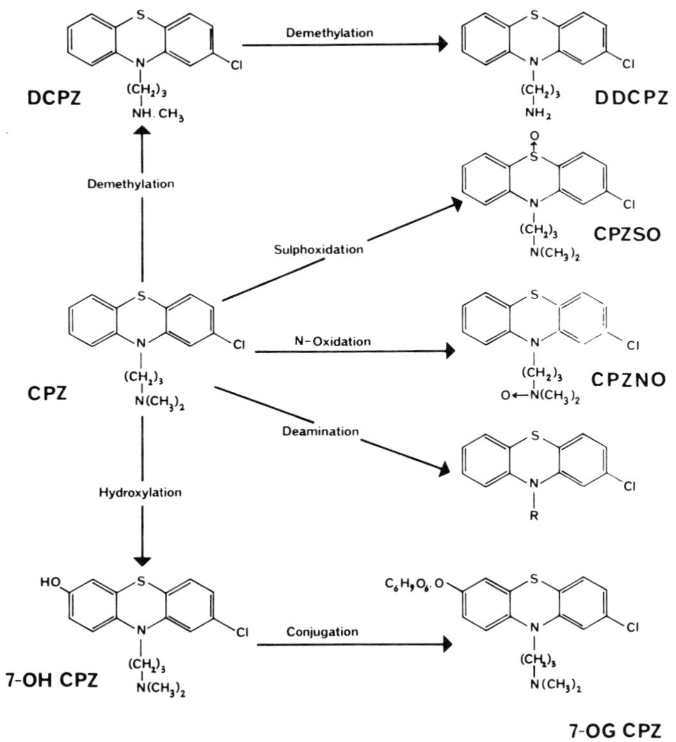

Fig. 1. Principal metabolic reactions of chlorpromazine (CPZ). DCPZ = demonomethylchlorpromazine; DDCPZ = dedimethylchlorpromazine; 7-OH-CPZ = 7-hydroxychlorpromazine; CPZSO = chlorpromazine sulphoxide; CPZNO = chlorpromazine *N*-oxide; 7-OG-CPZ = 7-hydroxychlorpromazine glucuronide. (Reprinted with permission, from Curry, 1976 b.)

The major metabolic pathways of chlorpromazine are summarized in Fig. 1. The reactions occur in various combinations to give a wide variety of compounds, and the reactions listed above could potentially lead to over 200 metabolites if all possible combinations occurred. In fact, thin layer chromatographic examination of urine leads to the belief that over 50 metabolites of chlorpromazine are certainly formed in the body. Furthermore, the figure of 200 assumes only one hydroxylation position in the phenothiazine ring. At one time considerable effort was expended to determine the site of hydroxylation. The primary site of hydroxylation is undoubtedly as shown in Fig. 1, but the other sites para to the ring nitrogen or sulphur may well be of some importance.

Phenothiazines other than chlorpromazine can undergo different reactions. For example, thioridazine forms both ring and side chain sulphoxides and sulphones, but probably no hydroxylated metabolites. The compounds with piperazine in the side chain, such as trifluoperazine, are partially metabolized by opening of the piperazine ring. The compounds with an alchoholic OH group at the ends of their side chains, such as fluphenazine and perphenazine, can undergo direct conjugation with glucuronic acid to form *O*-glucuronides. The formulae of thioridazine, trifluoperazine, and fluphenazine are shown in Fig. 2. The principal biotransformation reactions of fluphenazine are shown in Fig. 3.

Significance of metabolites of antipsychotic drugs

The complexity of the metabolic pathways leads to major problems in evaluating the importance of the metabolites. However, certain facts prevail. First, metabolism of phenothiazine drugs, like metabolism of almost all drugs, confers polarity. The products are almost always more polar than their precursors. The polarity of a large number of phenothiazine model metabolites has been assessed by measurement of the partition ratios of the compounds between a series of hexane/hexanol mixtures and phosphate buffer at pH 7.4. All the metabolites were more polar than chlor-

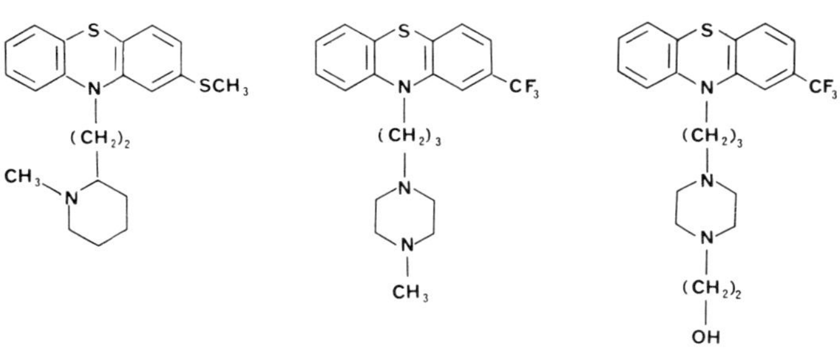

I II III

Fig. 2. Chemical formulae of thioridazine (I), trifluoperazine (II), and fluphenazine (III).

promazine (Table 1). Conferment of polarity reduces the likelihood of passage across the blood-brain barrier, increases the likelihood of renal excretion, and decreases the likelihood of extensive tissue binding, which can be a factor in long-term retention of drug-derived material in the body. It appears, also, that lipophilicity correlates well with binding to dopamine receptor of the D-1 type (Fig. 4). This relationship has not been studied with D-2 receptors.

A second important fact concerning the metabolites of phenothiazine relates to the absence of a common metabolic route among the compounds. At one time, a theory prevailed that the metabolic reaction per se was involved in the mediation of the effect at the biochemical level. The lack of a common metabolic pathway among such similar drugs is evidence against this theory.

Third, some of the metabolites undoubtedly possess pharmacological activity qualitatively comparable with that of chlorpromazine, and exemplified in vitro in tests which are thought to be models of the biochemical mechanism of action in

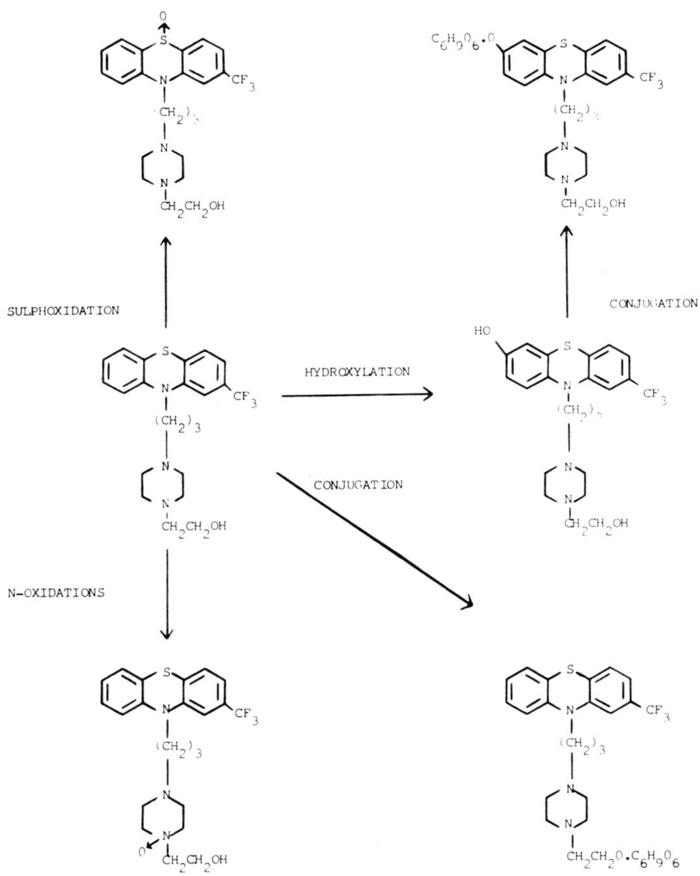

Fig. 3. Principal biotransformation reactions of fluphenazine.

TABLE 1

Relative polarity of chlorpromazine and 15 of its model metabolites.

No.	Compound	Polarity index
1.	Chlorpromazine	Approx. 1
2.	Demonomethylchlorpromazine	5
3.	Dedimethylchlorpromazine	35
4.	7-Hydroxychlorpromazine	50
5.	Chlorpromazine *N*-oxide	74
6.	3-(2-Chlorophenothiazinyl-10)-propionic acid	153
7.	7-Hydroxydemonomethylchlorpromazine	195
8.	7-Hydroxydedimethylchlorpromazine	334
9.	Chlorpromazine sulphoxide	781
10.	Sulphoxide of 4	1259
11.	Sulphoxide of 5	2553
12.	Sulphoxide of 2	4444
13.	Sulphoxide of 7	5036
14.	Sulphoxide of 3	5504
15.	Sulphoxide of 6	5665
16.	Sulphoxide of 8	6161

Partition coefficients were measured between equal volumes of 0.1 M phosphate buffer (pH 7.4) and light liquid paraffin (mineral oil)/hexanol mixtures. Graphs were plotted of percent in buffer against percent hexanol in solvent mixture for each compound. The polarity index is the multiple of the co-ordinates on this graph where the line for the compound crosses a construction line of identity (slope and intercept = 1). (For details, see Curry and Whelpton, 1974.)

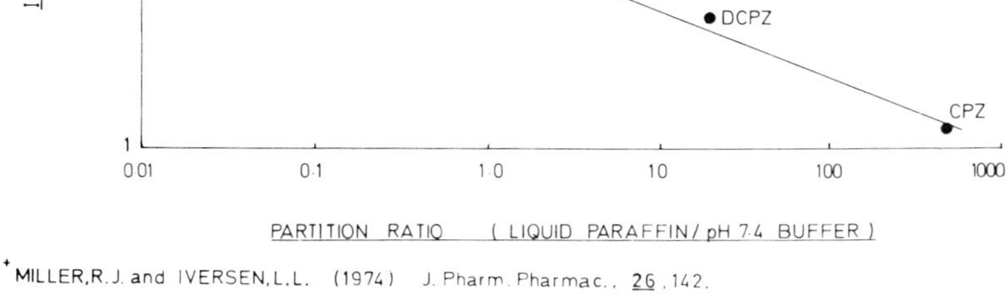

Fig. 4. Relation between IC_{50} for inhibition of dopamine-stimulated adenylate cyclase of rat striatum, and partition ratio between liquid paraffin (mineral oil) and pH 7.4 buffer. (Reprinted with permission, from Curry, 1981 b.)

vivo. However, this action is apparently restricted to the parent drug and the primary products of metabolism, such as chlorpromazine, desmonomethylchlorpromazine and 7-hydroxychlorpromazine, and to a lesser extent, chlorpromazine sulphoxide and chlorpromazine *N*-oxide. It seems that once more than one metabolic reaction has occurred, the compound loses its activity, possibly because of failure to bind to receptors, or possibly because of failure to cross the blood-brain barrier. The primary products of metabolism do indeed cross the blood-brain barrier. Whether or not the drug metabolites contribute to the pharmacological action of the phenothiazines is however dependent on more than whether or not they have activity in vitro, and are capable of crossing the blood-brain barrier. It is also dependent on whether they reach sufficient concentrations in the biophase when arising from the parent drug, and this is a pharmacokinetic issue considered later. The consensus view is that 7-hydroxychlorpromazine and desmonomethylchlorpromazine should be considered as playing a part in the action of chlorpromazine when present. Their formation is not however, essential to the action of chlorpromazine.

Fourth, the metabolites of phenothiazines are primarily formed in the liver. This can result from delivery through the hepatic artery or from delivery through the hepatic portal system. In the latter case it is a component of the first-pass effect, which is principally metabolism of orally-administered drug in the liver before it has a chance to reach the general circulation. This was discovered to be the major influence on chlorpromazine plasma levels as much as 15 years ago (Curry et al., 1970, 1971; Curry and Mould, 1975). Other sites of metabolism of phenothiazine drugs seem to include lung, brain, and the intestinal mucosa. In the case of lung and brain it is doubtful whether a major contribution is made. However, metabolism in the intestinal mucosa is probably a major part of the first-pass effect. This has been challenged (Taylor and Houston, 1983), but it should be noted that the intestinal mucosa was implicated as the result of: (1) the discovery of the necessary enzymes actually present in the intestinal mucosa; (2) comparative studies of plasma levels of chlorpromazine following intraperitoneal administration, as well as oral, intramuscular and intravenous administration, the significance being that the intraperitoneal doses are subject to the hepatic component of the first-pass effect, and a large difference between the orally and intraperitoneally induced plasma chlorpromazine was noted; and (3) metabolism of chlorpromazine was noted in living intestinal strips, without the liver present. The lack of intestinal metabolism has been claimed for promethazine, not for chlorpromazine, and in studies in herbivorous species not noted for their ability to metabolize drugs in intestinal tissue. Thus, there is no reason to dismiss the idea that chlorpromazine, and perhaps other antipsychotic phenothiazines, are at least partially metabolize in the intestinal mucosa, and are certainly metabolized in the liver before reaching the general circulation after oral dosing. The metabolic reactions of the first-pass effect appear particularly to be sulphoxidation and *N*-oxidation, whereas there is strong evidence that hydroxylation and demethylation prevail on systemic delivery to the liver. The status of *N*-

oxidation and demethylation is equivocal, as *N*-oxidation may be an intermediate reaction in demethylation.

Fluphenazine also has a major first-pass effect and in this case the metabolic reaction involved is probably direct glucuronidation (Curry et al., 1979). Other antipsychotic phenothiazines have not received the intensive investigation needed to fully characterize the first-pass effect.

PHARMACOKINETICS

History

The study of the pharmacokinetics of phenothiazine drugs dates back to approximately 1966, when it was first shown that chlorpromazine could be measured in plasma by gas chromatography with electron-capture detection (Curry and Brodie, 1967; Curry, 1968). This observation was quickly followed by the demonstration of wide interpatient variation in plasma levels of chlorpromazine in different patients treated with similar doses (Curry and Marshall, 1968). It was proposed then that levels below approximately 30 ng/ml were probably sub-therapeutic, and levels over 500 ng/ml were likely to be toxic. This 'therapeutic range', wide and approximate though it is, has been narrowed more recently to 35 – 350 ng/ml; but it remains basically valid. Other features of phenothiazine kinetics include: (1) the massive 'first-pass effect' mentioned previously; (2) production of the pharmacologically active metabolites mentioned earlier – their kinetics per se have never been studied; (3) double or triple exponential decay of plasma levels after intravenous injections; (4) long-term tissue retention; (5) considerable enzyme induction.

Pharmacokinetic models

Pharmacokineticists commonly draw figures with boxes representing compartments, and arrows representing transfer between the compartments. Pharmacokineticists also use equations. This is desirable but it need not become a burden. It is important however, to differentiate between the one-, two- and three-compartment models shown in Fig. 5. In the single compartment case, the drug is considered to be distributed homogeneously throughout the body. Input into the compartment is generally at a constant rate (k_0) by intravenous infusion, or by absorption (k_a) of doses placed in the gastrointestinal tract by swallowing. Absorption can follow intramuscular injection. Absorption processes are generally assessed by means of k_a values (exponential absorption rate constants). The single homogeneous compartment has an apparent volume (V) obtained by multiplying the concentration in plasma by the total body content, and the removal from the compartment is by elimination, an exponential process comprising metabolism, and ex-

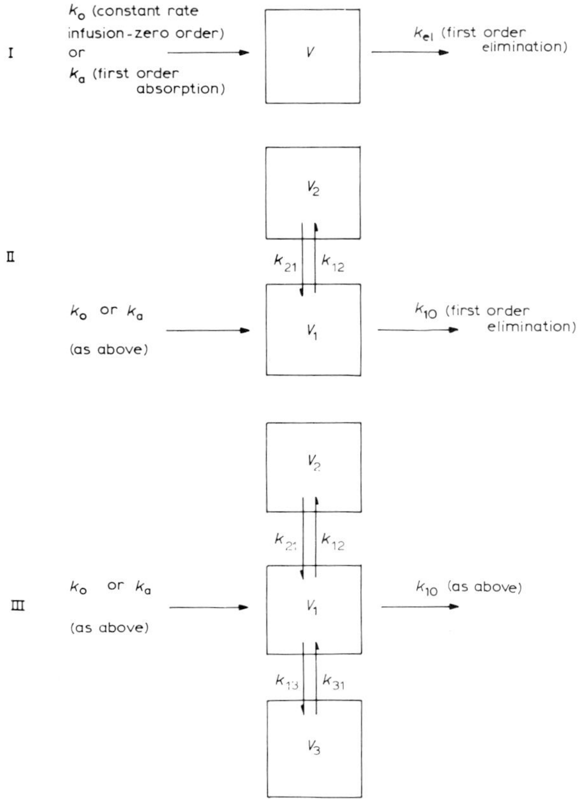

Fig. 5. The one (I), two (II), and three (III) compartment models.

cretion of the unchanged drug. This is assessed by k_{el}, the first order rate constant of elimination. The half-life of the drug ($t_{1/2}$) *is given by:*

$$t_{1/2} = \frac{0.693}{k_{el}}.$$

In the two-compartment case, the drug is distributed unevenly but to equilibrium, between two theoretical 'spaces', ' compartments' or areas of the body. These 'compartments' have theoretical volumes V_1 and V_2. Input is again by infusion or absorption, generally into the 'central' compartment (compartment 1) and output is by exponential elimination, from the central compartment. The rate constant of elimination from the central compartment is given the symbol k_{10} in this case. The transfer rate constants between the two compartments are k_{12} and k_{21}. The three-compartment case adds a third compartment to the two-compartment case.

After an intravenous bolus dose into a single compartment, the concentration of the drug declines exponentially with the same rate constant at all times and concentrations. The rate constant k_{el} represents loss of the drug from the body. Decline of the concentration in plasma within a two-compartment case is biphasic, fast at first, and slower later, with a transition point between the two parts of the decay curve being approximately identifiable. During the initial rapid phase (the equilibration phase), the drug decay is dominated by transfer of the drug from the central compartment, which includes plasma, into the peripheral compartment. The slower phase indicates decay of drug concentrations in the body as a whole. If there are three compartments, there are three phases of decay. In the two-compartment case, the rate constant of decline of drug concentration in the plasma in the slower phase (β) is the rate constant of decline of the drug amount in the body as a whole once equilibrium is reached, but it is not equal to k_{10}.

Comparisons between drug concentrations in plasma after intravenous, oral and

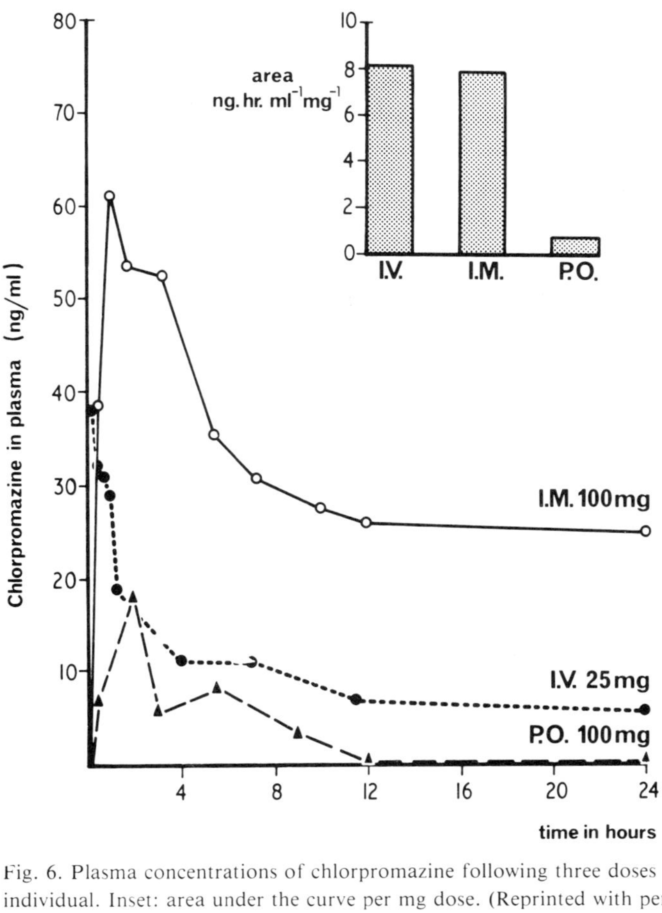

Fig. 6. Plasma concentrations of chlorpromazine following three doses in a single previously untreated individual. Inset: area under the curve per mg dose. (Reprinted with permission, from Curry, 1976 a.)

intramuscular doses lead to the realization that intravenous doses are unique in leading to an initial high concentration in the one-compartment system, or in the central compartment of the two-compartment system. Intramuscular doses generally lead to an area under the curve of a drug concentration diagram the same as that after a corresponding intravenous dose. Oral doses, like intramuscular doses, lead to a growth and decay pattern of drug concentration, but the area under the curve does not have to be the same as that after the injected doses because of the first-pass effect. This is shown for chlorpromazine in Fig. 6.

When second and later doses follow an initial dose, the doses build successively on the residues left from the previous doses. There is an overall rise in the mean concentration, but the rate of rise gradually decreases, so that the mean concentration tends to reach a plateau. It can be shown that, while the true plateau can only be reached if dosing continues for an infinite time, 90% of the plateau is reached by the time approximately four drug half-lives have elapsed, regardless of the frequency and magnitude of dosing. It is here that the concept of a steady state applies. True steady state is reached only at infinity, but the 90% point is a reasonable approximation. However, it must be noted that the pulsed nature of oral and intramuscular dosing causes a considerable fluctuation in the concentration both during the rise towards steady state, and at the steady state. This is shown for chlorpromazine in Fig. 7, with the added problem of enzyme induction being a considerable influence.

The last model to be considered relates to loading doses. If the initial dose of a multiple dosing regimen is higher than the ensuing doses, and if the relationship between the levels of the two doses is properly chosen then the steady state concentration is induced by the initial loading dose and maintained by the later doses. Generally speaking, if the dosage interval is equal to the half-life of the drug, the

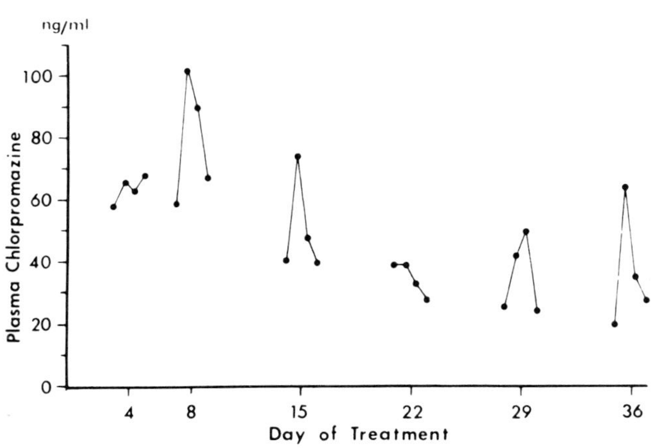

Fig. 7. Mean plasma concentrations of chlorpromazine in a group of patients treated for 36 days with 100 mg three times daily, and sampled at four times following the first dose on the days indicated. (From Sakalis et al., 1972.)

drug concentration will double after each dose, and fall by 50% from the peak by the time the next dose is due. More frequent dosing will lead to less fluctuation and less frequent dosing will lead to more fluctuation. This will be made more complex if doses are given on the equilibration phase of the biexponential decay in two-compartment cases when dosing is less frequent.

Specific examples of pharmacokinetics of phenothiazine drugs

It is clearly desirable in all circumstances to know the details of the drugs under study in regard to their many pharmacokinetic variables. These include whether a one- or two-compartment model is applicable, and if the latter whether the receptors, in the brain, are in the central or the peripheral compartment. Also, we need to know k_a values, especially if a rapid effect is sought. Whether or not a first-pass effect is prominent is also important, as is the activity of any metabolites. Also, the possibilities for enzyme induction, interpatient variation, dose relationships, and a host of other influences become important.

In considering specific examples, it is appropriate to stress that progress in pharmacokinetic studies of phenothiazines has been remarkably slow. Progress has in fact been so slow, that since investigators seem to be aware only of literature published during the 10 years previous to the time of their own interest in a particular problem, there is now a problem with investigators merely repeating earlier work.

Chlorpromazine is still the most widely studied drug. As mentioned earlier, prior to 1965, chlorpromazine had been studied extensively for its metabolic properties, but it had resisted plasma level studies. Gas chromatography with electron-capture detection revolutionized this research. The first-pass effect was demonstrated. The bi- or perhaps triexponential decay of intravenous doses was observed, with early phases lasting 6 to 8 hours. The time courses of effects and concentrations after single doses and during longer term treatment were studied, and the fact that enzyme induction occurred, reducing the plasma level induced per unit of dose was recognized as an important factor. Interaction studies followed. More recently, the multi-exponential decay has been re-emphasized, and multiple dosing clearly occurs on the equilibration phase. There is wide variation between patients. Intramuscular doses induce detectable concentrations rapidly, but absorption is still prolonged. Plasma and CSF levels are correlated but the distribution ratio varies between patients. Variation of single doses within individuals leads to a linear relationship between levels and dose, but when patients stabilized on different doses are studied, quite small increments of level per unit of dose are observed (Harmon et al., 1980; Loo et al., 1980; Van Putten et al., 1980, 1981; Alfredsson and Sedvall, 1981; Hershey et al., 1981; May et al., 1981; Midha et al., 1981; Sedvall, 1981; Wode-Helgodt and Alfredsson, 1981; Alfredsson et al., 1982; Murakami et al., 1982; Pantuck et al., 1982; Harris et al., 1983; Howes et al., 1983).

Multiple dosing with chlorpromazine every 6 – 8 hours is widely practised. The earliest half-life value given for chlorpromazine was approximately 6 hours, and this figure has found its way into textbooks of pharmacology. It is a valid figure for the fall from peak to trough levels within the pseudo-steady-state after long-term stabilization on chlorpromazine. However, it is an equilibration phase half-life, as tissue-to-plasma equilibration takes 8 or more hours. If the half-life of loss of the drug from the body were 6 hours, single doses would be 99% removed from the body within 48 hours, as would accumulated residues after cessation of dosing. It

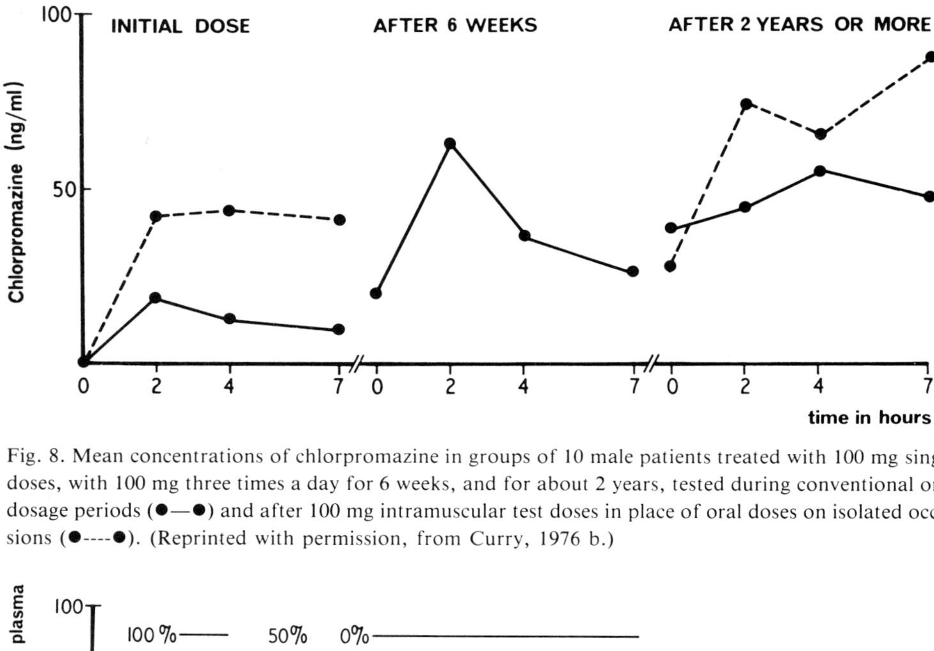

Fig. 8. Mean concentrations of chlorpromazine in groups of 10 male patients treated with 100 mg single doses, with 100 mg three times a day for 6 weeks, and for about 2 years, tested during conventional oral dosage periods (●—●) and after 100 mg intramuscular test doses in place of oral doses on isolated occasions (●----●). (Reprinted with permission, from Curry, 1976 b.)

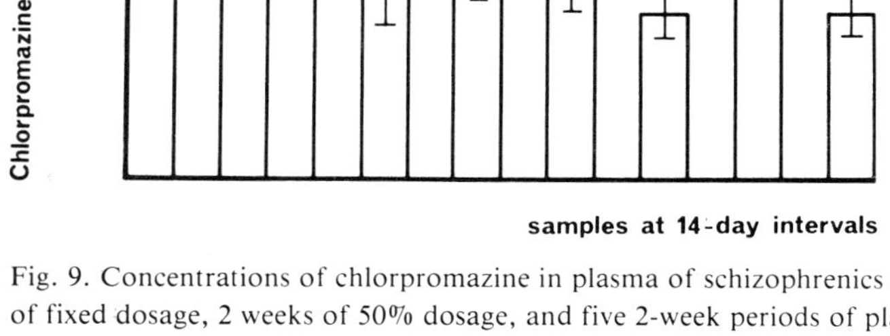

Fig. 9. Concentrations of chlorpromazine in plasma of schizophrenics at the end of two 2-week periods of fixed dosage, 2 weeks of 50% dosage, and five 2-week periods of placebo treatment. (Reprinted with permission, from Curry, 1976 b.)

is well known that chlorpromazine metabolites can be detected in urine up to 2 years after stopping dosing. When sufficiently sensitive assay techniques have been applied, and when trials have been dose and placebo controlled, plasma samples have provided evidence of a terminal phase half-life of chlorpromazine in the region of 60 days (see Figs. 8 and 9).

As mentioned earlier, fluphenazine also has a massive first-pass effect, with wide variations between individuals. There is little or no enzyme induction with this drug. Seven hydroxyfluphenazine is a controversial metabolite. The half-life of fluphenazine is approximately 16 hours. The depot intramuscular preparations are different. The enanthate leads to increasing plasma fluphenazine up to 2 – 3 days after the dose, after which it declines. The decanoate causes an initial sharp rise in plasma fluphenazine in the first 8 hours, after which the concentration drops to a level which persists almost unchanged for almost 2 weeks or perhaps longer.

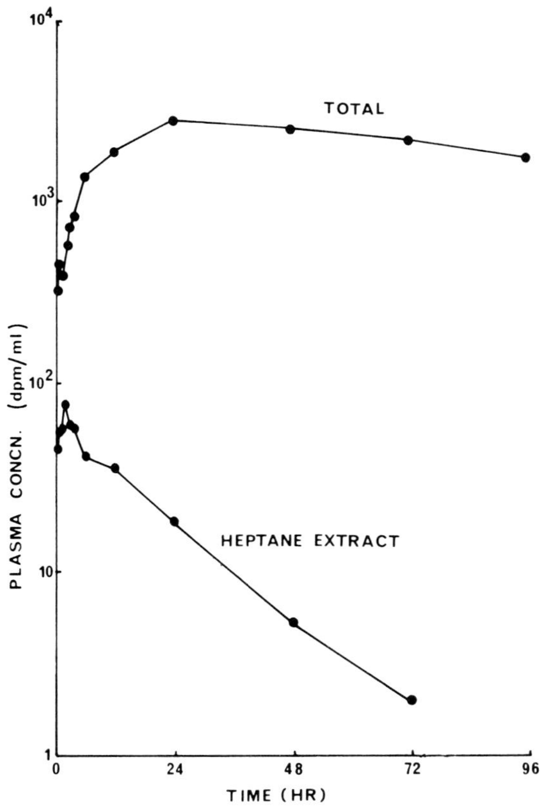

Fig. 10. Fluphenazine concentrations (in radioactivity units) (heptane extract) and total radioactivity (total) in plasma of a patient treated with 25 mg of radioactive fluphenazine (for details, see Curry et al., 1979).

Fluphenazine levels are not changed by antiparkinsonian drugs (see Figs. 10 – 12) (Heyes et al., 1980; Midha et al., 1980; Dysken et al., 1981; Goldstein and Van Vunakis, 1981; Javaid et al., 1981; Sakalis and Traficante, 1981; Davis and Fenimore, 1983).

Butaperazine shows immense variation in levels, as does thioridazine which has much higher levels than the other drugs. Thioridazine is complicated by having metabolites which have been proved to possess clinical activity, and by there being no injectable form of the drug. There is also a wide range in the non-protein bound fraction, which is also known to occur with chlorpromazine (Casper et al., 1980; Papadopoulos et al., 1980; Skinner et al., 1980; Crammer, 1981; Nyberg et al.,

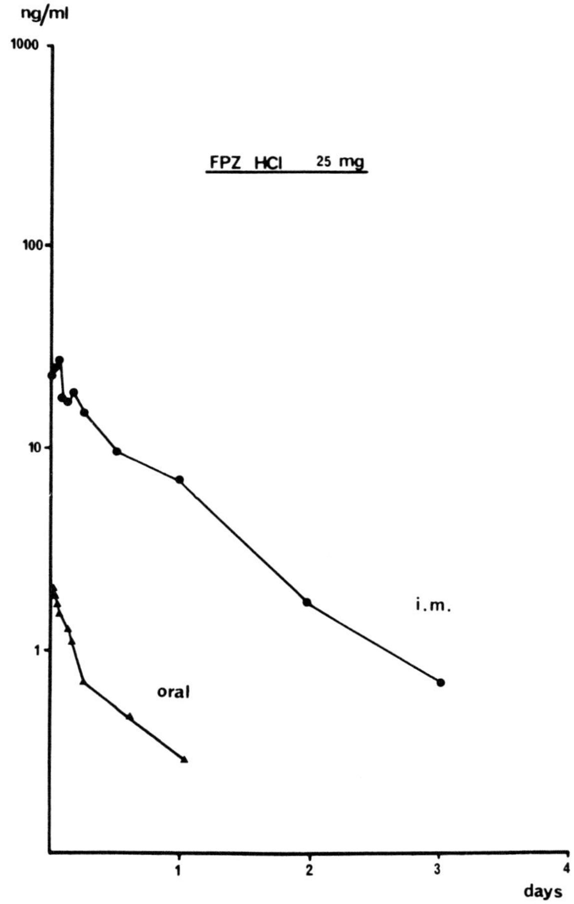

Fig. 11. Fluphenazine concentrations in plasma of a patient treated with fluphenazine hydrochloride orally and by intramuscular injection (both 25 mg) (for details see Curry et al., 1979).

1981; Vaisanen et al., 1981; Axelsson et al., 1982; Kilts et al., 1982; Nyberg and Martensson, 1982; Widerlov et al., 1982).

Trifluoperazine is one of the oldest of the drugs but one of the most recently studied. Its concentrations are proportional to dose, and its half-life is in the general region of seven to 20 hours after single doses. However, in one study, virtually no within-dose fluctuation was observed in a single patient treated long term (Gillespie and Sipes, 1981; Javaid et al., 1982; Midha et al., 1982; Whelpton et al., 1982). Perphenazine (Bolvig-Hanssen et al., 1981), perazine (Schley et al., 1981; Brinkschulte et al., 1982; Schley 1983), pipothiazine (Cooper and Lapierre, 1981) and levomepromazine (Dahl et al., 1982) have been the subject of isolated studies. Several studies have been non-specific (Cohen et al., 1980; Kurland et al., 1980;

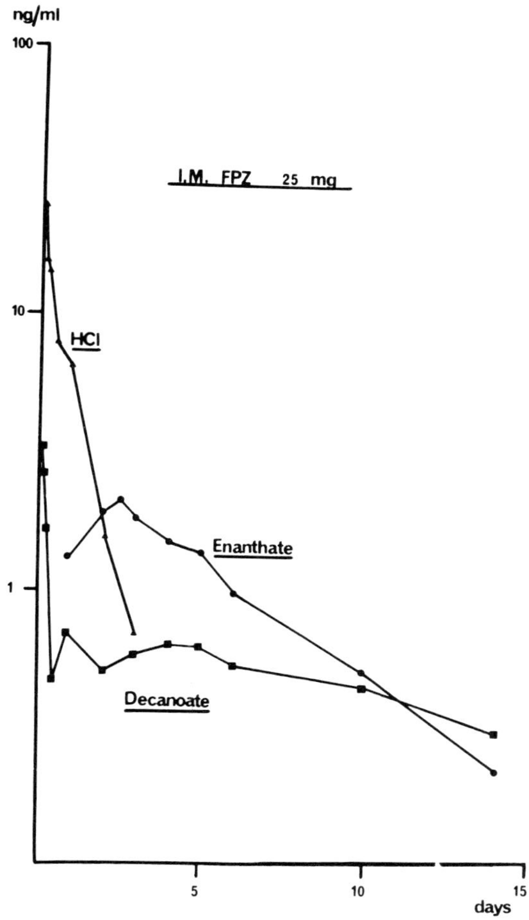

Fig. 12. Fluphenazine concentrations in a single subject treated with fluphenazine hydrochloride (i.m.), fluphenazine enanthate and fluphenazine decanoate (for details, see Curry et al., 1979).

Morselli and Zarifian, 1980; Meltzer et al., 1981; Tune and Coyle, 1981; Tune et al., 1981; Jeste et al., 1982).

CONCLUSION

It is apparent that any review of the metabolism and kinetics of phenothiazine drugs relies heavily on chlorpromazine data. This has resulted from methodological problems in the past. However, the application of liquid chromatography and other new techniques to the study of similar phenomena is currently leading to a considerable expansion of the data base for other phenothiazines (Stevenson and Reid, 1981; Curry et al., 1982; McKay et al., 1982a, b; Melethil et al., 1983). Much research is still needed, but the next 5 years should see a welcome escalation of the information available, and an adequate review of the applicability of principles observed with chlorpromazine to the other drugs of the phenothiazine group.

REFERENCES

Alfredsson, G. and Sedvall, G. (1981) Protein binding of chlorpromazine in cerebrospinal fluid and serum. Int. Pharmacopsychiatry 73, 55 – 62.

Alfredsson, G., Lindberg, M. and Sedvall, G. (1982) The presence of 7-hydroxychlorpromazine in CSF of chlorpromazine treated patients. Psychopharmacol. 77, 376 – 378.

Axelsson, R., Martensson, E. and Alling, C. (1982) Serum concentration and protein binding of thioridazine and its metabolites in patients with chronic alcoholism. Eur. J. Clin. Pharmacol. 23, 359 – 363.

Bolvig-Hanssen, L., Larsen, F. F. and Vestergard, P. (1981) Plasma levels of perphenazine (Trilafon) related to development of side effects. Psychopharmacology 74, 306 – 309.

Brinkschulte, M., Gaertner, H. J., Schied, H. W. and Breyer-Pfaff, V. (1982) Plasma protein binding of perazine and amitriptyline in psychiatric patients. Eur. J. Clin. Pharmacol. 22, 367 – 373.

Brodie, B. B. (1968) Physicochemical and biochemical aspects of pharmacology. J. Am. Med. Assoc. 202, 600 – 609.

Casper, R., Garver, D. L., Dekirmenjian, H., Chang, S. and Davis, J. M. (1980) Phenothiazine levels in plasma and red blood cells. Arch. Gen. Psychiatry 37, 301 – 305.

Cohen, B. M., Lipinski, J. F., Pope, H. G., Harris, P. O. and Altesman, R. I. (1980) Neuroleptic blood levels and therapeutic effect. Psychopharmacology 70, 191 – 193.

Cooper, S. F. and Lapierre, Y. D. (1981) Gas liquid chromatographic determination of pipotiazine in plasma of psychiatric patients. J. Chromatogr. 223, 95 – 102.

Crammer, J. L. (1981) Antipsychotic agents: thioridazine; pharmacokinetics, plasma levels, and clinical response. In: G. D. Burrows and T. R. Norman (Eds), Psychotropic Drugs: Plasma Concentration and Clinical Response. Marcel Dekker, New York, pp. 303 – 318.

Curry, S. H. (1968) Determination of nanogram quantities of chlorpromazine and some of its metabolites in plasma using gas-liquid chromatography with an electron capture detector. Anal. Chem. 40, 1251 – 1255.

Curry, S. H. (1976a) Metabolism and kinetics of chlorpromazine in relation to effect. In: G. Sedvall, B. Uvnas and Y. Zolterman (Eds), Antipsychotic Drugs: Pharmacokinetics and Pharmacodynamics. Pergamon Press, Oxford, pp. 343 – 352.

Curry, S. H. (1976b) Plasma level studies in psychotropic drug evaluation. Br. J. Clin. Pharmacol. 3, 20 – 28.

Curry, S. H. (1980) Methodological pitfalls; the influence of experimental design on results. In: Drug Concentrations in Neuropsychiatry (Ciba Foundation). Excerpta Medica, Amsterdam, pp. 35 – 49.

Curry, S. H. (1981a) Binding of psychotropic drugs to plasma protein and its influence on drug distribution. In: E. Usdin (Ed.), Clinical Pharmacology in Psychiatry. Elsevier, New York, pp. 213 – 223.

Curry, S. H. (1981b) Antipsychotic agents – chlorpromazine: pharmacokinetics, plasma levels and clinical response. In: G. D. Burrows and T. R. Norman (Eds), Psychotropic Drugs: Plasma Concentrations and Clinical Response. Marcel Dekker, New York, pp. 243 – 286.

Curry, S. H. and Brodie, B. B. (1967) Estimation of nanogram quantities of chlorpromazine (CPZ) in plasma using gas-liquid chromatography (GLC) with an electron capture director. Fed. Proc. 26, 761.

Curry, S. H. and Marshall, J. H. L. (1968) Plasma levels of chlorpromazine and some of its relatively non-polar metabolites in psychiatric patients. Life Sci. 7, 9 – 17.

Curry, S. H. and Mould, G. P. (1975) A microsomal oxidase system in rat intestinal mucosa. Br. J. Pharmacol. 54, 229P – 230P.

Curry, S. H. and Whelpton, R. (1974) Hydrophobic character of 15 model chlorpromazine metabolites determined from partition ratios in mixed solvents. Br. J. Pharmacol. 42, 143P – 144P.

Curry, S. H., Derr, J. E. and Maling, H. M. (1970) The physiological disposition of chlorpromazine in the rat and dog. Proc. Soc. Exp. Biol. Med. 134, 314 – 318.

Curry, S. H., D'Mello, A. and Mould, G. P. (1971) Destruction of chlorpromazine during absorption in the rat in vivo and in vitro. Br. J. Pharmacol. 42, 403 – 411.

Curry, S. H., Whelpton, R., de Schepper, P. J., Vranckx, S. and Schiff, A. A. (1979) Kinetics of fluphenazine after fluphenazine dihydrochloride, enanthate and decanoate administration to man. Br. J. Clin. Pharmacol. 7, 325 – 331.

Curry, S. H., Brown, E. A., Hu, O. Y-P. and Perrin, J. H. (1982) LC assay of phenothiazine, thiothixene, and butyrophenone neuroleptics and antihistamines in biological fluids with conventional and radial compression columns and UV and electro-chemical detection. J. Chromatogr. 231, 361 – 376.

Dahl, S. G., Johnsen, H. and Lee, C. R. (1982) Gas chromatographic mass spectrometric identification of O-demethylated and monohydroxylated metabolites of levomepromazine in blood from psychiatric patients by selected ion recording with high resolution. Biomed. Mass Spectrom. 9, 534 – 538.

Davis, C. M. and Fenimore, D. C. (1983) Determination of fluphenazine in plasma by high-performance thin-layer chromatography. J. Chromatogr. 272, 157 – 165.

Dysken, M. W., Javaid, J. I., Chang, S. S., Schaffer, C., Shaid, A. and Davis, J. M. (1981) Fluphenazine pharmacokinetics and therapeutic response. Psychopharmacology 73, 205 – 210.

Gillespie, T. J. and Sipes, I. G. (1981) Sensitive gas chromatographic determination of trifluoperazine in human plasma. J. Chromatogr. 223, 95 – 102.

Goldstein, S. A. and Van Vunakis, H. (1981) Determination of fluphenazine, related phenothiazine drugs and metabolites by combined high-performance liquid chromatography and radioimmunoassay. J. Pharmacol. Exp. Ther. 217, 36 – 43.

Harmon, A. W., Frewin, D. B. and Priestly, B. G. (1980) Comparative enzyme-inducing effects of chlorpromazine and fluphenazine therapies in psychotic patients. Psychopharmacology 69, 35 – 37.

Harris, J. P., Phillipson, O. T., Watkins, G. M. and Whelpton, R. (1983) Effects of chlorpromazine and promazine on the visual after effects of tilt and movement. Psychopharmacology 79, 49 – 57.

Hershey, L. A., Gift, T., Atkins, R. W. and Rivera-Calimlim, L. (1981) Effects of a drug holiday on plasma chlorpromazine levels in chronic schizophrenic patients. Psychopharmacology 73, 355 – 358.

Heyes, W. F., Salmon, J. R. and Marlow, W. (1980) High performance liquid chromatographic separation of the N- and S-oxides of fluphenazine decanoate. J. Chromatogr. 194, 416 – 420.

Howes, C. A., Pullar, T., Sourindhrin, I., Mistra, P. C., Capel, H., Lawson, D. H. and Tilstone, W.

J. (1983) Reduced steady-state plasma concentrations of chlorpromazine and indomethacin in patients receiving cimetidine. Eur. J. Clin. Pharmacol. 24, 99 – 102.

Javaid, J. I., Dekirmenjian, H. Liskevych, V., Lin, R-I. and Davis, J. M. (1981) Fluphenazine determination in human plasma by a sensitive gas chromatographic method using nitrogen detector. J. chromatogr. Sci. 19, 439 – 443.

Javaid, J. I., Dekirmenjian, H. and Davis, J. M. (1982) GLC analysis of trifluoperazine in human plasma. J. Pharmaceut. Sci. 71, 63 – 66.

Jeste, D. V., Linnoila, M., Wagner, R. L. and Wyatt, R. J. (1982) Serum neuroleptic concentrations and tardive dyskinesia. Psychopharmacology 76, 377 – 380.

Kilts, C. D., Patrick, K. S., Breese, G. R. and Mailman, R. B. (1982) Simultaneous determination of thioridazine and its S-oxidized and demethylated metabolites using high performance liquid chromatography on radially compressed silica. J. Chromatogr. 231, 377 – 391.

Kurland, A. A., Nagaraju, A. and Hanlon, T. E. (1980) The dopamine radioreceptor assay – a clinical application. J. Clin. Pharmacol. 20, 191 – 193.

Loo, J. C. K., Midha, K. K. and McGilveray, I. J. (1980) Pharmacokinetics of chlorpromazine in normal volunteers. Commun. Psychopharmacol. 4, 121 – 129.

May, R. R. A., Van Putten, T., Jenden, D. J., Yale, D. and Dixon, W. J. (1981) Chlorpromazine levels and the outcome of treatment in schizophrenic patients. Arch. Gen. Psychiatry 38, 202 – 207.

McKay, G., Cooper, J. K., Midha, K. K., Hall, K. and Hawes E. M. (1982a) Simple and sensitive high-performance liquid chromatographic procedure with electrochemical detection for the determination of plasma concentrations of trimeprazine following single oral doses. J. Chromatogr. 233, 417 – 422.

McKay, G., Hall, K., Cooper, J. K., Hawes, E. M. and Midha, K. K. (1982b) Gas-chromatographic-mass spectrometric procedure for the quantitation of chlorpromazine in plasma and its comparison with a new high-performance liquid chromatographic assay with electrochemical detection. J. Chromatogr. 232, 275 – 282.

Melethil, S., Dutta, A., Chungi, V. and Dittert, L. (1983) Liquid chromatographic assay for promethazine in plasma using electrochemical detection. Anal. Lett. 16 (B9), 701 – 709.

Meltzer, H. Y., Busch, D. A. and Fang, V. S. (1981) Effect of neuroleptics on serum prolactin levels in relation to clinical response and neuroleptic blood levels. In: E. Usdin (Ed.), Clinical Pharmacology in Psychiatry. Elsevier, New York, pp. 251 – 268.

Midha, K. K., Cooper, J. K. and Hubbard, J. W. (1980) Radioimmunoassay for fluphenazine in plasma. Commun. Psychopharmacol. 4, 107 – 114.

Midha, K. K., Cooper, J. K., McGilveray, I. J., Butterfield, A. G. and Hubbard, J. W. (1981) High-performance liquid chromatographic assay for nanogram determination of chlorpromazine and its comparison with radioimmunoassay. J. Pharmaceut. Sci. 70, 1043 – 1046.

Midha, K. K., Roscoe, R. M. H., Hall, K., Hawes, E. M., Cooper, J. K., McKay, G. and Shetty, H. V. (1982) A gas chromatographic mass spectrometric assay for plasma trifluoperazine concentrations following single doses. Biomed. Mass Spectrom. 9, 186 – 190.

Morselli, P. L. and Zarifian, E. (1980) Clinical significance of monitoring plasma levels of psychotropic drugs. In: Drug Concentrations in Neuropsychiatry (Ciba Foundation). Excerpta Medica, Amsterdam, pp. 115 – 139.

Murakami, K., Murakami, K., Veno, T., Hijikata, J., Shirasawa, K. and Muto, T. (1982) Simultaneous determination of chlorpromazine and levomepromazine in human plasma and urine by high-performance liquid chromatography using electrochemical detection. J. Chromatogr. 227, 103 – 112.

Nyberg, C. L. and Martensson, E. (1982) Binding of thioridazine and thioridazine metabolites to serum protein. Naunyn-Schmiedeberg's Arch. Pharmacol. 319, 189 – 196.

Nyberg, G. L., Axelsson, R. and Martensson, E. (1981) Cerebrospinal fluid concentrations of thioridazine and its main metabolites in psychiatric patients. Eur. J. Clin. Pharmacol. 19, 139 – 148.

Pantuck, E. J., Pantuck, C. B., Anderson, K. E., Conney, A. H. and Kappas, A. (1982) Cigarette smoking and chlorpromazine disposition and actions. Clin. Pharmacol. Ther. 31, 533 – 538.

Papadopoulos, A. S., Chand, T. G., Crammer, J. L. and Lader, S. (1980) A pilot study of plasma thioridazine and metabolites in chronically treated patients. Br. J. Psychiatry 126, 591 – 596.

Sakalis, G. and Traficante, L. (1981) Antipsychotic agents: fluphenazine. In: G. D. Burrows and T. R. Norman (Eds), Psychotropic Drugs: Plasma Concentration and Clinical Response. Marcel Dekker, New York, pp. 287 – 301.

Sakalis, G., Curry, S. H., Mould, G. P. and Lader, M. H. (1972) Physiologic and clinical effects of chlorpromazine and their relationship to plasma level. Clin. Pharmacol. Ther. 13, 931 – 946.

Schley, V. J. (1983) Uber die Bindung verschiedener Perazio-Metaboliten und Phenothiazine-Derivate an saures a_1-Glykoprotein. Arzneimittel-Forschung 33, 185 – 187.

Schley, V. J., Riedel, E. and Muller-Oerlinghausen, B. (1981) Metabolism and excretion of the neuroleptic drug perazine in healthy volunteers. Int. Pharmacopsychiatry 16, 201 – 205.

Sedvall, G. (1981) Correlations between clinical biochemical and pharmacokinetic data in chlorpromazine-treated patients. In: E. Usdin (Ed.), Clinical Pharmacology in Psychiatry. Elsevier, New York, pp. 243 – 249.

Skinner, T., Gochnauer, R. and Linnoila, M. (1980) Liquid chromatographic method to measure thioridazine and its active metabolites in plasma. Acta Pharmacol. Toxicol. 48, 416 – 420.

Stevenson, D, and Reid, E. (1981) Determination of chlorpromazine and its sulfoxide and 7-hydroxy metabolites by ion-pair high pressure liquid chromatography. Anal. Lett. 14 (B20), 1785 – 1805.

Taylor, G. and Houston, J. B. (1983) Determinants of systemic availability of promethazine in rabbits. J. Pharm. Pharmacol. 35, 284 – 288.

Tune, L. E. and Coyle, J. T. (1981) Acute extrapyramidal side effects: serum level of neuroleptics and anticholinergics. Psychopharmacology 75, 9 – 15

Tune, L. E., Creese, I., Depaulo, J. R., Slavney, P. R. and Snyder, S. H. (1981) Neuroleptic serum levels measured by radioreceptor assay and clinical response in schizophrenic patients. J. Nerv. Ment. Dis. 169, 60 – 63.

Vaisanen, K., Viukari, M., Rimon, R. and Raisanen, P. (1981) Haloperidol, thioridazine and placebo in mentally subnormal patients – serum levels and clinical effects. Acta Psychiatr. Scand. 63, 262 – 271.

Van Putten, T., May, P. R. A., Jenden, D. J., Cho, A. K. and Yale, C. (1980) Plasma and saliva levels of chlorpromazine and subjective response. Am. J. Psychiatry 137, 1241 – 1242.

Van Putten, T., May, P. R. A. and Jenden, D. J. (1981) Does a plasma level of chlorpromazine help? Psychol. Med. 11, 729 – 734.

Vierfond, J-M., Lehuede, J. and Miocque, M. (1983) Aminométhylation de la phénothiazine et de la phénoxazine. Eur. J. Med. Chem. Chim. Ther. 19, 35 – 40.

Whelpton, R., Curry, S. H. and Watkins, G. M. (1982) Analysis of plasma trifluoperazine by gas chromatography and selected ion monitoring. J. Chromatogr. 228, 321 – 326.

Widerlov, E., Haggstrom, J-E., Kilts, C. D., Andersson, V., Breese, G. R. and Mailman, R. B. (1982) Serum concentrations of thioridazine, its major metabolites and serum neuroleptic-like activities in schizophrenics with and without tardive dyskinesia. Acta Psychiatr. Scand. 66, 294 – 305.

Wode-Helgodt, B. and Alfredsson, G. (1981) Concentration of chlorpromazine and two of its active metabolites in plasma and cerebrospinal fluid of psychotic patients treated with fixed drug doses. Psychopharmacology 73, 55 – 62.

Burrows/Norman/Davies (eds) Antipsychotics

Chapter 8

Butyrophenones: Plasma level and clinical response

H. ITOH

Department of Neuropsychiatry, School of Medicine, Keio University, Tokyo, Japan

INTRODUCTION

Antipsychotic drug treatment forms the principal constituent of therapy for schizophrenia and other psychoses, but on the other hand, therapy-resistant cases are encountered in considerable proportions of psychotic patients. Moreover, clinical effects and adverse reactions associated with antipsychotic drug treatment vary markedly with the individual. It is not always easy, therefore, to predict whether and, if at all, to what extent a particular neuroleptic drug may afford clinical benefit and occurrence and degree of side effects in a patient.

Biological parameters that might be of use for such anticipation have been sought continually, especially by clinicians. Pharmacokinetic studies of neuroleptics have thus been acquiring increasing importance and arousing a great deal of interest.

Unlike antipsychotics such as chlorpromazine, the butyrophenone derivative haloperidol has a fairly simple metabolic pathway and does not yield any appreciable active metabolite, it may therefore be said to be a convenient drug for investigating the correlation of blood level and clinical effects.

For determining the concentration of haloperidol in the blood, improved assay methods have been successively introduced, viz. gas-liquid chromatography (GLC), radioimmunoassay (RIA) and radioreceptor assay (RRA). The clinical situations where the measurement of blood drug levels has noticeable practical value are listed on the basis of the published views of investigators as follows: 1) determination of the threshold value for therapeutic response, and as a guide for determining the optimal therapeutic dosage range; 2) measurement of blood drug concentration at which adverse reactions are evoked and as a guide for determining the safe dose range; 3) compliance; 4) identification of non-responders and modifying therapy; 5) factors which affect the blood drug concentration, including drug interaction, and establishment of appropriate measures to cope with them; 6) ascertaining diurnal variations in blood drug concentration, time required to attain a steady state concentration and biological half-life, and the adjustment or modification of dosage accordingly (the time and/or frequency of dosing, etc.); and 7) prediction of therapeutic effects and choice of drugs. A considerable amount of research has been reported on the blood concentration of haloperidol during the past decade. Besides haloperidol, a few studies on plasma level monitoring of other butyrophenone derivatives, such as pimozide and bromperidol were reported recently. But their clinical significance has not yet been fully investigated. At the present time, I would like to review the studies reported including the author's own with particular reference to: 1) interrelation between the concentration in blood and clinical effects of the drug; 2) clinical implication of the blood level in non-responders; 3) the blood level of haloperidol during therapy with depot haloperidol (decanoate); 4) relation between the blood level and side effects of the drug; and 5) drug interactions.

INTERRELATION BETWEEN HALOPERIDOL BLOOD LEVELS AND CLINICAL EFFECTS

The relationship between psychic symptoms and blood levels of haloperidol in patients with psychoses undergoing treatment with the drug has been described by several investigators.

In the early period, Zingales et al. (1971) measured the plasma level of haloperidol by GLC in 14 psychotic patients receiving the drug orally in doses of 9 – 15 mg/day, among whom one displaying very poor therapeutic response had the highest plasma level. From the results it was inferred that the dosage need not be necessarily high to attain clinical benefit.

The use of the more sensitive gas-chromatographic techniques developed later, yielded findings somewhat inconsistent with what had previously been reported (Forsman et al., 1974).

Attempts were made to correlate the plasma haloperidol level with symptomatic changes in psychotic patients by Forsman and Öhman (1977), Ericksen et al. (1978), Takahashi et al. (1979), Yoshimoto et al. (1979, 1980), Morselli et al. (1979, 1980), Smith et al. (1979) and Moulin et al. (1982). In all these studies fasting blood specimens withdrawn in the morning were analyzed by GLC, and the clinical assessments were based on global clinical judgment and/or the total and individual symptom item scores on the Brief Psychiatric Rating Scale (BPRS).

The subsequent development of RIA led to investigations of the plasma level/clinical response relations of haloperidol using this technique (Ericksen et al., 1978; Bjørndal et al., 1980; Rama Rao et al., 1980; Itoh et al., 1980, 1983 a, b; Rimón et al., 1981). Forsman (1977) suggested a therapeutic blood level of haloperidol might be between 3 and 10 ng/ml for most patients. Takahashi and Yoshimoto et al. (1979, 1980) compared the blood haloperidol concentration in 54 schizophrenic inpatients receiving haloperidol alone who were classified into three groups according to degree of therapeutic response, i.e. improved, slightly improved and unchanged. The results failed to reveal any significant inter-group difference in mean blood haloperidol level (Fig. 1).

However, when compared in terms of relation between the dose per kilogram of body weight and the blood level of haloperidol, the 'improved' group displayed a significantly higher blood level than the 'unchanged' group (Fig. 2).

Radioreceptor assay has been adopted as the latest laboratory tool for measuring the concentration of haloperidol and other dopamine receptor-blocking neuroleptics in biological materials. It was first introduced as an antipsychotic drug assay in clinical specimens by Creese and Snyder (1977).

In RRA, both parent compound in a given specimen together with metabolites capable of binding to dopamine receptors, are quantitated.

Calil et al. (1979) observed that the blood haloperidol concentrations measured by RRA, showed a significant positive correlation with their BPRS total scores. Among the individual BPRS items, scores for thinking disturbance and paranoid disturbance correlated best with the blood concentration of haloperidol.

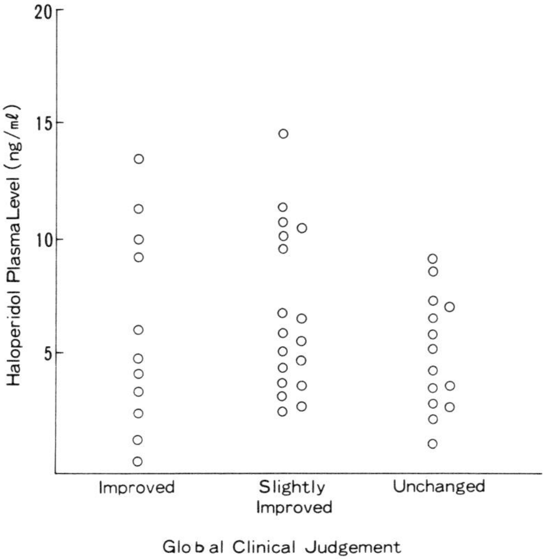

Fig. 1. Plasma concentration of haloperidol and clinical effect. (Reproduced with permission from: Yoshimoto et al., 1979.)

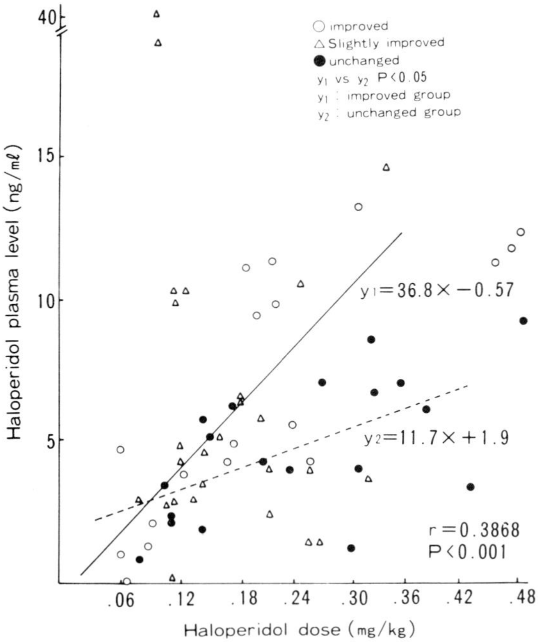

Fig. 2. Haloperidol dose, its plasma level and clinical effect. (Reproduced with permission from: Yoshimoto et al., 1979.)

A positive correlation ($r = 0.402$, $p < 0.05$) was also demonstrated between blood levels (mean ± S. E.: 16.52 ± 2.23 ng/ml) and psychiatric morbidity (BPRS score) in a study conducted by Rama Rao et al. (1980).

In the meantime, there exists a view that the relationship between therapeutic response to psychotropic drugs and blood concentration can be graphically depicted as an inverted U-shaped curve response (the 'therapeutic window').

Tune et al. (1980) reported that, in 30 schizophrenic patients receiving haloperidol, chlorpromazine, or other neuroleptics, the most favorable therapeutic responses were seen in patients with blood levels of 100 – 200 ng/ml as chlorpromazine equivalents, measured by RRA. Dunlop et al. (1982) also reported that: 1) in a group of 25 chronic patients, plasma level was significantly curvilinearly related to total BPRS; 2) for subjects with plasma levels below 25 ng haloperidol/ml, BPRS total and thought disorder subscores were negatively correlated to plasma level.

At the ACNP Meeting in 1981, Extein and co-workers presented a paper dealing with the interrelation of plasma haloperidol level and clinical effects observed in a series of patients with acute schizophrenia. Of 12 defined as responders by changes in BPRS score at 2 – 4 weeks, 10 had haloperidol levels in the proposed therapeutic range of 5 – 15 ng/ml. Extein concluded that these findings were consistent with the concept of a 'therapeutic window' for haloperidol in schizophrenia.

Smith et al. (1982) measured microquantities of haloperidol in plasma and in erythrocytes from 26 schizophrenics by GLC during a 24-day period of treatment with the drug at constant dose levels. Analysis of the data in terms of drug concentrations and improvement of BPRS total score disclosed a significantly greater rate of symptomatic amelioration in patients showing moderate drug concentrations (2.4 – 5.4 ng/ml) in red blood cells, compared to those showing higher or lower RBC concentrations. It also revealed a significantly greater improvement rate (37.5%) in patients with plasma haloperidol levels of 5 – 14 ng/ml than patients with plasma levels of 0 – 4.9 ng/ml (12%) and those with values of ≧ 14.1 ng/ml (23%). The report stresses the presence of a 'therapeutic window' in the haloperidol concentration and indicates that the drug concentration in red cells has a better correlation with the clinical response. But Ericksen (1978) reported a different finding. In his study, 42 acutely decompensated schizophrenic patients were divided at random into two groups and received haloperidol at high and standard dose levels. The high-dose

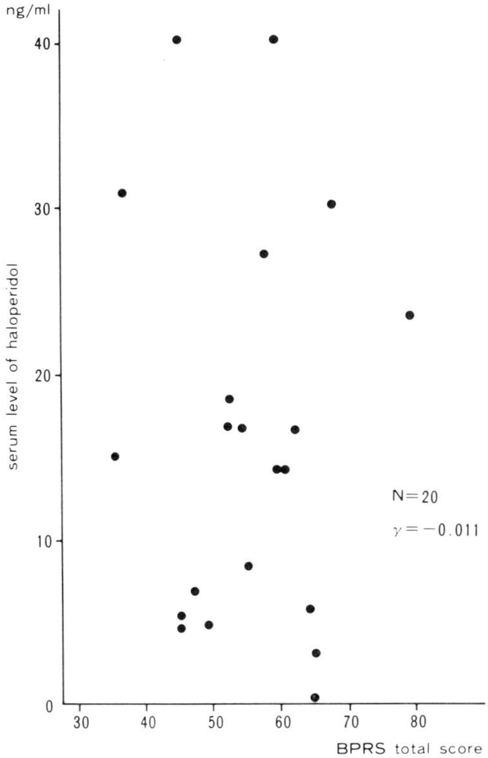

Fig. 3. Relationship between BPRS total score and serum level of haloperidol.

group showed higher blood levels than the standard-dose group but there was practically no inter-group difference in degree of improvement of psychotic symptoms rated on the BPRS.

The results of our 1981 investigation also failed to show any definite correlation between the BPRS total score and the serum basal level of haloperidol in a series of 20 cases under treatment. That is, the patients with lower BPRS total scores did not necessarily show higher serum levels of the drug, nor did those with higher scores display lower serum concentration (Itoh et al., 1983 a), (Fig. 3).

Further studies are needed to clarify the interrelation of blood drug concentrations and clinical effects of haloperidol.

PLASMA HALOPERIDOL LEVELS IN NON-RESPONDERS

In a study by Itoh et al. (1983 b), 11 schizophrenics treated with oral haloperidol (fixed dose of 6 mg/day) were divided into two groups according to their changes in BPRS total scores. Seven of them showed improvement in BPRS ratings during the 4 weeks of the trial.

Trends of mean changes of BPRS total scores and blood levels of haloperidol dur-

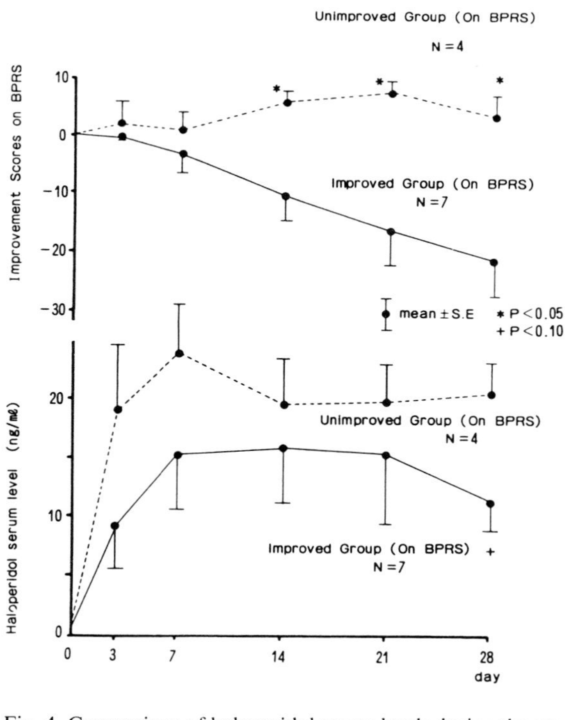

Fig. 4. Comparison of haloperidol serum levels during the course of treatment between the improved and unimproved cases group on BPRS total scores.

ing treatment in each group are shown in Fig. 4. In the improved group, a lower level of haloperidol was maintained throughout the 4-week treatment period. Improvement of psychopathology as shown in BPRS scores was also obtained as the serum concentration of haloperidol increased. Furthermore, the blood concentrations of haloperidol in the 'BPRS unimproved cases' group were always higher than those in the 'BPRS improved cases' group throughout the treatment. That is, in the 'Improved Cases' group, an inverse relationship was observed between the decrease of BPRS scores and the increase of the blood levels. Improvement of psychopathology by means of a decrease of the BPRS total score was still found after blood levels reached a plateau.

The subjects were also classified into two groups in accordance with the duration of the current hospitalization; one was 'more-than-one-year' group (4 cases), and the other was the 'less-than-one-year' group (7 cases).

Trends of mean changes of BPRS total scores and serum levels of haloperidol during the treatment in each group are shown in Fig. 5.

Four cases out of seven in the 'less-than-one-year' group showed improvement in BPRS total scores, and, in this group, the mean total score improved by 20 points

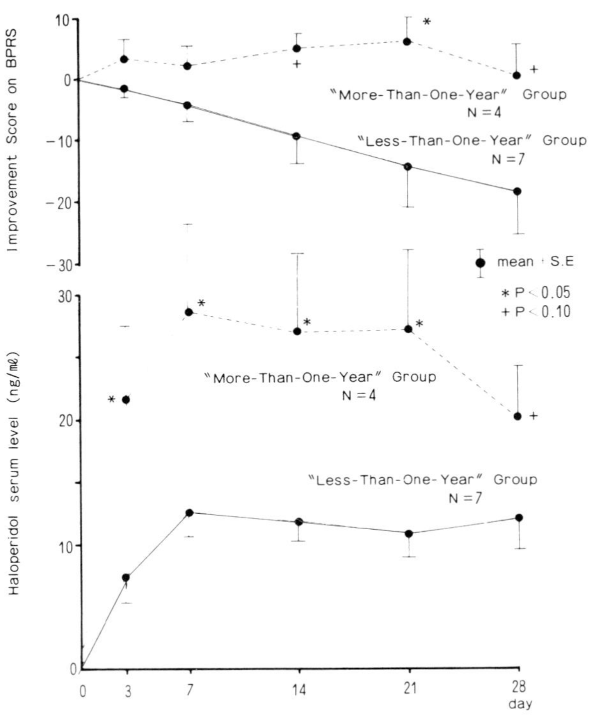

Fig. 5. Comparison of improvement scores and haloperidol serum levels between the two groups classified by duration of hospitalization.

at the end of the 4-week treatment period. But mean serum concentrations of haloperidol at each day of sampling in this group were significantly lower than those in the 'more-than-one-year' group.

Our results showed that, among schizophrenic patients under lower-dose haloperidol treatment, cases having a short duration of illness and higher total pretreatment total scores on the BPRS showed positive therapeutic responses to the drug despite their lower blood levels of haloperidol.

The results did not support the view that high blood concentrations of haloperidol might contribute to clinical effects. The presence of refractory schizophrenics is becoming one of the major problems in the practice of psychiatry.

Smith (1979) investigated blood concentrations of butaperazine, thioridazine and haloperidol in clinical responders and non-responders to these neuroleptics. With haloperidol, non-responders receiving greater doses (20 – 60 mg/day) than responders treated with oral haloperidol (15 mg/day) exhibited far lower steady-state blood levels of drug (mean, 4.0 ng/ml; range, 0 – 9 ng/ml) as compared to the responders (10 ± 1.0 ng/ml).

According to Smith, problems concerned with the absorptive phase of drugs would account for poor clinical responses to neuroleptic treatment, e.g. augmented drug-metabolizing activity in the intestinal wall and increased excretion via the bile duct.

This hypothesis was refuted by Rimón et al. (1981) on the grounds of their own findings. Namely, 12 chronic schizophrenic patients with active psychotic symptoms despite usual neuroleptic treatment were given haloperidol in doses of 60 mg/day for one month and subsequently in doses of 120 mg/day. All the patients receiving 60 mg of haloperidol daily showed higher blood levels (mean ± S.D.: 86 ± 46 ng/ml by RIA) than those observed by Smith in the responder group. After a dosage increase to 120 mg/day, the blood concentration became elevated in all the cases as measured by RRA (132 ± 64 ng/ml) and significantly by RIA (149 ± 43 ng/ml). Drug concentrations in the CSF of patients also showed elevation following the dosage increase, and this increase correlated significantly with the elevation of blood concentration. No significant change in psychotic symptoms, assessed on the BPRS, was observed although the concentration of haloperidol in body fluids increased with the elevation of dose level. Rimón concludes that treatment failure in chronic schizophrenia is not usually due to poor absorption of neuroleptic into blood or poor penetration into CSF. In three patients with delusional schizophrenia who had failed to respond to various medical treatments and were receiving high doses of haloperidol (for 6 weeks with gradual dosage increase to a maximum of 200 mg/day), the plasma level of the drug (peak concentration: 140 – 250 ng/ml) correlated with dosage but the medication did not produce any noticeable symptomatic improvement in respect to hallucination and delusion (Scatton et al., 1982).

Morselli and Zarifian (1980) reported the results of their clinical study. In six chronically ill, 'unresponsive' paranoid schizophrenics, oral haloperidol was administered daily over a period of 45 days with gradual dosage increase at weekly intervals from 20 to 150 mg/day. Although their blood levels of haloperidol reached maximum concentrations of 150 – 170 ng/ml, no appreciable clinical improvement could be attained as assessed by observation of ward behavior and by rating on the BPRS.

It may be of value to administer haloperidol by a parenteral route, if non-responders fail to attain sufficient blood levels due to any difficulty in absorption, as suggested by Smith. However we must remember that not only the blood concentration or pharmacokinetics, but also the pharmacodynamics of drugs, are important factors in the pharmacotherapy of psychotic disorders.

HALOPERIDOL PLASMA LEVELS DURING HALOPERIDOL DECANOATE TREATMENT

Several long-acting neuroleptics have been developed in recent years, most of which are effective for one to a few weeks following a single intramuscular injection. Depot haloperidol is one of these long-acting preparations.

It was reported by Niemegeers (1979) that single intramuscular doses of haloperidol decanoate produced pharmacologic effects, which were sustained for a minimum of one month. Deberdt et al. (1980) investigated interrelations of efficacy, dosage schedule and blood levels of haloperidol in neuroleptic maintenance therapy, using intramuscular haloperidol decanoate. The study was as follows.

A dosage scheme was devised based on the observations by Forsman and Öhman (1977), that the bioavailability of an oral dose of haloperidol is about 60 – 70%. This would correspond to a monthly dose of haloperidol decanoate of about 20 times the daily oral dose. Twenty-eight patients were placed on a 3-month schedule of study treatment with intramuscular haloperidol decanoate, injected in a dose 20-fold of the daily oral dose at 4-week intervals. Their blood levels of haloperidol were monitored by RIA over the 3-month period. A small rise in blood level was noted in some patients only during the first few days post-injection, but subsequently the levels were remarkably stable. The patients generally showed blood levels of haloperidol comparable to those during the preceding therapy with an oral preparation.

The interval mean blood levels of haloperidol after an initial dose (30 – 300 mg) ranged from 0.8 to 3.2 ng/ml in the patients. After the second dose, their blood levels were between about 2 and 8 ng/ml, significantly higher than those after the first injection ($p < 0.001$). The patients displayed essentially the same blood levels after the third dose as after the second, that is, a steady state of blood concentration was achieved following the first two doses.

All patients were well stabilized symptomatically on their optimal doses of intramuscular haloperidol decanoate, besides the remarkably stable blood levels. Further amelioration occurred in several symptoms during the treatment, and no increase in incidence or degree of extrapyramidal or other side effects was observed at all. There was no clinical evidence of accumulation of haloperidol. The results indicate the potential usefulness of blood level monitoring for haloperidol in treatment with intramuscular depot preparations.

Roose et al. (1981) and De Buck et al. (1981) also reported that haloperidol decanoate was highly efficacious and well-tolerated for long-term treatment of chronic psychoses, with an improvement in the overall clinical picture as well as the safety results.

According to a report of Aschauer et al. (1981), the blood levels of haloperidol after injection of the drug as decanoate vary considerably with the individual. Of 10 patients given an i.m. injection of haloperidol decanoate, (25 – 200 mg/month), the blood level of haloperidol at 14 days after administration was more than 250% of that within the first week post-injection in one patient, between 50 and 150% in 7 patients and less than 50% in 2 patients.

More studies are needed on the measurement of blood levels of haloperidol and on the blood level/clinical response relationship. At all events, it is now recognized that regular monitoring of the blood concentration of haloperidol is of great value for successful haloperidol therapy with an intramuscular depot preparation.

INTERRELATION BETWEEN HALOPERIDOL BLOOD LEVELS AND SIDE-EFFECTS

In case of antipsychotic drugs such as haloperidol with profound activity toward the striatum, great importance is placed on the relationship of the development of extrapyramidal symptoms (EPS) to the blood concentration.

Forsman and Öhman (1978) measured the blood levels of haloperidol by GLC in 12 patients with chronic schizophrenia receiving haloperidol orally at progressively increasing dose levels (3 – 90 mg/day) for 4 weeks after a drug-free period of 4 weeks. During the study treatment, the patients were observed for EPS, using various assessment instruments that included the Simpson's EPS rating scale, the handwriting test, a brachiokinesiometer, a pedometer, the step-length test and the salivation test. The mean of total haloperidol concentrations in serum was 6.3 ng/ml (at one week of medication), 9.3 ng/ml (at 2 weeks) and 21.2 ng/ml (at 4 weeks), and the mean of free haloperidol concentrations 0.5 ng/ml (at one week), 0.7 ng/ml (at 2 weeks) and 1.5 ng/ml (at 4 weeks). Analysis of these serum concentration data revealed decreased spontaneous motility associated with development and/or enhancement of EPS at high serum concentrations of haloperidol.

The present author and associates investigated the relation between the plasma level of haloperidol and the development of EPS in 135 patients receiving the drug over extended periods.

Blood haloperidol levels were determined in two groups of subjects stratified ac-

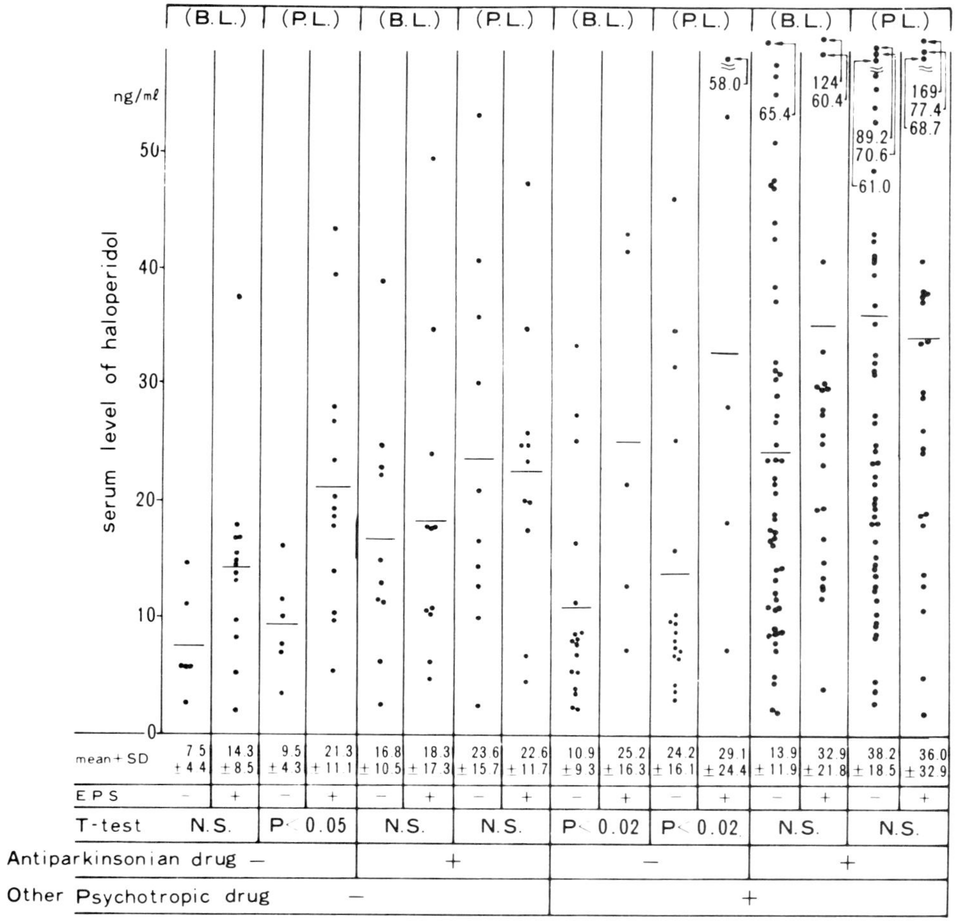

Fig. 6. Serum levels of haloperidol in relation to the incidence of extrapyramidal symptoms in patients receiving long-term administration of haloperidol. B.L. = basal level; P.L. = peak level.

cording to the presence of EPS. (Mainly dystonia, akathisia and parkinsonism.) The results are shown in Fig. 6. In the group receiving haloperidol alone, the mean basal blood concentration of the drug was 7.5 ± 4.4 ng/ml in the absence of EPS and 14.3 ± 8.5 ng/ml in the presence of EPS; the difference is not significant but subjects with EPS tended to show higher blood levels. The peak blood level averaged 9.5 ± 4.3 ng/ml for subjects without EPS and 21.3 ± 11.0 ng/ml for those with EPS, the difference being significant. Where haloperidol was combined with antiparkinsonian drugs, no such difference existed in either the basal or the peak level between subjects with or without EPS. In the group receiving haloperidol with another psychotropic drug, the mean basal blood concentration was 10.9 ± 9.3 ng/ml for the subgroup without EPS and 25.2 ± 16.3 ng/ml for the one with EPS

($p < 0.02$). The mean peak blood level was 13.9 ± 11.9 ng/ml for the subgroup without EPS and 32.8 ± 21.8 ng/ml for the one with EPS ($p < 0.02$) (Fig. 6).

Longitudinal observation of the blood level, clinical effects and EPS in patients receiving repeated doses of haloperidol was also performed.

EPS developed in all of these patients. Figure 7 illustrates basal and peak serum haloperidol levels up to the onset of EPS. The time elapsing before the development of EPS averaged 8.4 ± 5.3 days (3 – 16 days). EPS developed at a mean basal serum level of 10.7 ± 3.3 ng/ml and a mean peak serum level of 20.6 ± 3.0 ng/ml.

Our study confirms that there is a definite relationship between the development of EPS and the serum level of haloperidol, unless haloperidol is given in combination with an antiparkinsonian drug and that EPS often develops at a basal serum haloperidol level of 10 ng/ml or over and at a peak level of 20 ng/ml or over.

It was pointed out by McCreadie et al. (1977) that EPS developed less frequently with high doses of antipsychotics, and Zarifian et al. (1979) found that EPS disappeared as the blood haloperidol concentration reached the level of 200 ng/ml in patients receiving progressively increasing dosage up to 200 mg/day, but reappeared as it fell below a level of 100 ng/ml.

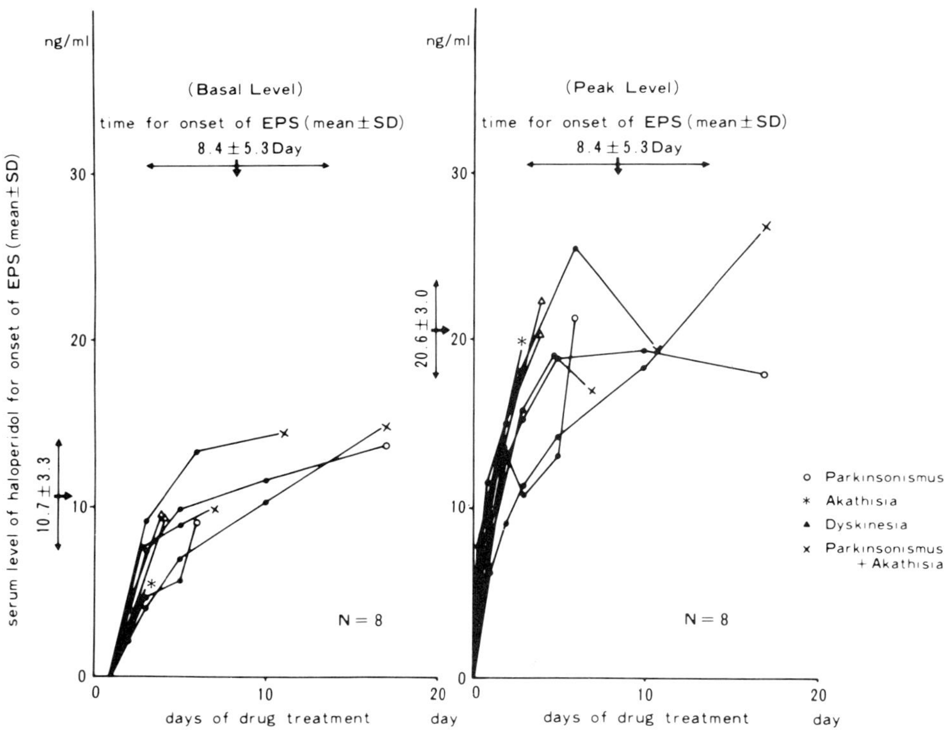

Fig. 7. Serum levels of haloperidol in patients after successive oral administration in relation to the time for onset of extrapyramidal symptoms. Left side shows basal level. Right side shows peak level.

Meanwhile, Bjørndal et al. (1980) showed that practically no difference in incidence of EPS was observed between a standard dosage group (12 – 36 mg/day; mean, 15 mg q.d.) and a high dosage group (10 – 240 mg/day; mean, 103 mg q.d.) but there was a greater incidence of side effects in the latter group. They included, mainly, sedation, aggressive episodes, muscular weakness and tendency to fall and, in one patient, epileptic attacks. These, along with the finding of a positive correlation between the dosage and blood concentration of haloperidol, suggested an interrelationship between blood concentration and the incidence of side effects. Bjørndal et al. (1980) and Neborsky et al. (1981) have issued a warning against the increased risk of evoking tardive dyskinesia by prolonged treatment with high dosage of neuroleptic drugs.

A survey on tardive dyskinesia made by the present authors, nevertheless, did not show any significant interrelation between the occurrence of this complication and the plasma level of haloperidol.

DRUG INTERACTION

In clinical practice haloperidol is usually prescribed in combination with other psychotropic drugs, antiparkinsonian drugs and/or hypnotics. In such combined therapy regimens drug interactions may cause alterations in plasma haloperidol concentration, thereby affecting the clinical effects and development of adverse reactions.

However, it appears from data reported to the present time that concomitantly administered antipsychotic drugs, antianxiety drugs or antidepressants rarely or, if at all, only modestly affect the plasma haloperidol concentration. Our previous study in 135 patients showed no significant difference in plasma haloperidol level between a group receiving haloperidol alone and other groups receiving the drug in combination with other psychotropic agents such as chlorpromazine, levomepromazine or perphenazine (Itoh et al., 1980). However, in eight schizophrenic patients Hayashi et al. (1982) observed that combined haloperidol-levomepromazine regimens yielded higher plasma concentrations of the former drug, yet with a reduced frequency and severity of EPS, compared with those during treatment with haloperidol alone.

Some articles purported to demonstrate that concomitantly administered antiparkinsonian drugs had no appreciable influence on the plasma level of haloperidol (Forsman and Öhman, 1977; Linnoila et al., 1980; Itoh et al., 1980; Tune et al., 1980; Oka et al., 1981). Gautier and co-workers (1977) reported that on withdrawal of a concomitant antipsychotic medication the plasma concentration of antipsychotic drug was elevated, though the elevation had little or no effect on psychotic symptoms.

Of particular note is the depression of the plasma haloperidol level seen in patients given barbiturates during haloperidol therapy, as reported by Forsman and

Öhman (1977) and many others. The depression stems from accelerated metabolic breakdown of haloperidol in the liver due to enzyme induction by barbiturates. It would be of great value to monitor the blood levels of haloperidol in such cases, while observing clinical manifestations.

CONCLUSION

The interrelationships between the plasma level and therapeutic and adverse effects of haloperidol, a butyrophenone derivative, have been discussed above on the grounds of facts proven to date. Nevertheless, a number of problems remain to be resolved.

In our daily practice in pharmacotherapy for schizophrenic patients, we have frequently experienced satisfactory clinical effects in some cases using the lowest doses of antipsychotics, while in other cases, psychotic symptoms persisted despite high doses of neuroleptic medication. Hence, these cases require prolonged psychiatric hospitalization as non-responders.

The diverse problems concerned with antipsychotic drug treatment including non-response to therapy may find solution with the development and general application of more accurate, simplified laboratory methods for measurement of microquantities of the drug in clinical specimens.

REFERENCES

Aschauer, H., Langer, G., Schonbeck, G. and Kinig, G. (1981) Further neuro-endocrine studies on the pharmacodynamics of haloperidol in psychotic patients. III World Congress of Biological Psychiatry, Stockholm, June 30.

Bjørndal, N., Bjerre, M., Gerlach, J., Kristjansen, P., Magelund, G., Oestrich, I. H. and Waehres, J. (1980) High-dosage haloperidol therapy in chronic schizophrenic patients: a double-blind study of clinical response, side effects, serum haloperidol, and prolactin. Psychopharmacology 67, 17 – 23.

Calil, H. M., Avery, D. H., Hollister, L. H., Creese, I. and Snyder, S. H. (1979) Serum levels of neuroleptics measured by dopamine radioreceptor assay and some clinical observations. Psychiatry Res. 1, 39 – 44.

Creese, I. and Snyder, S. H. (1977) A simple and sensitive radioreceptor assay for antischizophrenic drugs in blood. Nature (London) 270, 180 – 182.

Deberdt, R., Elens, P., Bergmans, W., Heykants, J., Woestenborghs, R., Driens, F., Reyntjens, A. and Van Wijngaarden, I. (1980) Intramuscular haloperidol decanoate for neuroleptic maintenance therapy. Efficacy, dosage schedule and plasma levels. An open multicenter study. Acta Psychiatr. Scand. 62, 356 – 363.

De Buck, R. P., Zelaschi, N. and Gilles, C. (1981) Haloperidol plasma levels during haloperidol decanoate treatment: correlation with CEEG and clinical data. III World Congress of Biological Psychiatry, Stockholm, June 29.

Dunlop, S. R., Shea, P. A. and Hendrie, H. C. (1982) The relationship between plasma and red cell neuroleptic levels, oral and clinical parameter in a chronic schizophrenic population. Biol. Psychiatry 17, 929 – 935.

Ericksen, S. E., Hurt, S. W., Chang, S. et al. (1978) Haloperidol dose, plasma levels and clinical response: a double-blind study. Psychopharmacol. Bull. 14, 15 – 16.

Forsman, A. and Öhman, R. (1977) Applied pharmacokinetics of haloperidol in man. Curr. Ther. Res. 21, 396 – 411.

Forsman, A. and Öhman, R. (1978) On the objective evaluation of haloperidol effects in man. Curr. Ther. Res. 24, 179 – 191.

Forsman, A., Martensson, E., Nyberg, G. and Öhman, R. (1974) A gas chromatographic method for determining haloperidol. Naunyn-Schmiedeberg's Arch. Pharmacol. 286, 113 – 124.

Gautier, J., Jus, A., Villeneuve, A., Jus, K., Pires, P. and Villeneuve, R. (1977) Influence of the antiparkinsonian drugs on the plasma level of neuroleptics. Biol. Psychiatry 12, 389 – 399.

Hayashi, O., Miyoshi, S., Higashimura, T., Miyoshi, C., Nakata, S., Ohya, F. and Aoyama, H. (1982) Blood concentration and clinical effects of haloperidol in combination with levomepromazine. Jpn. J. Neuropsychopharmacol. 5, 41 – 47.

Itoh, H., Yagi, G., Ohtsuka, N., Iwamura, K. and Ichikawa, K. (1980) Serum level of haloperidol and its clinical significance. Prog. Neuro-Psychopharmacol. 4, 171 – 183.

Itoh, H., Yagi, G., Tateyama, M., Fujii, Y., Iwamura, K. and Ichikawa, K. (1983a) Monitoring of haloperidol serum levels and it's clinical significance. Prog. Neuro-Psychopharmacol. Biol. Psychiatr. 8, 51 – 62.

Itoh, H., Yagi, G., Fujii, Y., Iwamura, K. and Ichikawa, K. (1983b) The relationship between haloperidol blood levels and clinical responses. Prog. Neuro-Psychopharmacol. Biol. Psychiatr. 8, 285 – 292.

Kubokura, A., Tomita, K., Ara, M. and Iizuka, R. (1974) Blood concentration level of neuroleptics in schizophrenic patients. Annual Report of the Pharmacopsychiatry Research Foundation (Japanese) 5, 190 – 194.

Linnoila, M., Viukari, M., Vaisanen, K. and Auvinen, J. (1980) Effect of anticonvulsants on plasma haloperidol and thioridazine levels. Am. J. Psychiatry 137, 819 – 821.

McCreadie, R. G. and MacDonald, I. M. (1977) High dosage haloperidol in chronic schizophrenia. Br. J. Psychiatry 131, 310 – 316.

Moulin, M. A., Davy, J. P., Debruyne, D., Anderson, J. C., Bigot, M. C. and Poilpré, E. (1982) Serum level monitoring and therapeutic effect of haloperidol. Psychopharmacology 76, 346 – 350.

Morselli, P. L., and Zarifian, E. (1980) Clinical significance of monitoring plasma levels of psychotropic drugs. In: R. Porter, J. Rivers and J. Whelan (Eds), Drug Concentration in Neuropsychiatry. Excerpta Medica, Oxford, pp. 115 – 139.

Morselli, P. L., Bianchetti, G., Durand, G., Le Heuzey, M. F., Zarifian, E. and Dugas, M. (1979) Haloperidol plasma level monitoring in pediatric patients. Ther. Drug Monit. 1, 35 – 46.

Neborsky, R., Janowsky, D., Munson, E. and Depry, D. (1981) Rapid treatment of acute psychotic symptoms with high- and low-dose haloperidol. Behavioral consideration. Arch. Gen. Psychiatry 38, 195 – 199.

Niemegeers, C. J. E. (1979) The antiemetic activity of haloperidol decanoate in dogs. Preclinical research report R- 1625 Deca/1. Janssen Pharmaceutica, Beerse, Belgium.

Oka, I., Koyama, T., Matsubara, S., Mikuni, M., Saito, Y. and Yamashita, I. (1981) Effects of longterm haloperidol treatment on dopaminergic, adrenergic and cholinergic activities in schizophrenic patients. Annual Report of the Pharmacopsychiatry Research Foundation (Japanese), 12, 62 – 67.

Rama Rao, V. A., Bishop, M. and Coppen, A. (1980) Clinical state, plasma levels of haloperidol and prolactin: a correlation study in chronic schizophrenia. Br. J. Psychiatry 137, 518 – 521.

Rimón, R., Averbuch, I., Rozick, P., Fijiman-Damilovich, L., Kara, T., Dasberg, H., Ebstein, R. P. and Belmaker, R. H. (1981) Serum and CSF levels of haloperidol by radioimmunoassay and radioreceptor assay during high-dose therapy of resistant schizophrenic patients. Psychopharmacology 73, 197 – 199.

Roose, K. (1981) Monthly haloperidol decanoate as a replacement for maintenance therapy with intramuscular fluphenazine decanoate: clinical, pharmacokinetic and safety evaluation after one year of treatment. III World Congress of Biological Psychiatry, Stockholm, June 30.

Scatton, B., Zarifian, E., et al. (1982) Utilisation de l'halopéridol á forte dose dans la schizophrénie. Etude clinique, biochimique et pharmacocinétique. Encephale 8, 1 – 8.

Smith, R. C., Crayton, J., Dekirmenjian, H., Klass, D. and Davis, J. M. (1979) Blood levels of neuroleptic drugs in nonresponding chronic schizophrenic patients. Arch. Gen. Psychiatry 36, 579 – 584.

Smith, R. C., Vroulis, G. et al. (1982) Rbc and plasma levels of haloperidol and clinical response. Am. J. Psychiatry 139, 1054 – 1056.

Takahashi, R., Yoshimoto, H. and Matsumoto, H. (1979) Implication of plasma level of neuroleptics in the treatment and pathophysiological research of schizophrenia. 1-er Colloque Franco-Japonais de Psychopharmacologie, Paris, 4 – 6 Oct. INSERM (ed), pp. 337 – 370.

Tomita, K., Kubokura, A., Inoue, R. and Iizuka, R. (1975) On the relation of clinical feature of schizophrenia and EEG under pharmacotherapy. Annual Report of the Pharmacopsychiatry Research Foundation (Japanese) 6, 110 – 116.

Tune, L. E., Creese, I., Depaulo, J. r., Slavney, P. R., Coyle, J. T. and Snyder, S. H. (1980) Clinical state and serum neuroleptic levels measured by radioreceptor assay in schizophrenia. Am. J. Psychiatry 137, 187 – 190.

Yoshimoto, S., Matsumoto, H., Nakahara, T., Sakurai, Y. and Takahashi, R. (1979) Clinical significance of haloperidol plasma level in the treatment of schizophrenia (Japanese). Neuropsychopharmacology (Japan) 5, 67 – 74.

Yoshimoto, S., Matsumoto, H., Minami, H. and Takahashi, R. (1980) The significance of haloperidol plasma level in the treatment and pathogenesis of schizophrenia (Japanese). Clin. Psychiatr. 22, 1159 – 1165.

Zarifian, E., Cottereau, M. J., Cuche, H., Loo, H. and Deniker, P. (1979) Interet des donnees pharmacocinetiques an cours des traitements des psychoses par l'haloperidol. Encephale 3, 197 – 204.

Zingales, I. N. (1971) A gas chromatographic method for the determination of haloperidol in human plasma. J. Chromatogr. 54, 15 – 24.

Burrows/Norman/Davies (eds) Antipsychotics

Chapter 9

Thioxanthenes: Measurement, kinetics and clinical response

L. K. OYEWUMI

and

Y. D. LAPIERRE

Department of Psychiatry, University of Ottawa, and The Royal Ottawa Hospital, 1145 Carling Ave., Ottawa, Ontario, Canada KlZ 7K4

DISCOVERY, CHEMISTRY AND SYNTHESIS OF THE THIOXANTHENES

The advent of chlorpromazine into clinical psychiatry in the early fifties stimulated further research for other pharmacological agents with superior therapeutic efficacy and with fewer side effects. Petersen et al. (1958) developed the thioxanthenes, a group of psychotropics of similar structure to the phenothiazines.

The thioxanthenes have a tricyclic nucleus which differs from that of the phenothiazines in that the central nitrogen atom (position 10 of the phenothiazine nucleus) is replaced by a carbon atom (position 9 of the thioxanthene nucleus) with a double-bond attachment to the side chain. There is thus a structural difference in the attachment of the side chain to the tricyclic nucleus (Fig. 1). The side chain of thioxanthenes is attached to the tricyclic core by a double bond. This prevents rotation of the first carbon in the chain (Nielsen et al., 1962). The thioxanthenes thus have limited configurational changes. Two stable geometric isomers (*cis*- and *trans*-) are possible when the symmetry of the nucleus is offset by further substitu-

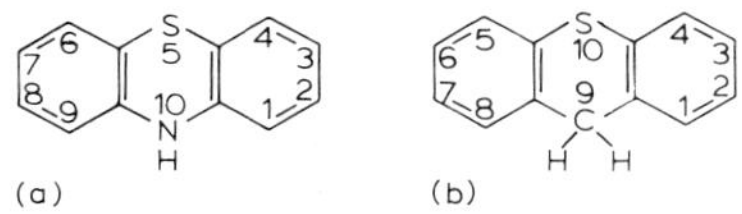

Fig. 1. The phenothiazine and thioxanthene nucleus. (a) Phenothiazine; (b) thioxanthene.

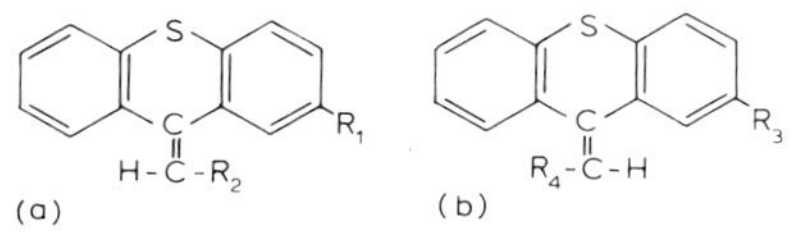

Fig. 2. Geometric isomerism in thioxanthenes. (a) *Cis*-configuration; (b) *trans*-configuration.

tion, usually in the 2-position (Fig. 2). These two stereoisomers possess different physicochemical properties and differ in their infra red absorption spectra and X-ray crystallography. The biological activity of the *cis*-isomer of the currently known thioxanthenes is consistently several times greater than that of the *trans*-isomer.

Unsaturated 9-amino alkylene thioxanthenes bear greater similarity to the corresponding phenothiazine preparations in their biological activity than saturated 9-aminoalkyl thioxanthenes. This was borne out by similarities between the unsaturated compounds and the corresponding phenothiazines as shown by the π-electron distribution, the infra red and ultra violet absorption curves spectra. Ravn (1970) showed that the double bond between the carbon atom of the thioxanthene ring (position 9) and the first carbon atom of the side chain seems to be prerequisite for any appreciable neuroleptic activity of the thioxanthenes. The nuclear substitution in position 2 of the unsaturated thioxanthenes leads to increased CNS activity as it does for corresponding phenothiazines.

Several techniques have been used in the synthesis of thioxanthenes in general. These included the methods of Petersen and Nielsen (1964), and their modification in 1971 by Fontanella et al. These methods are based on the reaction of 2-substituted thioxanthene with a Grignard reagent; or an allylmagnesium halide or a substituted propynylamine in the presence of lithium amide and *N*-methyl pyrrolidone. Fontanella et al. (1971) used the reaction of a ω-aminoketone with sulfuric or polyphosphoric acid. With these methods, a mixture of *cis*- and *trans*-isomers of the psychoactive thioxanthene is formed. Separation of the geometric isomers is accomplished by crystallization from a suitable agent.

To date, many thioxanthene derivatives have been synthesized and tested in animal pharmacological studies. Of these, chlorprothixene, clopenthixol, flupenthixol and thiothixene progressed from the preclinical to the clinical stage and are now available for clinical use (Ravn, 1970). Figure 3 shows the corresponding phenothiazine analogues of these thioxanthenes. Chlorprothixene was the first to be used clinically.

THIOXANTHENES

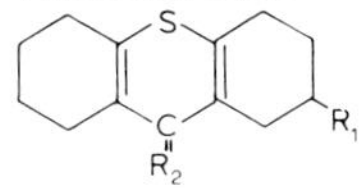

PHENOTHIAZINES

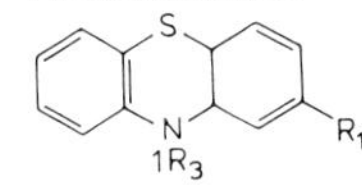

Chemical structure		Generic name	Average daily oral dose (mg)	Chemical structure		Generic name	Average daily oral dose (mg)
R_1	R_2			R_1	R_3		
Cl	$= CH(CH_2)_2$-$N(CH_3)_2$	Chlorprothixene	45 – 400	Cl	$(CH_2)_3$-$N(CH_3)_2$	Chlorpromazine	150 – 600
Cl	$CH(CH_2)_2$-N N-$(CH_2)_2OH$	Clopenthixol	30 – 150	Cl	$(CH_2)_3$-N N-$CH_2)_2OH$	Perphenazine	6 – 32
CF_3	$CH(CH_2)_2$-N N-$(CH_2)_2OH$	Flupenthixol	6 – 18	CF_3	$(CH_2)_3$-N N-$(CH_2)_2OH$	Fluphenazine	1 – 10
SO_2-N $(CH_3)_2$	$CH(CH_2)_2$-N N-CH_3	Thiothixene	20 – 60	SO_2N $(CH_3)_2$	$(CH_2)_3$-N N-CH_3	Thioproperazine	20 – 60

Fig. 3. Clinically available thioxanthenes and their phenothiazine analogues.

PHARMACOLOGY OF THE THIOXANTHENES

Although the study of animal behaviour has not yet produced much information concerning the mode of action of drugs in abnormal human behaviour, such studies have led to screening procedures for the selection of drugs in the treatment of mental illness. Like all neuroleptics, the thioxanthenes, in low doses in animals and in man, reduce operant behaviour but spinal reflexes are unchanged. Exploratory behaviour is diminished and responses to a variety of stimuli are fewer, slower and smaller, although the ability to discriminate stimuli is retained. Conditioned avoidance behaviours are selectively inhibited while unconditioned escape or avoidance responses are not. The highly reinforcing self-stimulation of the animal brain (median forebrain bundle) is blocked, although the capacity to press the stimulation-inducing lever is not lost. The following activities are either blocked or inhibited: behavioural activation stimulated environmentally or pharmacologically, feeding, emesis, and aggression induced by apomorphine. Apomorphine is a dopamine agonist. At high doses, the thioxanthenes like most neuroleptics induce characteristic catalepsy. Many learned tasks are performed if sufficient stimulation and motivation are provided. Very high doses do not induce coma and the lethal dose is extraordinarily high (Fielding and Lal, 1978).

Scheckel (1969) adequately summarized the pharmacological actions of chlorprothixene as a typical thioxanthene of the aliphatic series. The neuroleptic action of chlorprothixene was first seen in mice where its action resembled that of chlorpromazine. Similar effects were observed in rats, rabbits, cats, dogs and monkeys. Chlorprothixene is a potent sedative in a variety of animal species. Pharmacologically, it blocks the autonomic effects of acetylcholine and the adrenergic agents. Biochemically, it enhances tyrosine hydroxylase and increases the concentration of homovanillic acid in brain. It has no effect on the absolute brain levels of norepinephrine, dopamine or serotonin. Behavioural studies indicate that it specifically disrupts active avoidance, having no significant effect on passive avoidance behaviour.

Comparing the psychopharmacological actions of thiothixene, chlorprothixene and clopenthixol in rats, Weissman (1969) found that thiothixene displayed considerable selectivity. It disrupts conditioned avoidance behaviour in the rat at low doses, produces catalepsy and blocks the stereotyped symptoms caused by amphetamine. In dogs, it has strong antiemetic effects. In each of the above actions, thiothixene is more potent than chlorprothixene or clopenthixol, however, both chlorprothixene and clopenthixol are more potent in blocking thermoregulation, disrupting escape behaviour, potentiating hexobarbital or eliciting flaccidity in rats. Generally, clopenthixol has strong sedative effects. It produces potent cataleptic action and inhibits conditioned avoidance response and antiemetic effect (Nielsen, 1969). It has weak anticholinergic effects in contrast to chlorprothixene.

Kato et al. (1969) reported that chlorprothixene, clopenthixol and thiothixene strongly inhibit the vascular response induced by histamine in the rat. They found that these thioxanthene derivatives have a similar inhibiting effect on catecholamine reuptake into the storage granules as does imipramine. They thus concluded that the peripheral vascular effects of the thioxanthene derivatives are related to their effect on the catecholamine inactivating mechanism.

KINETICS OF THIOXANTHENES

Metabolism

Pharmacokinetic and metabolic studies of thioxanthenes have yet to be demonstrated as clinically applicable. This is due to the complex metabolism of these compounds as well as to the difficulties inherent in the measurement of clinical effect. As with most antipsychotics, oral administration results in erratic and unpredictable absorption. Parenteral administration increases bioavailability 4 to 10-fold.

In animal isotope studies, rats and dogs absorb and metabolize thioxanthenes rapidly. Thirty minutes after oral or intraperitoneal administration, the bile contains all identifiable thiothixene metabolites (Ban, 1978). Since thiothixene is rapidly and extensively metabolized, only an insignificant portion of the administered drug is excreted unchanged. Hobbs (1968) demarcated a number of thiothixene metabolites but only the *N*-demethylthiothixenes were clearly identifiable. The metabolism of these drugs does not result in the breakdown of the thioxanthene nucleus.

The thioxanthenes are lipophilic and membrane or protein bound. They accumulate in the brain, lungs, liver and other tissues with a high blood supply. The affinity of chlorprothixene for melanin was found to be considerably higher than that of thiothixene (Potts, 1962).

In human pharmacokinetic studies, Lauffer et al. (1969), using five healthy volunteers, administered 20 mg of thiothixene orally and found that a peak plasma concentration above 40 ng/ml was achieved in all cases. They were able to identify two metabolites of thiothixene. These include thiothixene sulfoxide and *N*-demethylthiothixene. Hobbs et al. (1974) carried out clinical metabolic studies on 15 chronic schizophrenics who had been treated with thiothixene for periods ranging from 1 to 25 months, at individually adjusted dosage for control of psychopathology. In spite of the wide variation of individual dosage requirements (15 – 60 mg) the therapeutically effective plasma levels of thiothixene varied only between 10.0 ng/ml and 22.5 ng/ml. Peak plasma levels were at 1 – 3 hours after the administration during maintenance treatment. Thiothixene absorption half time is estimated at 0.5 hour; the early elimination half-life at 3.5 hours and a late elimination half-life at 34 hours. Hobbs et al. (1974) also observed appreciable levels of thiothixene in the plasma 24 hours after administration, suggesting that daily administration is sufficient during maintenance therapy. The absorption of the tablets of thioxanthenes is more erratic resulting in less bioavailability than with liquid concentrates.

The main metabolic routes of the thioxanthenes are oxidation, glucuronidation, *N*-demethylation, sulfoxidation and *N*-oxidation. The conjugated metabolites are excreted in urine as well as bile. The presently known metabolites are inactive. In contrast to phenothiazines, no ring hydroxylation metabolites are seen (Peterson et al., 1977). A specific radioimmunoassay may detect thioxanthenes to a sensitivity of 0.3 ng/ml (Jorgensen, 1978).

Intramuscular injection of flupenthixol decanoate in oil produces maximum serum concentrations at 7 days after injection and a factor of two fluctuation in serum level in a 2-week dosage interval.

Biochemistry

The psychoactive thioxanthenes are antiadrenergic centrally and antiserotonergic and anticholinergic peripherally (Petersen and Neilsen, 1964). They are also antihistaminic (Itoh et al., 1969; Shibuya et al., 1969).

Roos (1965) found an increase in concentration of homovanillic acid, a dopamine metabolite, in the corpus striatum of rabbits 3 hours after the administration of thioxanthenes. Similar findings were reported in rats and mice (Pletscher and Da Prada, 1967; Lahti et al., 1972). These findings led to the hypothesis that thioxanthenes probably produce a postsynaptic dopamine receptor blockade, leading to a compensatory increase in dopamine synthesis and turnover rate.

Hollister (1968), administered 5 – 40 mg of thiothixene orally to 10 normal volunteer subjects and measured free fatty acid and glucose concentrations in the plasma prior to and after drug administration. He also measured vanilmandelic acid (VMA) excretion in a 6-hour collection of urine. Thiothixene did not produce significant changes in the three parameters measured.

MEASUREMENT OF THIOXANTHENES

There is no consistent evidence of a correlation between plasma levels of thioxanthenes and therapeutic response in psychotic patients. Several factors may contribute to this. These include the use of chronically hospitalized patients or subjects in whom clinical changes can be expected to be minimal. There may also be a metabolic explanation as some patients convert the active *cis*-isomer of thioxanthenes to the relatively inactive *trans*-isomer. Reifler et al. (1981) studied thiothixene plasma levels and clinical response in acute schizophrenia administering *cis*-thioxanthene. Subsequently, plasma levels of both *cis*- and *trans*-isomers of thiothixene were determined and these findings suggest that change in plasma concentration to *trans*-thiothixene may be more predictive of clinical response than absolute plasma levels.

A cross-over study by Stauning et al. (1979) compared serum levels of 2 and 10% *cis*-flupenthixol decanoate intramuscularly. No statistically significant difference between the pharmacokinetics of the two preparations was found. The maximum serum concentrations was seen at 4 or 7 days after injection.

In summary, presently available methodology does not allow the establishment of a sufficiently clear relationship between clinical efficacy and plasma levels to justify its use as a routine clinical procedure.

CLINICAL STUDIES WITH THIOXANTHENES

Four thioxanthenes are presently available for clinical use. These are chlorprothixene, an aliphatic derivative, thiothixene, clopenthixol and flupenthixol which are of the piperazine derivatives. They are available in oral (capsules, tablets and liquid) and in parenteral preparations. The parenteral preparations are short-acting hydrochloride salts (thiothixene, chlorprothixene, clopenthixol and flupenthixol) or the long-acting ester (flupenthixol and clopenthixol). The long-acting flupenthixol or clopenthixol are esterified with decanoic or palmitic acid. The clinical effectiveness of the esters has a duration of between 2 and 4 weeks. Table 1 summarizes the dose, dosage forms and trade names of the available thioxanthenes for clinical use.

Thioxanthenes have been used in a number of psychiatric and medical disorders in both adults and children (Ban, 1978). Generally the therapeutic dosage of the thioxanthenes depends on the diagnosis, severity of illness and physical conditions, taking into consideration the age and sex of the patient. As with any phar-

TABLE 1

The clinically available thioxanthenes

Thioxanthene derivative		Dose			Dosage forms	
Generic name	Trade name	Antipsychotic dosage range (daily dosage)		Single i.m. dose	Oral	Injectable
		Usual (mg)	Extreme (mg)			
1. Chlorprothixene	Taractan Truxal	50–400	30–600	25 –50	T, OC	S
2. Thiothixene	Navane Orbinamon	6– 30	6– 60	2 – 6	C, OC	S
3. Clopenthixol	Ciatyl Sordinol	30–150	30–200	12.5–25	T	S, LA
4. Flupenthixol	Fluanxol	6– 18	6– 25	1 – 5	T	S, LA

Abbreviations: C = capsule; T = tablet; OC = oral concentrate; S = short acting; LA = long acting.

macotherapeutic agent, dosage is gradually adjusted to the optimum therapeutic index balancing the desired and undesired effects.

THIOXANTHENES IN MAJOR PSYCHIATRIC SYNDROMES

Schizophrenia

A bimodal action for thioxanthenes was observed clinically quite early after they became available. It was felt that small doses were accompanied by an elevation of mood when the patient showed signs of depression and at higher doses, antipsychotic activity took place. A 1967 study by Angus et al. involving thiothixene on chronic schizophrenics supported this observation. Similar findings occurred with flupenthixol (Young et al., 1976) clopenthixol (Okasha et al., 1978) and chlorprothixene (Hagopian and Crossfield, 1963). A review of the then available literature on thiothixene by Gardos and Cole (1973), also supported this dual action hypothesis. Barsa (1975) suggested that this may be a feature of most neuroleptics.

To test the 'dual action' hypothesis, Gardos et al. (1974) administered thiothixene in 'high' (40 mg/day) and 'low' (10 mg/day) dosages to 40 chronically hospitalized schizophrenic patients over a 16-week period. Using several parameters (clinical, psychometric and neurophysiological measures), they found significant differences between the two groups of patients. The low dose group had a greater frequency of insomnia and excitement, variable resting electroencephalographic pattern of higher average frequency; and improvement in the depression factor of the Brief Psychiatry Rating Scale (BPRS), while the group treated with the high dose showed more of tremor and akathisia; an increase in the alpha and a decrease in the beta bands of the 'attentive electroencephalogram' and they made significantly fewer incorrect responses on the paced digit symbol test (a complex attention task). These findings supported the hypothesis of an 'activating-stimulating' effect of the thiothixene at low doses. In the group treated with high doses, the therapeutic effects equalled the therapeutic effects of other antipsychotic drugs.

Numerous clinical evaluations of the clinically available thioxanthenes have confirmed their effects as potent antipsychotic drugs in the acute, chronic and maintenance therapy of schizophrenics. The intramuscular administration of the short-acting preparations of fluphenazine, thiothixene and haloperidol, in acute schizophrenia results in rapid remission of the symptoms at an equally efficacious rate (Levenson et al., 1976). In a double-blind comparison of flupenthixol decanoate and fluphenazine decanoate in the treatment of chronic schizophrenia, Pinto et al. (1979), studying 64 chronic stabilized schizophrenics for 18 months, were unable to demonstrate any significant differences between the two drugs in overall antipsychotic effect. However, more patients on fluphenazine required additional therapy for depression or anxiety. Other studies supported the equal therapeutic efficacy of both fluphenazine decanoate and flupenthixol decanoate in maintenance therapy of chronic schizophrenics. However, Kelly et al. (1977) found fewer extrapyramidal side effects with flupenthixol ($p < 0.05$). Johnson and Malik (1975) also found both depot neuroleptics equally effective in the treatment of acute schizophrenia but noted that flupenthixol resulted in more mood elevation.

Several studies (Gottfries, 1971; Hall and Coleman, 1972) have suggested that flupenthixol possesses some activating properties and may be of particular value in the treatment of schizophrenic patients showing features of apathy, anergia and withdrawal (the negative symptoms of schizophrenia). A number of studies (Reiter, 1969; Merskey, 1971; Hall and Coleman, 1972; Frolund, 1974; Young et al., 1976; Johnson, 1979) suggest that flupenthixol may be an effective antidepressant. However, others failed to bring out a difference between the effect of fluphenazine decanoate and flupenthixol decanoate on depression (Haslam et al., 1975; Johnson and Malik, 1975; Kelly et al., 1977; Hirsch et al., 1978). At this time, the consensus of research findings suggests that flupenthixol may have some antidepressant effect in schizophrenia and is probably equivalent to fluphenazine in antipsychotic potency and extrapyramidal activity. This is illustrated in a recent study by Hamilton et al. (1979) where the decanoate of flupenthixol was equivalent to that of fluphenazine in antipsychotic and extrapyramidal activity but superior in the improvement of affective symptoms.

In addition to flupenthixol, the other thioxanthenes have been studied as antipsychotics, usually in samples of acute and chronic schizophrenic patients. Also, reports of studies comparing these drugs with phenothiazines and haloperidol have consistently indicated equal antipsychotic efficacy provided equivalent doses are used. Particularly notable is the ability of the thioxanthenes to improve alertness and increase the degree of purposeful activity in chronically ill apathetic patients. Sugarman (1969) indicated the usefulness of thiothixene in reducing hallucinatory behaviour, tension, suspiciousness, manifest psychosis and irritability, while increasing cooperation and social competence. As far as the drug of choice is concerned, thioxanthenes with an aromatic side chain are considered to be more suitable for the maintenance therapy of schizophrenics than thioxanthenes with an aliphatic side chain; being less sedative, less hypotensive and less likely to be deposited in tissues. However, they may produce more extrapyramidal side effects (Abuzzahab, 1969).

Major affective illnesses

Filotto et al. (1969) treated nine first-admission patients in acute mania with thiothixene. They reported good clinical response to thiothixene in eight of the nine patients. The daily dosage of thiothixene which they used varied between 20 and 60 mg. Thiothixene, like other neuroleptics, induces extrapyramidal symptoms. At these doses the drug is relatively safe. Ginestet (1969) also found thiothixene to be effective in the control of mania in the higher dosage range of 30 – 60 mg/day in four manic patients. Others however, could not replicate these favorable observations in mania (Delay et al., 1966; Clavier, 1969). In fact, Delay and Deniker reported thiothixene as being ineffective in manic states and in severely agitated psychotics. In schizo-affective psychosis flupenthixol decanoate may exert a mood stabilizing effect. This finding has not been subjected to controlled studies (Kielholz et al., 1979).

The prophylactic effect of flupenthixol decanoate in endogenous depression had been a matter of speculation for some time. Kielholz et al. (1979) treated 30 patients with periodical and cyclic depressions with flupenthixol decanoate over 2 to 3 years in an open study. Flupenthixol was found to reduce the number and severity of cycling as would be expected from lithium – this, again, was not controlled. Merskey (1971) noted a 'worthwhile sustained improvement' in 24 out of 53 patients with affective disorders. Frolund (1974) found flupenthixol effective in a trial with 231 patients suffering from anxiety and depression. Flupenthixol was given for only 2 weeks, however, and the drop-out rate was high. Young et al. (1976), in a controlled comparison of flupenthixol and amitriptyline in depressed out-patients, found that flupenthixol effectively relieves mild or moderate symptoms of depression associated with anxiety. Flupenthixol was as effective as amitriptyline as an antidepressant and as an anxiolytic and was less likely to produce side effects. There was no difference between the drugs in rapidity of onset of action. It was suggested that flupenthixol may be a useful alternative antidepressant with rapid action, higher potency and relatively few side effects.

Thioxanthenes in neurotic disorders

Most thioxanthenes have some antidepressant plus anxiolytic properties. Several studies have attempted to explore this further. In a double-blind placebo controlled study of 155 anxious neurotic out-patients, Rickels et al. (1974) compared the anxiolytic properties of thiothixene and thioridazine. There was little evidence for the superiority of thiothixene and thioridazine over placebo. However, some degree of antidepressant properties was found with both active drugs. They both exerted some weak anxiolytic effect at the initial 2 weeks of treatment but this dissipated after 4 weeks. In this study, 6 – 12 mg/day of thiothixene and 75 – 150 mg/day of thioridazine were used.

The therapeutic dosage of thiothixene for this diagnostic category has not been established. Raab and Mariategui (1968) used 3 mg/day of thiothixene while Simeon et al. (1970) used a dose of 8 – 14 mg/day in neurotic children.

Johnson (1979) reported on a double-blind comparison of flupenthixol, nortriptyline and diazepam in neurotic depression using flexible dose schedules. He suggested that each drug is an efficient treatment for neurotic depression although the patterns of response and prevalence of side effects varied. He found no significant differences on rating scales of depression and anxiety, between flupenthixol, nortriptyline and diazepam, but trends favored flupenthixol. Flupenthixol resulted in fewer side effects than nortriptyline. Doses of 1.5 – 3 mg/day of flupenthixol, 75 – 150 mg/day of nortriptyline and 7.5 – 15 mg/day of diazepam were used.

While several reports have acknowledged the usefulness of the thioxanthenes, especially thiothixene and flupenthixol in neurotic depression and anxiety, the fear of serious late-appearing neurologic effects such as tardive dyskinesia has restricted their use as primary therapeutic agents in this area.

Other clinical used of thioxanthenes

Thioxanthenes have been used in the treatment of various types of organic brain syndromes and in geriatric, child and adolescent patients. The therapeutic dosage of thioxanthenes in these populations and in the diagnostic category of organic brain syndrome has not been established. Most reports are anecdotal and no controlled studies have yet been done.

Treatment schedules

As with most psychotropic medications, the thioxanthenes are administered in divided doses 3 or 4 times daily during the initial, or acute phase of treatment. This dosage schedule can gradually be replaced by 1 or 2 daily doses during maintenance or during the chronic phase of treatment (Hollister, 1972). Donlon and Tupin (1974) have used thiothixene at a daily dose of 50 or 100 mg in divided doses for rapid tranquillization. Ayd (1972) emphasized the need to decrease the frequency of drug administration to improve compliance with simpler schedules of once- or twice-a-day dose. In a 24-week double-blind comparative clinical study of 38 schizophrenic patients, Lee et al. (1974) found no significant difference in improvement between the group that took a once-a-day dose of thiothixene and the group that took the thiothixene in divided doses of 3 times daily. There was a somewhat faster therapeutic response to thrice-a-day administration of medication than the once-a-day administration but this resulted in a slightly higher incidence of extrapyramidal manifestations. Generally, for improved compliance and equal therapeutic efficacy, an accepted treatment schedule is to use divided dose in the acute phase of the illness.

ADVERSE DRUG REACTIONS INVOLVING THIOXANTHENES

Generally, the incidence of adverse drug reactions (ADR) with thioxanthenes in the treatment of schizophrenic patients has been found to be comparable to that encountered with the other commonly used neuroleptic drugs. These ADRs include: 1) behavioural (anxiety, confusional state, delirium, drowsiness and insomnia, exacerbation of psychosis, mood changes, sleep disturbances and suicidal attempts); 2) neurological (ataxia, cerebral seizures, EEG changes, extrapyramidal effects); 3) autonomic (blurred vision, perspiration, salivation, nasal congestion); and 4) other effects involving the endocrinological, cardiovascular, haematological systems.

REFERENCES

Abuzzahab, Sr., F. S. (1969) Psychopharmacologic agents in the prevention of psychiatric disorders. Postgrad. Med. J. 46, 141 – 144.

Angus, J. W. S., Iqbal, F., Iqbal, J. and Simpson, G. M. (1967) A year's trial of thiothixene in chronic schizophrenia. Int. J. Neuropsychiatry 3, 408 – 412.

Ayd, Jr., F. J. (1972) Effects of the withdrawal of neuroleptics from psychotic children. Int. Drug Ther. Newsletter 7, 29 – 32.

Ban, T. A. (1978) Psychopharmacology of Thiothixene. Raven Press, New York, pp. 39 – 46.

Barsa, J. A. (1975) The dual action of tranquilizers. Am. J. Psychiatry 114, 74 – 75.

Clavier, L. C. (1969) Navane in psychosis. Arch. Ven. Psiquiatr. Neurol. 15, 71 – 78.

Delay, J., Deniker, P., Ginestet, D., Perier, M., Peron-Magnan, P. and Dalle, B. (1966) Short range clinical evaluation of a new neuroleptic agent, thiothixene. Ann. Med. Psychol. (Paris) 2, 196 – 202.

Donlon, P. T. and Tupin, J. P. (1974) Rapid 'digitalization' of decompensated schizophrenic patients with antipsychotic agents. Am. J. Psychiatry 131, 310 – 312.

Fielding, S. and Lal, H. (1978) Behavioral actions of neuroleptics. In: L. L. Iversen, S. D. Iversen and S. H. Snyder (Eds), Handbook of Psychopharmacology, Vol. 10. Plenum Press, New York, pp. 91 – 128.

Filotto, J. Bordeleau, J. M. and Tetreault, L. (1969) Thiothixene in treatment of affective psychoses: pilot study. In: F. A. Freyman, N. Petrilowitsch and P. Pichot (Eds), Modern Problems of Pharmacopsychiatry: The Thioxanthenes, Vol. 2. Karger, Basel and New York, pp. 55 – 63.

Fontanella, L., Mariani, L., Occelli, E., Rosselli del Turco, B. and Diena, A. (1971) Nuovi del tioxanthen attivi sul sistens nervosa centrale. Farmaco (Sci) 26, 489 – 511.

Frolund, F. (1974) Treatment of depression in general practice – a controlled study of flupenthixol (Fluanxol). Curr. Med. Res. Opin. 2, 78 – 89.

Gardos, G. and Cole, J. O. (1973) The dual action of thiothixene. Arch. Gen. Psychiatry 29, 222 – 225.

Gardos, G., Orzack, M. H., Finn, G. and Cole, J. O. (1974) High and low dose thiothixene treatment in chronic schizophrenia. Dis. Nerv. Syst. 35, 53 – 58.

Ginestet, D. (1969) Studies with the thioxanthenes. In: H. E. Lehmann and T. A. Ban (Eds), The Thioxanthenes. Karger, Basel and New York, pp. 111 – 112.

Gottfries, C. G. (1971) Klinisk provning av flupenthixoldecanoat son depa neuroleptikum, Nord. Psykiatr. Tidsski. 25, 296 – 303.

Hagopian, P. B. and Crossfield, R. M. (1963) Experiences with chlorprothixene in a State Hospital. Dis. Nerv. Syst. 24, 6, 1 – 4.

Hall, P. and Coleman, J. (1972) Flupenthixol in the treatment of schizophrenia. (Letter to the Editor). Br. J. Psychiatry 120, 241 – 244.

Hamilton, M., Card, I. R., Wallis, G. G. and Mahmoud, M. R. (1979) A comparative trial of the decanoates of flupenthixol and fluphenazine. Psychopharmacologia 64, 225 – 229.

Haslam, M. T., Bromham, B. M. and Schiff, A. A. (1975) A comparative trial of fluphenazine decanoate and flupenthixol decanoate. Acta Psychiatr. Scand. 51, 92 – 100.

Hirsch, S. R., Knights, A., Okash, M. S. and Salih, M. A. (1978) Maintenance therapy in out patient schizophrenics, a report of a double-blind trial comparison of fluphenazine decanoate and flupenthixol decanoate. Br. J. Psychiatry 133, 371.

Hobbs, D. C. (1968) Metabolism of thiothixene. J. Pharm. Sci. 57, 105 – 111.

Hobbs, D. C., Welch, W. M., Short, M. J., Moody, W. A., and Van der Velde, C. D. (1974) Pharmacokinetics of thiothixene in man. Clin. Pharmacol. Ther. 16, 473 – 478.

Hollister, L. E. (1968) Some human pharmacological studies of three psychotropic drugs, thiothixene, molindone, and W-1867. J. Clin. Pharmacol. 9, 95 – 101.

Hollister, L. E. (1972) Drug therapy. N. Engl. J. Med. 286, 984 – 987.

Itoh, H., Sato, A., Horiguchi, Y., Tamura, M., Ozawa, K. and Harada, S. (1969) The effects of the antipsychotic drug thiothixene (Navane). On the circulatory and respiratory systems and on smooth muscle organs. Yokohoma Igaku 20, 214 – 225.

Johnson, D. A. W. (1979) A double blind comparison of flupenthixol, nortriptyline and diazepam in neurotic depression. Acta Psychiat. Scand. 59, 1 – 8.

Johnson, D. A. W. and Malik, N. A. (1975) A double-blind comparison of fluphenazine decanoate and flupenthixol decanoate in the treatment of acute schizophrenia. Acta Psychiat. Scand. 51, 257 – 267.

Jorgensen, A. (1978) A sensitive and specific radioimmunoassay for Cis (z)- flupenthixol in human serum. Life Sci. 23, 1533 – 1542.

Kato, L., Gozsy, B., Roy, P. B. and Trsic, T. (1969) Peripheral vascular effects of thioxanthenes. In: F. A. Freyman, N. Petrilowitsch and P. Pichot (Eds), Modern Problems of Pharmacopsychiatry, The Thioxanthenes. S. Karger, Basel and New York, pp. 30 – 39.

Kelly, H. B., Freeman, H. L., Banning, B. and Schiff, A. A. (1977) Clinical and social comparison of fluphenazine decanoate and flupenthixol decanoate in the community maintenance therapy of schizophrenia. Int. Pharmacopsychiatry 12, 54 – 64.

Kielholz, P., Terzani, S. and Poldinger, W. (1979) The long term treatment of periodical and cyclic depressions with flupenthixol decanoate. Int. Pharmacopsychiatry 14, 305 – 309.

Lahti, R. A., McAllister, B. and Wozniak, J. (1972) Apomorphine antagonism of the elevation of homovanillic acid induced by antipsychotic drugs. Life Sci. 11, 605 – 613.

Lauffer, S., Schmid, E. and Weist, F. (1969) Dunnschichtchromatographische Trennung und Spectro photo fluometrischer Nachweis psychotroper Pharmaka. Arzneim-Forsch. 19, 1965 – 1971.

Lee, J. H., Branchey, M., Hahler, E. J., Varga, E. and Simpson, G. M. (1974) Once versus thrice daily thiothixene in the treatment of schizophrenic inpatients. Br. J. Psychiatry 125, 73 – 78.

Levenson, A. J., Barnett, G. B., Nottingham, J. D., Sermas, C. E. and Thornby, J. I. (1976) Speed and rate of remission in acute schizophrenia. A comparison of intramuscularly administered fluphenazine HCL with thiothixene and haloperidol. Curr. Ther. Res. 20, 5, 695 – 700.

Merskey, H. (1971) Flupenthixol (Fluanxol). Br. J. Psychiatry 119, 230.

Nielsen, I. M. (1969) Pharmacology of clopenthixol. In: F. A. Freyman, N. Petrilowitsch and P. Pichot (Eds), Modern Problems of Pharmacopsychiatry. The Thioxanthenes. Karger, Basel and New York, pp. 23 – 29.

Nielsen, I. M. and Neuthold, K. (1959) The comparative pharmacology and toxicology of the trans-isomere of 2-chloral-9-(3,dimethylaminopropyledene)-thioxanthene HCL (chlorprothixene) = N 714 tran and chlorpromazine. Acta Pharmacol. Toxicol. 15, 335 – 359.

Okasha, M. S., Hirsch, S. R., Knights, A. and Salih, M. A. (1978) Flupenthixol and fluphenazine decanoate. A comparative review. Psychiatr. Annals 8, 51 – 67.

Petersen, P. V. and Nielsen, I. M. (1964) Thioxanthene derivatives. In: M. Gordon (Ed.), Psychopharmacological Agents, Vol. 1. Academic Press, New York, pp. 301 – 324.

Petersen, P. V., Lassen, N., Holm, T., Kopf, R. and Nielsen, I. M. (1958) Chemische Konstitution und pharmakologische Wirkungen einiger Thioxanthenanaloge zu Chlorpromazin, Promazin und Mepazin. Arzneim-Forsch. 8, 395 – 397.

Petersen, P. V., Nielsen, I. M., Pedersen, V., Jorgensen, A. and Lassen, N. (1977) Thioxanthenes. In: E. Usdin and I. S. Forrest (Eds), Psychotherapeutic Drugs, Part 2: Applications (Psychopharmacology series 2). Marcel Dekker, N.Y., pp. 857 – 867.

Pinto, R., Bannergee, A. and Ghosh, N. (1979) A double blind comparison of flupenthixol decanoate and fluphenazine decanoate in the treatment of chronic schizophrenia. Acta Psychiatr. Scand. 60, 313 – 322.

Pletscher, A. and Da Prada, M. (1967) Mechanism of action of neuroleptics. In: H. Brill, J. C. Cole, P. Beniker, H. Hippius and P. B. Bradley (Eds), Proceedings of the 5th Congress of the Collegium Internationale Neuropsychopharmacologicum. International Congress Series No. 129. Excerpta Medica Foundation, Amsterdam.

Potts, A. M. (1962) Uveal pigment and phenothiazine compounds. Trans. Am. Ophthalmol. Soc. 60, 517 – 552.

Raab, E. S. and Mariategui, J. (1968) Thiothixene in the treatment of psychoneurotic outpatients. Rev. Neuropsiquiatr. 31, 104 – 110.

Ravn. J. (1970) The history of thioxanthenes. In: F. J. Ayd, Jr. and B. Blackwell (Eds), Discoveries in Biological Psychiatry. Lippincott, Philadelphia, pp. 180 – 193.

Reifler, B. V., Ward, N., Davis, C. M. and Friedel, R. O. (1981) Thiothixene plasma levels and clinical response in acute schizophrenia. J. Clin. Psychiatry 42, 207 – 211.

Reiter, P. (1969) On flupenthixol, an antidepressant of a new chemical group. Br. J. Psychiatry 115, 1399 – 1422.

Rickels, K., Weise, C. C., Clark, E. L., Jenkins, B. W., Rose, C. K., Rosenfeld, H. and Gordon, P. E. (1974) Thiothixene and thioridazine in anxiety. Br. J. Psychiatry 125, 79 – 87.

Roos, B. E. (1965) Effects of certain tranquilizers on the level of homovanillic acid in the corpus striatum. J. Pharm. Pharmacol. 17, 820 – 821.

Scheckel, C. L. (1969) Pharmacology and chemistry of the thioxanthenes with special reference to chlorprothixene. In: F. A. Freyman, N. Petrilowitsch and P. Pichot (Eds), Modern Problems of Pharmacopsychiatry. The Thioxanthenes. S. Karger, Basel and New York, pp. 1 – 14.

Shibuya, T., Horibe, M., Sasaki, Y., Matsuda, H., Matsumiya, T. and Nakada, K. (1969) Pharmacological studies on psychotropic drugs – the pharmacological action of thiothixene (Navane). Tokyo Ika Daigaku Zasshi 27, 839 – 957.

Simeon, J., Saletu, B., Saletu, M., Itil, T. M., and DaSilva, J. (1974) thiothixene in childhood psychoses. In: I. S. Forrest, C. J. Carr and E. Usdin (Eds), Phenothiazines and Structurally Related Drugs. Raven Press, New York, pp. 519 – 534.

Stauning, J. A., Kirk, L. and Jorgensen, A. (1979) Comparison of serum levels after intramuscular injections of 2% and 10% Cis (z)-Flupenthixol decanoate in viscoleo to schizophrenic patients. Psychopharmacology 65, 69 – 72.

Sugarman, A. A. (1969) Studies with the thioxanthenes. In: H. E. Lehmann and T. A. Ban (Eds), The Thioxanthenes. S. Karger, Basel and New York. pp. 80 – 84.

Weissman, A. (1969) A psychopharmacological comparison of thiothixene, chlorprothixene and clopenthixol in rats. In: F. A. Freyman, N. Petrilowitsch and P. Pichot (Eds), Modern Problems of Pharmacopsychiatry. The Thioxanthenes. Karger, Basel and New York, pp. 15 – 22.

Young, J. P. R., Hughes, W. C. and Lader, M. H. (1976) A controlled comparison of flupenthixol and amitriptyline in depressed outpatients. Br. Med. J. 1, 1116 – 1118.

Burrows/Norman/Davies (eds) Antipsychotics

Chapter 10

Clozapine and loxapine – measurement, pharmacokinetics and therapeutic levels

EDMOND H. PI.

and

GEORGE M. SIMPSON

Department of Psychiatry, Medical College of Pennsylvania/EPPI, 3200 Henry Avenue, Philadelphia, PA 19129, U.S.A.

INTRODUCTION

The dibenzoxazepines, discovered in the 1960's, are a class of neuroleptics, eight of which have been investigated in humans. All but two have neuroleptic or antipsychotic properties. Amoxapine and dibenzepine have antidepressant properties. Clozapine is a dibenzodiazepine compound closely related to loxapine succinate and metiapine as shown in Fig. 1. Further information on these agents can be found in the review by Simpson and Lee (1978). Despite the fact that loxapine has been investigated and used for more than 15 years, there is still a lack of knowledge regarding its pharmacokinetics and therapeutic plasma levels. In the case of clozapine, information is even more sparse.

CLOZAPINE

Introduction

Clozapine differs from the other members of this group in a variety of ways (Bente et al., 1966). It depresses spontaneous activity in the mouse, rat and cat, but does not block apomorphine-induced gnawing in the rat. In this respect it is similar to thioridazine but differs from it, having weak or absent cataleptic effects in the rat. In addition, it has a powerful anticholinergic effect (Stille et al., 1971). The ability to produce catalepsy and to block apomorphine are generally associated with neuroleptic activity. Further studies on clozapine revealed that there was no difference in regard to turnover of noradrenaline in the brainstem and dopamine in the corpus striatum as compared to other neuroleptics. However, clozapine increased HVA content in the corpus striatum (Bartholini et al., 1972) but selectively more so in the limbic system (Anden and Stock, 1973).

Another interesting property of clozapine is that despite its powerful anticholinergic effect, it produces hypersalivation in animals and in humans (Gross and Langner, 1970; Stille et al., 1971; Simpson and Varga, 1975). It also produces marked sedation, tachycardia and lowering of blood pressure (Berzewski et al., 1969). Delirium has also been reported to occur in humans when administered clozapine (Gross and Langner, 1966). All neuroleptics produce elevation in serum prolactin indicative of dopamine receptor blockade in the pituitary gland (Meltzer et al., 1978). Kane et al. (1981) reported that despite good therapeutic response and substantial blood levels obtained 11 – 12 hours after the last oral dose of clozapine, prolactin levels were not affected or only insignificantly elevated. The above effects may be related to the surprising claims that clozapine had an antipsychotic effect but did not produce any extrapyramidal effects (Gross and Langner, 1966; Matz et al., 1974; Simpson and Varga, 1974). These findings suggest that the antipsychotic action of clozapine may be dependent on more than blockade of dopamine receptors or on a selective effect outside the striatal area. The unique properties of clozapine immediately called into the question the animal models used for screening for neuroleptics and the conventional idea of what is a 'neuroleptic' (Stille and Hippius,

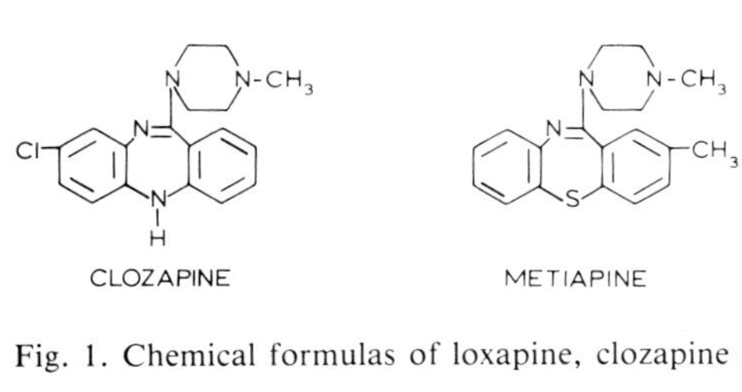

Fig. 1. Chemical formulas of loxapine, clozapine and metiapine.

1971), and led to use of the term 'atypical' neuroleptics (Pi and Simpson, 1983). It is still unclear why or how the decision was made to test the drug in schizophrenic patients. It is also unclear as to why a drug, developed as early as 1962, had no reports on its activity published until 1966. Indeed, a few more years were to pass before substantial reports were available to confirm these claims (Berzewski et al., 1969; Angst et al., 1971; Gerlach et al., 1974; Gerlach et al., 1975). Thereafter, claims appeared for its use in a variety of conditions, e.g. insomnia, depression, mania, psychopathy, etc. (Ayd, 1974). In all of the studies carried out, the absence of EPS was consistently reported.

Clozapine was found to suppress symptoms of tardive dyskinesia (Ruther, 1974; Simpson and Varga, 1974; Simpson et al., 1978b). The latter authors also reported a rebound of abnormal movements when clozapine was discontinued. On the basis of the biochemical effects, namely the effect on HVA and 5-HIAA in the CSF, it was also suggested that clozapine would not produce tardive dyskinesia (Gerlach al., 1975). It is not surprising that this agent was thought to be the drug of choice in treating psychotic patients who also suffer from tardive dyskinesia (Simpson et al., 1978b). However, the high incidence of agranulocytosis reported in Finland has hindered its wide usage (Idanpaan-Heikkila et al., 1975). It appears to be less of a problem in some countries than in others, e.g. it did not produce notable white cell depression in Central Europe as it did in Finland, and is reported as being widely used in China.

Measurement

Plasma levels of clozapine were monitored using a gas-liquid chromatography (GLC) method with an electron capture detector and later a nitrogen detector. The method is sensitive enough to detect as little as 1 ng/ml when a 3 ml sample is extracted (Simpson and Cooper, 1978; Kane et al., 1981).

Pharmacokinetics and clinical response

Significant amounts of clozapine were present 11 – 12 hours after the last dose in two schizophrenic patients who received maximum doses of clozapine, i.e. 450 mg b.i.d., p.o. (Kane et al., 1981). In one study using a single dose of 100 mg clozapine, the mean half-life was reported to be 6 hours. The peak plasma level was reached after 2 – 4 hours and exceeded 300 ng/ml. During chronic treatment with clozapine, steady state was reached after 6 – 10 days (Ackenheil and Hippius, 1977).

Clozapine is extensively metabolized in humans. Both conjugated and unconjugated metabolites were present in human urine, but the latter was present in very small amounts. However, most of the metabolites have not been identified (Gauch and Michaelis, 1971). The principle metabolite of clozapine in humans is the *N*-oxide. The *N*-desmethyl derivative and unidentified metabolites are found in smaller amounts (Ackenheil and Hippius, 1977). The possible dehalogenation of clozapine was also considered (Usdin, 1978).

There is little information about therapeutic plasma levels of clozapine, although in one study the mean plasma therapeutic range was reported as 150 – 300 ng/ml (Ackenheil and Hippius, 1977). They claimed that the actual plasma level required depended on the acute symptomatology of the patient.

Kane et al. (1981) reported on a patient whose plasma levels were up to 200 ng/ml on doses of up to 300 mg/day; 329 – 558 ng/ml on doses of up to 500 – 700 mg/day and over 1000 ng/ml on doses higher than 700 mg/day. Simpson and Cooper (1978) reported that steady state plasma levels of clozapine in treated patients ranged from 15 to 879 ng/ml (dose ranges 100 – 900 mg/day). They proposed that levels of less than 600 ng/ml should be adequate for most patients. Two patients developed grand mal seizures when receiving clozapine; their plasma levels were 1313 ng/ml and above 2000 ng/ml, respectively.

Conclusion

Clozapine is a unique antipsychotic agent because of its lack of EPS and its unusual neuroendocrine profile which will undoubtedly be the forerunner of many similar type agents. Despite the difficulties produced by agranulocytosis and little information regarding its kinetics and therapeutic levels, many experienced investigators think that it has a place for the selective treatment of patients sensitive to conventional neuroleptics or young people who show dyskinetic symptoms on conventional neuroleptics. Whatever the future of clozapine will be, it obviously opens a new era in neuropsychopharmacology and continues to stimulate interest in biological aspects and treatment of the major psychiatric illnesses.

LOXAPINE

Introduction

Loxapine is distinct from the conventional neuroleptics by having a 7-membered heterocyclic central ring in a tricyclic structure instead of the 6-membered ring (Fig. 1).

Loxapine produces catalepsy and blocks apomorphine-induced vomiting in animals. As would be expected in a neuroleptic that produces catalepsy, loxapine also blocks striatal dopamine receptors. In man, the usual maintenance dosage is in the range of 60 – 100 mg/day. Many schizophrenics have been successfully maintained with dosages between 20 and 60 mg/day. Pharmacologically, this agent falls somewhere between chlorpromazine and trifluoperazine in terms of potency per milligram, sedative, cardiovascular and neurological properties. In earlier studies it was suggested that the onset of action of loxapine was slower than with other neuroleptics (Bishop and Gallant, 1970; Clark et al., 1972). Later studies showed that loxapine was equally effective in treating both acute and chronic patients (Simpson and Cuculic, 1976; Paprocki and Versiani, 1977; Denber, 1980).

Measurement

Loxapine has fewer metabolites than many conventional neuroleptics. This may be considered an advantage from both a research and clinical point of view when measuring plasma levels. Several methods have been used with the suggestion that the radioreceptor assay method may be a favorable one (Creese et al., 1976; DePaulo and Ayd, 1982). Gas-liquid chromatography has been used most commonly. Cooper and Kelly (1979) described methods for the quantitation of loxapine, amoxapine and their 7- and 8-hydroxylated metabolites using GLC following trifluoroacetylation of the secondary amine functions and trimethylsilylation of the phenolic group. Vasiliades et al. (1979) used a gas-liquid chromatographic procedure for the determination of therapeutic and toxic serum levels of loxapine using a nitrogen-phosphorus-sensitive detector. An advantage of this procedure is the small amount of plasma required for analysis and the sensitivity of the detector. Gas chromatography-mass spectrometry (GC-MS) was also used for the identification and confirmation of loxapine. Cooper et al. (1979) also used a gas-liquid chromatographic method for pharmacokinetic studies and identified the major urinary metabolic products by GC-MS.

Pharmacokinetics and clinical response

After the administration of oral or intravenous labelled loxapine, it disappeared rapidly from the plasma and redistributed to organs. After 30 minutes in rats, brain and lung contained the highest concentration with lesser amounts in the pancreas, spleen, liver and other organs. The diencephalic and mesocephalic regions contained about twice the concentration of the neocortex one hour after i.v. injection.

No unmetabolized drug was found in the feces or urine and only traces were found in plasma one hour after administering 30 mg of loxapine to three healthy volunteer subjects (Lederle Laboratories, 1975). Conjugated hydroxy loxapine accounted for over 50% of the excreted radioactivity, 70% of the radioactivity was recovered in the urine and 15 – 22% in the feces within 144 hours of administering a single dose of 25 mg to six healthy volunteers (Lederle Laboratories, 1979). Loxapine is extensively metabolized after oral administration. The major metabolites in plasma are 8-hydroxy loxapine which appears rapidly (within an hour) and 8-hydroxy desmethyl loxapine (8-hydroxy amoxapine), which appears a little later but is present in measurable amounts at one hour. The *N*-oxide is also detectable in plasma. The 7-hydroxy and 7-hydroxy desmethyl loxapine are present in very small quantities in plasma but are not found in urine. While the *N*-oxide is present in minimal amounts in humans, it is a major metabolite in the serum of the dog (Cooper and Kelly, 1979). In steady state studies of loxapine, the presence of loxapine, 8-hydroxy loxapine and 8-hydroxy amoxapine were found. This, plus the limited number of metabolites, suggests that loxapine could simplify the study of both therapeutic and side effects in relation to plasma levels (Fig. 2) compared to phenothiazines.

Figure 3 details the differences between the oral and intramuscular administration of loxapine. Given orally, loxapine peaks in one hour and thereafter falls off. The 8-hydroxy loxapine peaks at a much higher level at 2 hours; thereafter it falls off gradually. Given intramuscularly, loxapine peaks around 2 hours and falls off slowly, whereas the 8-hydroxy loxapine gradually builds up over a 24-hour period. Small amounts of the 8-hydroxy amoxapine are found rapidly after oral administration,

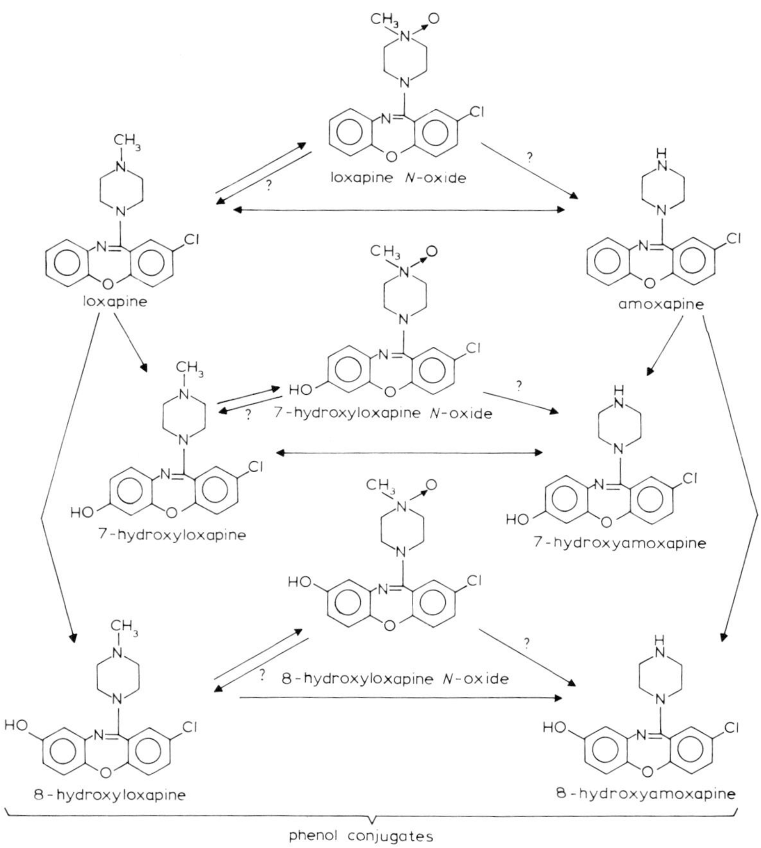

Fig. 2. Metabolic pathways of loxapine. (Reproduced with permission of the editor of the Journal of Pharmaceutical Sciences. 68, 216–219, 1979.)

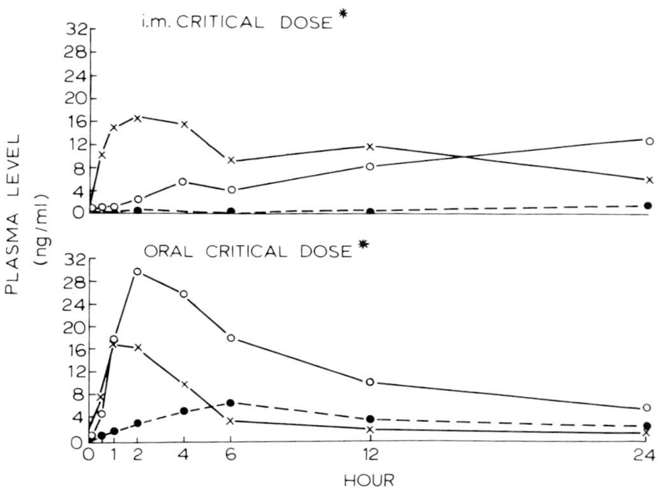

Fig. 3. Plasma levels of loxapine (x – x), 8-OH loxapine (○ – ○) and 8-OH amoxapine (●----●) after individual critical doses of i.m. and oral forms. * Critical dose equals amount of loxapine required to produce a defined amount of sedation. (Reproduced with permission of the editor of Psychopharmacology 56, 225 – 232, 1978.)

but are slow to appear and never reach readily quantifiable amounts with the intramuscular preparation. Information on the activity of the 8-hydroxy loxapine is not available but the high quantities present led one observer to postulate that the antipsychotic activity may be correlated with the hydroxylated metabolites (Simpson et al., 1978a). However, at this stage further information is required.

Cooper et al. (1979) reported that the steady state concentration of five hospitalized non-schizophrenic psychotic patients treated with loxapine ranged from 1 to 8.8 ng/ml using the GLC method. Differences were noted in the time course of plasma concentrations in the various patients. This was partially attributed to the 'first-pass' effect as described by Simpson et al. (1978). The maximum plasma levels were obtained within 2 to 4 hours after administration; thereafter, loxapine disappears from plasma. The authors suggested that the serum half-life of loxapine ranged from 1.3 to 3.5 hours and indicated that dosage intervals of 12 hours may not be suitable for all patients. Interestingly, loxapine was undetectable 6 hours after administration in one patient and a resurgence of plasma concentration was observed in two patients, possibly indicating enterohepatic circulation of the drug. Only very small amounts of loxapine were found in the urine indicating that the drug is rapidly and extensively metabolized, 50% of the dose is excreted within the first 24 hours after administration (Lederle Laboratories, 1979).

Cooper et al. (1981) found the concentration of loxapine in the plasma in a postmortem case was from 70 to 1000 times greater than concentrations reported following therapeutic use of the drug and was similar to the magnitude reported in other fatal cases (Reynolds et al., 1979). The concentrations of 8-hydroxy loxapine and of 8-hydroxy amoxapine were approximately 100 times greater than those reported following therapeutic usage. They also found significant amounts of amoxapine in the postmortem specimen of an overdose case. The authors postulated that metabolism of loxapine may be different in an overdose situation from that following therapeutic use of the drug. This might be explained by the oversaturation of microsomal hydroxylases and desmethylation thus becoming a viable alternative metabolic pathway.

A correlation between daily dosage and therapeutic effect for loxapine has been demonstrated. An attempt to establish a correlation between plasma levels and therapeutic effect for loxapine (Simpson et al., 1978) was unsuccessful but the methodology used is open to criticism and as with most neuroleptics, there is insufficient data to make definitive statements.

Conclusion

Loxapine, despite its chemical differences, behaves in most ways similar to conventional neuroleptics. Because of its limited metabolic profile, it may offer some advantages over phenothiazines for studying plasma levels. However, other agents, e.g. haloperidol, have more limited metabolism and would have a further advantage. If the receptor assays are standardized, of course, all of this becomes unimportant. In the meantime, gas-chromatography methods have permitted the evaluation of loxapine in clinical and toxicological situations in both animals and man. While the serum half-life is short, perhaps under 4 hours, it is possible that the 8-hydroxy loxapine is active since twice daily dosing seems to be adequate.

As with most neuroleptics, further systematic work is required to define an upper therapeutic or beginning toxicity range as well as a lower range for beginning activity.

REFERENCES

Ackenheil, M. and Hippius, H. (1977) Clozapine. In: E. Usdin and I. S. Forrest (Eds), Psychotherapeutic Drugs, Part II: Applications. Marcel Dekker, Inc., New York and Basel, pp. 923–956.

Anden, N. E. and Stock, G. (1973) Effect of clozapine on the turnover of dopamine in the corpus striatum and in the limbic system. J. Pharm. Pharmacol. 25, 346–348.

Angst, J., Bente, D., Berner, P., Helmann, H., Helmchen, H. and Hippius, H. (1971) Das klinische wirkungsbild von clozapin. Pharmacopsychiatry 4, 201–211.

Ayd, Jr., F. J. (1974) Clozapine: a unique new neuroleptic. Int. Drug Ther. Newslett. February and March Vol. IX, Nos. 2 and 3.

Bartholini, G., Haefely, W., Jalfre, M., Keller, H. H. and Pletscher, A. (1972) Effects of clozapine on cerebral catecholaminergic neurone systems. Br. J. Pharmacol. 46, 736–741.

Bente, D., Engelmeier, M-P., Heinrich, K., Hippius, H. and Schmitt, W. (1966) Clinical studies on a new group of tricyclic neuroleptics. CINP Neuro-Psycho-Pharmacology, 5th, Washington, DC, pp. 977–983.

Berzewski, H., Helmchen, H., Hippius, H., Hoffmann, H. and Kanowski, S. (1969) The clinical spectrum of activity of a new dibenzodiazepine derivative. Arzneim.-Forsch. (Drug Res.) 19, 495 – 496.

Bishop, M. P. and Gallant, D. M. (1970) Loxapine: a controlled evaluation in chronic schizophrenic patients. Curr. Ther. Res. 12, 594 – 597.

Clark, M. L., Huber, W. L., Sullivan, J., Wood, F. and Costilde, S. P. (1972) Evaluation of loxapine succinate in chronic schizophrenia. Dis. Nerv. Sys. 33, 783 – 791.

Cooper, S. F., Dugal, R. and Bertrand, M. J. (1979) Determination of loxapine in human plasma and urine and identification of three urinary metabolites. Xenobiotica 9, 405 – 414.

Cooper, T. B. and Kelly, R. G. (1979) GLC analysis of loxapine, amoxapine and their metabolites in serum and urine. J. Pharmaceut. Sci. 68, 216 – 219.

Cooper, T. B., Bost, R. and Sunshine, I. (1981) Postmortem blood and tissue levels of loxapine and its metabolites. J. Anal. Toxicol. 5, 99 – 100.

Creese, I., Burt, D. R. and Snyder, S. H. (1976) Dopamine receptor binding predicts clinical and pharmacological potencies of antischizophrenic drugs. Science 192, 481 – 483.

Denber, H. C. B. (1980) Efficacy of loxapine administered parenterally and orally to acute and chronic schizophrenic patients. Curr. Ther. Res. 28, 777 – 783.

DePaulo, Jr., J. R. and Ayd, Jr., F. J. (1982) Loxapine: fifteen years' clinical experience. Psychosomatics 23, 261 – 271.

Gauch, R. and Michaelis, W. (1971) The metabolism of 8-chloro-11-(4-methyl-1-piperazinyl)-5H-dibenzo(b.e)(1,4)diazepine (clozapine) in mice, dogs and human subjects. Farmaco. Ed. prat. 26, 667 – 681.

Gerlach, J., Koppelhus, P., Helweg, E. and Monrad, A. (1974) Clozapine and haloperidol in a single-blood cross-over trial: therapeutic and biochemical aspects in the treatment of schizophrenia. Acta Psychiatr. Scand. 50, 410 – 424.

Gerlach, J., Thorsen, U. and Fog. R. (1975) Extrapyramidal reactions and amine metabolites in cerebrospinal fluid during haloperidol and clozapine treatment of schizophrenic patients. Psychopharmacologia 40, 341 – 350.

Gross, H. and Langner, E. (1966) The activity profile of a novel broad-spectrum neuroleptic of the benzodiazepine group. Wien. Med. Wochenschr. 40, 814 – 816.

Gross, H. and Langner, E. (1970) The neuroleptic 100-129/HF-1854 (Clozapine) in psychiatry. Int. Pharmacopsychiatry 4, 220 – 230.

Idanpaan-Heikkila, J., Alhava, E., Okinoura, M. and Ilmari, P. (1975) Clozapine and agranulocytosis. Lancet 2, 611.

Kane, J. M., Cooper, T. B., Sachar, E. J., Halpern, F. S. and Bailine, S. (1981) Clozapine: plasma levels and prolactin response. Psychopharmacology 73, 184 – 187.

Lederle Laboratories (1975) Loxitane. Lederle Laboratories, Pearl River, New York, pp. 17 – 18.

Lederle Laboratories (1979) Loxitane: formulary and bioavailability information. Lederle Laboratories, Pearl River, New York, p. 3.

Matz, R., Rick W., Oh, D., Thompson, H. and Gershon, S. (1974) Clozapine: a potential anti-psychotic agent without extrapyramidal manifestation. Curr. Ther. Res. 16, 687 – 695.

Meltzer, H. Y., Goode, D. J. and Fang, V. S. (1978) The effects of psychotropic drugs on endocrine function. I. Neuroleptics, precursors and agonist. In: M. A. Lipton, A. DiMascio and K. Killam (Eds), Psychopharmacology: A Generation of Progress. Raven Press, New York, p. 509.

Paprocki, J. and Versiani, M. (1977) A double-blind comparison between loxapine and haloperidol by parenteral route in acute schizophrenia. Curr. Ther. Res. 21, 80 – 100.

Pi, E. H. and Simpson, G. M. (1983) Atypical neuroleptics: clozapine and the benzamides in the prevention of tardive dyskinesia. In: J. Bannet and R. H. Belmaker (Eds), New Directions in Tardive Dyskinesia Research. Karger Press, Basel and New York, pp. 80 – 86.

Reynolds, P. C., Som, C. W. and Herrmann, P. W. (1979) Loxapine fatalities. Clin. Toxicol. 14, 181 – 185.

Ruther, E. (1974) Leponex-rundtischgesprach. Psychiatrische Klinik der Fu, Berlin, 14, 12.

Simpson, G. M. and Cooper, T. B. (1978) Clozapine plasma levels and convulsions. Am. J. Psychiatry 135, 99 – 100.

Simpson, G. M. and Cuculic, Z. (1976) A double-blind comparison of loxapine succinate and trifluoperazine in newly admitted schizophrenic patients. J. Clin. Pharmacol. 16, 60 – 65.

Simpson, G. M. and Lee, J. H. (1978) A ten-year review of antipsychotics. In: M. A. Lipton, A. DiMascio and K. Killam (Eds), Psychopharmacology: A Generation of Progress. Raven Press, New York, pp. 1131 – 1138.

Simpson, G. M. and Varga, E. (1974) Clozapine: a new antipsychotic agent. Curr. Ther. Res. 16, 679 – 686.

Simpson, G. M. and Varga, E. (1975) Clozapine: a new and unusual antipsychotic agent. Psychopharmacol. Bull. 11, 14 – 15.

Simpson, G. M., Cooper, T. B., Lee, J. H. and Young, M. A. (1978a) Clinical and plasma level characteristics of intramuscular and oral loxapine. Psychopharmacology 56, 225 – 232.

Simpson, G. M., Lee, J. H. and Shrivastava, R. K. (1978b) Clozapine in tardive dyskinesia. Psychopharmacology 56, 75 – 80.

Stille, G. and Hippius, H. (1971) A critical assessment of the concept of neuroleptics. Pharmakopsychiatrie 4, 182 – 191.

Stille, G., Lauener, H. and Eichenberger, E. (1971) The pharmacology of 8-chloro-11-(4-methyl-1-piperazinyl)5H-dibenzo(b.e)(1,4)diazepine (clozapine). Farmaco. Ed. prat. 26, 603 – 625.

Usdin, E. (1978) Metabolic pathways of antipsychotic drugs. In: M. A. Lipton, A. DiMascio and K. Killam (Eds), Psychopharmacology: A Generation of Progress. Raven Press, New York, pp. 895 – 903.

Vasiliades J., Sahawneh, T. M. and Owens, C. (1979) Determination of therapeutic and toxic concentrations of doxepin and loxapine using gas-liquid chromatography with a nitrogen-sensitive detector and gas chromatography-mass spectrometry of loxapine. J. Chromatogr. 164, 457 – 470.

Section IV

CLINICAL APPLICATIONS

Burrows/Norman/Davies (eds) Antipsychotics

Chapter 11

Choice of antipsychotic drugs

LEO E. HOLLISTER

Veterans Administration Medical Center, 3801 Miranda Avenue, Palo Alto, CA 94304, U.S.A.

CHOICE OF DRUGS TO MASTER

The number of antipsychotic drugs available to the clinician increases every year. Even those expert in the field have difficulty remembering the various trade and generic names of the drugs, not to mention their doses and dosage forms. How should the average practitioner choose from such a bewildering array those drugs they might learn to use well? The usual dictum, whenever a great variety of different agents of a therapeutic class is available, is to learn to use a few drugs well rather than to use them all poorly.

One of the most rational ways would be to narrow the choice by mastering the use of one drug from each distinctive chemical type. Two assumptions would be made: a) that drugs within a chemical type are more similar than they are different; b) that major pharmacological differences between drugs are more likely among different chemical types. With a proper choice, a few drugs might provide all the potential benefits of the entire group.

Various members of different chemical classes of antipsychotics are shown in Table 1. Even with this incomplete list, both the number of different chemical classes as well as the members of each is much too large to allow all to be chosen. We shall have to prune first at the level of the different chemical classes.

I would eliminate the aliphatic phenothiazines. Chlorpromazine was an epoch-

TABLE 1

Various members of different chemical classes of antipsychotic drugs.

Phenothiazines	*Butyrophenones*
Aliphatic series	haloperidol, droperidol, bromperidol
chlorpromazine, triflupromazine	*Diphenylbutylpiperidines*
Piperidine series	pimozide, penfluridol, fluspiriline
thioridazine, mesoridazine, piperacetazine	*Dihydroindolone*
Piperazine series	molindone
trifluoperazine, perphenazine, fluphenazine,	*Dibenzoxazepine*
thioproperazine, butaperazine,	loxapine
acetophenazine	*Dibenzodiazepine*
Thioxanthenes	clozapine
Aliphatic series	*Benzamide*
chlorprothixine	sulpiride
Piperazine series	
thiothixene, flupenthixol	

making drug, but after more than three decades it would have been most surprising had it not been surpassed by newer agents. One thinks in this context of sulfanilamide among antibacterials or cortisone among corticosteroids. Many reasons exist for considering chlorpromazine to be obsolete. First, it is one of the least specific antipsychotic drugs, having substantial amounts of other pharmacological actions that produce unwanted effects: sedation, blurred vision, constipation, dry mouth, orthostatic hypotension, tachycardia, among others. Second, it presents a greater peril for severe side effects than any other drug. Such side effects as cholestatic jaundice, agranulocytosis, seizures, opacities of cornea and lens and skin pigmentation are virtually unknown with more modern agents. Finally, antipsychotic doses of this drug are severely limited by these side effects, so that doses can rarely exceed 1000 mg/day. Such a dose would be equivalent to 20 mg/day of haloperidol, a rather small dose for this drug. Although chlorpromazine can be administered parenterally, it is quite irritating when given this way. The only advantage the drug has is that it is cheap due to loss of patent protection. To save money by prescribing a drug with the potential for causing so many costly side effects may be false economy.

Other drugs might also be eliminated from our restricted choice. The homologue of chlorpromazine in the thioxanthene series, chlorprothixene, does not possess the strong claim to obsolescence of chlorpromazine, but other members of the thioxanthene group have greater advantages. Clozapine, the most atypical antipsychotic, is also difficult to manage clinically and has the potential for a fatal adverse reaction. It must be used under exceedingly limited conditions, so it does not fit our needs. The benzamide, sulpiride, is undoubtedly effective, but offers no major advantages

TABLE 2

Possible selection of antipsychotics to be mastered.

Drug class	Drug	Advantages	Disadvantages
Phenothiazine			
Piperidine	thioridazine	slight Parkinson syndrome	dose limit of 800 mg/day; no parenteral form; not very specific
Piperazine	fluphenazine	depot form available	
Thioxanthene	thiothixene	specific, high doses well-tolerated	
Butyrophenone	haloperidol	specific, high doses well-tolerated; depot form available	
Diphenylbutylpiperidine	penfluridol	long-acting orally	
Dihydroindolone	molindone	? less weight gain	
Dibenzoxazepine	loxapine	uncertain	

over other drugs that have been more widely used. Thus, we have reduced to seven the number of chemical classes from which to choose.

Table 2 shows a possible selection of drugs from these seven chemical classes. Other drugs might have been selected from some of these classes and would have been equally acceptable.

With the exception of thioridazine, all drugs listed in Table 2 are available as tablets or liquid preparations for oral use or in some parenteral form for intramuscular administration. Some have specific advantages and disadvantages, which have been noted.

CHOICE OF DRUG FOR INDIVIDUAL PATIENTS

Trying to find the right drug for the right patient has been an elusive goal. A number of investigative groups have spent considerable effort trying to determine the clinical characteristics of patients that might predict a favourable outcome from specific antipsychotics. Initial studies have seemed to point to promising leads, not subsequently replicated, which is why so much effort has been spent on this endeavour.

The best method by far is to rely on the past experience of the patient with these drugs. Whenever such information is available, the wise clinician will heed it well. It is not at all clear why some patients respond to one drug and not to another, but this phenomenon has been observed ever since more than one antipsychotic was available. Perhaps it has to do with side effects. Some patients might prefer haloperidol to thioridazine because the former interferes less with their sexual capacity. The converse might be true for patients who are disturbed by akathisia or the Parkinson syndrome. One can speculate that perhaps patients metabolize drugs differently so that one drug may attain more effective brain concentrations than another, but to date no evidence supports this assumption.

No differences in overall efficacy have been definitely documented for any of the widely used antipsychotics. One also assumes a common basic mode of antipsychotic action. Despite these observations, some clinicians still believe that certain drugs are more effective for specific symptoms or signs of psychosis. This erroneous assumption no doubt explains the great difficulty in suiting drugs to patients. Antipsychotic drugs do not treat specific symptoms but rather treat an illness. We do not treat pneumonia with a melange of drugs for every symptom; aspirin for fever, codeine for cough and potassium iodide for expectoration. Rather, we treat the illness with an antibiotic appropriate to the infecting organism. The illness is treated and individual symptoms and signs regress at somewhat different rates. Similarly when antipsychotic drugs are used, the illness is treated (albeit not optimally) and various manifestations of schizophrenia resolve to differing degrees and at different rates.

A simplistic model for choosing an antipsychotic drug is based entirely upon theory. Highly agitated patients were presumed to respond better to drugs such as chlorpromazine and thioridazine, with a marked sedative effect in relation to their antipsychotic action. Withdrawn, retarded patients with primarily thought disorder were thought to be better treated with drugs, such as fluphenazine, haloperidol or thiothixene, with a higher ratio of antipsychotic to sedative action. Such specificity of action has never been proved.

CHOICE OF DOSAGE PREPARATION

Conventional tablets are preferred whenever it is possible to use them. Although the bioavailability of drug from these preparations may be slightly less than for liquid concentrates and markedly less than from parenteral preparations, the dosage ranges for these drugs are so large that it really does not matter. Conventional tablets are almost universally cheaper than any other dosage form. Liquid concentrates have been preferred for those patients who may 'cheek' or otherwise fail to swallow conventional tablets.

Parenteral dosage forms have become increasingly popular in recent years. Actually, the initial studies with antipsychotic drugs in the 1950's almost always started treatment with parenteral medication. Reserpine was well tolerated in this form, but soon became obsolete. Chlorpromazine was rather poorly tolerated parenterally, leading to its abandonment. With the development of highly tolerable parenteral forms of high-potency neuroleptics, such as fluphenazine hydrochloride, haloperidol and thiothixene, this route of administration became preferred by many clinicians for the initiation of therapy. The advantages are that one can more rapidly titrate the required dose of drug and that one can be certain that the drug is fully bioavailable. No patients should be deemed as having failed to respond to a drug if the drug has only been given orally. A course of parenteral medication should be tried to assure that adequate amounts of drug enter the body.

The use of depot preparations has been surrounded by some controversy. Civil libertarians maintain that it is unethical to use these preparations as once given the patient has lost control over the decision about taking drugs. On the other hand, for the patient who is unreliable about drug-taking, depot preparations offer a distinct advantage. Just how often poor compliance is a problem is somewhat uncertain. Studies assessing the depot preparations against orally administered drug in randomly assigned, unselected patients have usually failed to show any superiority of the depot dosage forms. However, few doubt that for selected patients with known poor compliance, these preparations are useful. The fatty acid used for the ester can be of almost any carbon length, the decanoate being most widely used. Such preparations are available for fluphenazine, haloperidol and flupenthixol, among others. Although depot preparations have been used effectively for the initial treatment of schizophrenics, this practice is unwise. One wishes in this case to obtain a more rapid feedback of response in relation to dose than is possible with depot dosage forms. They should be used only for maintenance therapy of selected patients.

SUMMARY

By making a considered choice among the large group of antipsychotic drugs, the wise clinician can reduce to a manageable number the number of drugs that should be mastered. Nonetheless, the selection of a particular drug for a particular patient remains largely empirical. Initiation of treatment with parenteral medication is becoming more popular, with continuation of treatment using conventional tablets. Depot preparations should be used for maintenance therapy of patients with established poor compliance.

Burrows/Norman/Davies (eds) Antipsychotics

Chapter 12

New antipsychotic agents: Clinical studies

MAMOUN DABBAGH[1], MICHAEL STANLEY[1,2]
and
SAMUEL GERSHON[1]

Departments of [1]Psychiatry and [2]Pharmacology, Wayne State University School of Medicine, and Lafayette Clinic, Detroit, Michigan, U.S.A.

INTRODUCTION

The number of drugs that are thought to have antipsychotic effects has increased dramatically during the last decade. This chapter is an attempt to review several of the newer antipsychotics, with an emphasis on clinical aspects, although the theoretical implication of the 'newer' antipsychotics are also of considerable interest. Because of the availability of many 'me too' drugs, and the space limitation, we are not able to present an encyclopedic review of the available data.

Newer antipsychotic drugs are of interest because of the well-documented inadequacies of the currently available antipsychotics. Familiar shortcomings are the lack of effectiveness on 'negative symptoms', the lack of specificity of the site of action and subsequently numerous extrapyramidal side effects, the numerous non-extrapyramidal side effects and perhaps the most significant problem of irreversible tardive dyskinesia. Thus, the mandate for new drugs is that they will be at least as clinically useful as the compounds already in use and that they have a side effect profile that offers clear advantages over currently available drugs.

The theoretical implication of newer antipsychotics may be as important as the clinical aspects. By using these new compounds which may act by blocking receptors other than the dopamine or may be selective on specific subtypes of dopamine receptors, our understanding of the etiology of schizophrenia could be enhanced.

Newer antipsychotic drugs include compounds that are structurally, and often pharmacologically different from standard antipsychotics; new compounds of the old generation; and known drugs used for non-psychiatric purposes that are not generally thought of as antipsychotics.

DIHYDROINDOLONES

Molindone, a new antipsychotic, belongs to a chemical class not previously used for such treatment – a hydroindolone, an indole category and not related structurally to other antipsychotics. Its efficacy as an antischizophrenic is well-established. In one study (Clark et al., 1970), molindone was reported to be clearly superior to placebo in schizophrenics. In another study (Gallant and Bishop, 1968), molindone was found to be slightly less effective than trifluoperazine on the Global Rating Scale as scored by nurses, however, the difference was not statistically significant. Another investigation (Freeman and Frederick, 1969) found that trifluoperazine's efficacy was equal to molindone, whereas Simpson et al. (1971) reported slight superiority of molindone to trifluoperazine. In sum, the controlled studies, which included about 200 patients, permit us to conclude that molindone is approximately equal to the standard antipsychotics. Its range of side effects is similar to that of high-potency phenothiazines, except for its unique property of causing weight reduction (Gallant and Bishop, 1968; Clark et al., 1970; Gallant et al. 1973). Gardos and Cole (1977) studied two underweight and seven obese severely ill, hospitalized, chronic schizophrenics receiving the conventional antipsychotic medication (chlorpromazine, thioridazine, mesoridazine, fluphenazine, thiothixene, or haloperidol) in therapeutic doses. They substituted molindone (20 – 60 mg/day) for 3 months, after which the patients were put back on their previous antipsychotic medication. All nine patients lost weight, 0.9 – 16.8 kg (mean 7.6 kg, or 8.5% of their initial weight) during molindone treatment; most of the weight loss occurred during the first month. About half of the patients followed regained the lost weight in the post-molindone period. Eight of the nine patients were either clinically stable or improved during the molindrone trial. The mechanism of this weight loss is unknown and it could be due to central anorexogenic effect (Gallant et al., 1973). The rapid initial loss noted by Gardos and Cole (1977) is similar to the type of weight loss frequently seen with stimulants. Since many drug-treated patients are overweight (Gordon et al., 1960), this unique property of molindone may be advantageous in some instances.

BUTYROPHENONES

Several new butyrophenones have been tested, and one of the more interesting is lenperon. Early testing has suggested that the drug not only possessed antipsychotic activity but also that it is associated with few extrapyramidal side effects (Denber, 1973). However, reversible electrocardiographic abnormalities were noted with higher doses. Subsequent evaluation in chronic schizophrenia confirms the efficacy of lenperon as an antipsychotic agent with paucity of extrapyramidal side effects (Mielke et al., 1975).

Haloperidol decanoate injectable has become available in Europe and can be administered once monthly. Roose (1981) has reported that monthly injections of haloperidol decanoate in 34 psychotic patients who had previously received biweekly injections of fluphenazine decanoate were of similar or superior efficacy. Subsequently, two open studies have reported that haloperidol decanoate monthly injections were at least as effective as oral haloperidol (Darondel and Fengler, 1981; Meco et al., 1981). The dosage of haloperidol decanoate used in the three studies was 75 – 200 mg every 4 weeks.

THIOXANTHENE

Flupenthixol is a new antipsychotic from the thioxanthene series. It is an interesting compound in that it has antidepressant properties as well as antipsychotic activity in its short-acting form (Young et al., 1976). The long-acting form (decanoate) has been claimed to produce less depression and fewer extrapyramidal side effects (Gottfries, 1971). However, no significant difference has been found in its efficacy as an antipsychotic agent in a double-blind crossover study comparison to fluphenazine. Unlike most antipsychotic medications a certain activating effect has been described, and accordingly, it is not indicated in hyperactive patients.

BENZAMIDES

As with phenothiazines, which were first used in anesthesiology, the benzamide role as psychotropic agent came to us through a chance discovery. In 1968, Borenstein et al. reported antidepressant and antipsychotic efficacy for the benzamide, sulpiride, a derivative of para-aminosalicylic acid. A short time thereafter a number of benzamides (e.g. metoclopramide, sultopride, and tiapride) had been examined in a variety of psychiatric disorders.

The benzamides are a group of compounds structurally similar to procainamide with known dopamine antagonist properties but without a well-defined mechanism of action. They share the same distinct character of classical antipsychotic agents (e.g. release prolactin, increase dopamine turnover, antagonize the stereotyped behavior induced by dopamine agonists, cause catalepsy in rats, induce behavioral supersensitivity and receptor proliferation). However, they differ in their inactivity or lack of potency as inhibitors of the dopamine-sensitive adenylate cyclase and in displacing radiolabelled ligand from 'dopamine/neuroleptic' binding sites. This unique property makes this agent a very interesting tool for the study of dopamine receptors (Wazer et al., 1982).

Sulpiride

Of the currently available benzamides, sulpiride has been the most extensively tested in psychiatric disorders. Sulpiride has been tested on an open basis in several studies as an antipsychotic in schizophrenics. Though the methodological designs varied and the studies had numerous flaws (i.e. lack of standardized objective rating scales), there was a reported global improvement in approximately 75% of the subjects (Peselow and Stanley, 1982).

The clinical impressions of the open studies were confirmed in several double-blind trials comparing sulpiride with a reference antipsychotic or against placebo. Sulpiride was found to be superior over placebo in reducing psychotic behavior in double-blind randomized trial (Blanco et al., 1972) and in double-blind crossover design (Bellomo et al., 1977). Two studies (Toru et al., 1972; Bratfos and Haig, 1979) noted that sulpiride was essentially equivalent to chlorpromazine in antipsychotic efficacy and in one such study, certain target symptoms, such as verbal aggressiveness, aggressive behavior, and hyperactivity were reduced to a greater degree by sulpiride than by chlorpromazine (Toru et al., 1972).

Two Japanese studies compared the efficacy of sulpiride versus perphenazine (Amakusa et al., 1973; Asada et al., 1976). Clinical impressions seem to indicate that sulpiride was equivalent to perphenazine in a combined total of 140 schizophrenic patients.

Cassano et al. (1975) compared the efficacy of low dose of haloperidol (0.5 – 10.5 mg/day) versus sulpiride (100 – 2300 mg/day). Clinical improvement based on Brief Psychiatric Rating Scale (BPRS) and Inpatient Multidimensional Psychiatric Scale (IMPS) were essentially equal for the two drugs. In another study, Taverna et al. (1972) claimed superiority of sulpiride over haloperidol on global impression and on such factors as thought content and mood state. It must be pointed out that the dose of haloperidol used for acute psychosis in this study was low (1 – 4 mg/day). In a study by Edwards et al. (1980), it was noted that 600 – 1000 mg of sulpiride was equivalent in antipsychotic efficacy to 15 – 45 mg of trifluoperazine with no significant differences either in extrapyramidal symptoms or other side effects.

Although the open studies reported low incidence of side effects, the double-blind studies comparing sulpiride with other antipsychotics demonstrated that the side effects spectrum of sulpiride is not significantly different than other standard medication (i.e. chlorpromazine and haloperidol). There is an average 30% incidence of extrapyramidal symptoms and a 25% incidence of sedation.

Metoclopramide

Metoclopramide was one of the first benzamides to be used in psychiatry. The initial trial of low doses (20 – 100 mg/day) noted little antipsychotic efficacy (Borenstein and Bles, 1965). However, Stanley et al. (1979a) reported a significant decrease in BPRS score in an open evaluation of eight male chronic schizophrenics with acute exacerbations of their illness. The patients were treated for 8 – 22 days and the dose was administered up to 1000 mg/day. The open study of metoclopramide's efficacy as an antipsychotic requires further evaluation in the form of controlled double-blind studies.

The range of side effects is similar to standard antipsychotic medications; extrapyramidal symptoms are frequent when the drug is given in efficacious antipsychotic doses. Sedation, dry mouth, muscle weakness, and hypertension were observed in low dose. Also, a number of cases of tardive dyskinesia associated with the use of metoclopramide have been reported (Peselow and Stanley, 1982).

DIPHENYLBUTYLPIPERIDINE

Penfluridol is a unique drug and belongs to the diphenylbutylpiperidine group, a new chemical class found to have antipsychotic properties. Penfluridol is an orally administered long-acting antipsychotic, usually given weekly in doses ranging from 20 to 160 mg. It was found to be effective in patients with acute psychosis (Van Praag et al., 1971) and in chronic schizophrenia (Boban et al., 1970; Gallant et al., 1974; Jus et al., 1974; Quitkin et al., 1978). Its range of side effects, however, seems to be the same as with standard antipsychotics. A once-weekly oral dose may be a great advantage in obtaining the compliance of the patient.

Penfluridol has been reported recently to have some toxicity in animals. A significant increase in pancreatic tumors and nonsignificant increase in mammary tumors were found in rats treated 24 months at doses relatively higher than those proposed for use in humans. This finding has delayed penfluridol's approval in the U.S., however, the drug is marketed in Europe.

Fluspirilene (a fluorophenyl-butyl-triazaspirodecane) differs from other long-acting agents in that its formulation for injection is a micronized suspension rather than a fatty acid ester. The usual duration of action of this compound is one week, and tolerance seems to be adequate (Stermans et al., 1969). A controlled study by Bankier (1973) found that fluspirilene had equal clinical efficacy to trifluoperazine. A median dose of 6.5 mg fluspirilene was used; the trifluoperazine median dose was 40 mg/day. At this dosage, fewer extrapyramidal side effects were found in the fluspirilene group. It remains to be demonstrated whether such drugs are more effective or associated with less side effects than the currently available agents.

Pimozide is one of the purest dopamine antagonistic drugs available. It is one of the diphenylbutyryl-piperidine representatives. It has been included in the long-acting category based more on its pharmacokinetic characteristics than on its duration of action. It is administered orally, and peak plasma level occurs within 3 to 6 hours, followed by an initial rapid decline, then a subsequent very slow terminal phase. Pimozide accordingly has a very long plasma half-life of about 50 hours in man (McCreadie et al., 1979). Pimozide has been shown to be as effective in outpatient schizophrenics as standard neuroleptic maintenance therapy (Sterkmans et al., 1968; Anderson et al., 1971; Chouinard et al., 1971; Falloon et al., 1978). Pimozide was given on a once-a-day dose regimen. The usual dose range is 2 – 20 mg daily. Pimozide was found to be as effective as fluphenazine decanoate when given 4 days weekly, with a subsequent 3 day 'drug holiday' (McCreadie et al., 1980). A more recent study by McCreadie et al. (1982) has been done to examine the possibility of using pimozide as a single-once-weekly dose for maintenance therapy versus fluphenazine decanoate. There was no difference in relapse rates over 9 months. However, three quarters of the patients on pimozide who completed the trial developed at least mild tardive dyskinesia. While more studies are needed to confirm the reported clinical efficacy of pimozide, the unusually high reported incidence of tardive dyskinesia may limit its clinical use.

TREBENZOMINE

Trebenzomine (*N,N*,2-trimethyl-3-chromanamine) is a centrally acting psychotropic drug structurally distinct from currently available agents. Preclinical studies indicated that trebenzomine, unlike most psychotropic drugs, has both neuroleptic and stimulant profiles (Borgin, 1979). Further evaluation of the dopaminergic pharmacology of this compound revealed a mixed profile (Stanley et al., 1979b). Trebenzomine has been reported to lack potency in displacing [^{3}H]spiroperidol from striatal membranes. In spite of its mixed preclinical profile preliminary clinical reports indicate that trebenzomine is an effective antipsychotic that does not produce extrapyramidal side effects (Meltzer et al., 1978; Borgen, 1979). The clinical antipsychotic efficacy of trebenzomine was reevaluated by Georgotas et al. (1981) in a double-blind randomized study. Forty schizophrenics were randomly assigned to treatment either with trebenzomine or thioridazine for 3 weeks. The thioridazine was superior in reducing the symptomatology as rated by BPRS and CGI. The only reported side effects of trebenzomine were confusion, hypotension and urinary retention with no EPS reported. This trial failed to confirm the antipsychotic efficacy of trebenzomine.

BUTACLAMOL

Butaclamol is from a new chemical class having benzocycloheptapyridisoquinoline ring. Butaclamol appears to be a potent antipsychotic but also with a high level of extrapyramidal side effects. Open studies in chronic schizophrenic patients in dosage range of 20 to 100 mg have shown it to be efficacious as an antipsychotic (Gallant et al., 1975; Hollister et al., 1975). More data is needed for further evaluation of this compound.

BETA-BLOCKERS

These agents have had many uses in general medicine and more recently in psychiatry. The first report that propranolol might have a potential usefulness in the treatment of schizophrenia (Atsmon et al., 1971, 1972) aroused great interest, because propranolol does not significantly block dopamine receptors (Bremner et al., 1978) and does not induce tardive dyskinesia with long-term use. Since this initial report, a number of studies have been conducted and reported mixed results. Most studies of propranolol in schizophrenia have lacked a control group. Results of open studies have been equivocal. While there have been some enthusiastic positive reports (Atsmon et al., 1972; Orkston et al., 1974; Ridges et al., 1977; Elizur et al., 1979; Sheppard et al., 1979; Hanssen et al., 1980), others have found propranolol to be devoid of efficacy in schizophrenia (Stam, 1971; Gardos et al., 1973; Von Zerssen, 1976; Belmaker et al., 1979). There has been one small double-blind placebo-controlled study in which propranolol showed no advantage over placebo in the treatment of chronic schizophrenia (King et al., 1980). Yorkston et al. (1981) compared propranolol (670 mg) to chlorpromazine (300 mg) in double-blind randomized study. The authors have found that the two drugs were of similar overall efficacy, however, there were significant differences favoring chlorpromazine over propranolol on a number of measures. Another study (Peet et al., 1981a) or 53 hospitalized chronic schizophrenics who were treated with either propranolol, chlorpromazine or placebo in a double-blind randomized trial for up to 3 months did not show any improvement in propranolol-treated group (640 mg/day) relative to placebo, although the effects of chlorpromazine were small and inconsistent.

There have been two placebo-controlled studies in which propranolol appeared to have an antipsychotic effect, but the propranolol was given in addition to existing antipsychotic treatment rather than as sole agent (Yorkston et al., 1977; Lindstrom and Persson, 1980). One interpretation of the results of combined trials of propranolol and antipsychotics is that propranolol has pharmacokinetic interaction with chlorpromazine which increases markedly the plasma levels of chlorpromazine and its active metabolites (Peet et al., 1980, 1981b).

Data, thus, are insufficient to justify a nonresearch use of propranolol, but they do warrant further evaluation.

GABA AGONISTS

Putative gamma-aminobutyric acid (GABA)-ergic drugs have been tried in the treatment of schizophrenia following the proposal that schizophrenia was associated with a deficiency in GABA, resulting in dopaminergic hyperactivity (Robert, 1972). Generally, the results concerning specific antipsychotic effects have been equivocal or disappointing.

Benzodiazepine: Conflicting results have been reported about the efficacy of benzodiazepine in schizophrenia. Some authors have found that diazepam in high doses up to 600 mg/day was effective in eliminating both positive and negative symptoms in schizophrenics (Nestoros et al., 1982). Lingjaerde (1982) has reported that estazolam (as an addition to neuroleptics) had a significantly better effect than placebo on global clinical state, on the frequency of, and attitude towards the hallucinations with few additional side effects (see Chapter 13, this volume).

These results have not been confirmed by other investigators using diazepam (Jimerson et al., 1982) or clonazepam (Karson et al., 1982). Moreover, they have been reported to have potential for exacerbating aggressive behavior.

Baclofen: Another drug, which has GABA-ergic activities, has been claimed to be effective in the treatment of schizophrenic patients (Frederiksen, 1975). However, two further studies have not substantiated its antipsychotic efficacy (Hollister et al., 1976; Simpson et al., 1976); in fact these studies reported a worsening of psychotic symptoms.

Sodium valproate: A GABA agonist was reported to improve the schizophrenic symptoms in double-blind crossover trial in 16 of 32 patients (Linnoila et al., 1976). In this study, patients received 900 mg daily. Nagai et al. (1979) reported also an improvement in 3 of 7 patients in tardive dyskinesia and symptomatology. However, in contrast to previous reports, Lautin et al. (1980) reported a marked deterioration in the clinical status of schizophrenic patients receiving a higher dose of sodium valproate (750 – 3000 mg/day).

DOPAMINE AGONIST

It has been proposed that supersensitivity of the dopamine (DA) receptors in specific areas in the brain might be implicated in the etiology of psychosis especially schizophrenia (Snyder, 1980). This 'dopamine hypothesis' has led to speculation that a therapy which could down-regulate the sensitivity of the postsynaptic DA receptors or stimulate the inhibitory presynaptic receptors (autoreceptors) should improve the clinical symptoms of schizophrenia. The results of acute and chronic administration of DA agonists or precursors to schizophrenic patients have been contradictory and mixed results have been obtained (Bunney et al., 1979).

Recently, two types of treatment have been administered with different aims. In the first approach, low dose of apomorphine (a DA agonist) was given, either acutely or repeatedly (Corsini et al., 1977; Smith et al., 1977; Tamminga et al., 1978), in an attempt to stimulate the inhibitory presynaptic DA receptors, and thus to decrease tyrosine hydroxylase activity, and consequent DA synthesis and presynaptic impulse firing (Meltzer, 1982). Using this treatment strategy, Tamminga reported a transient rapid improvement of psychotic symptomatology in subgroups of subjects.

Tamminga et al. (1978) have also reported that administration of apomorphine

(3 mg S.C.) produced improvement in 9/18 antipsychotic-treated chronic schizophrenics. Cutler et al. (1982) reported that a dose of 0.005 mg/kg apomorphine produced significant improvement in the BPRS in 2 of 5 chronic schizophrenic patients receiving a daily dose of the equivalent of chlorpromazine, 1.1 g. Further studies seem to be needed to verify these results. If they can be replicated this would indicate the possibility of utilizing dopamine presynaptic agonists as complementary treatment to antipsychotics, rather than as a substitute (Meltzer, 1982).

The second type of treatment involves the production of increased dopaminergic activity by the administration of dopaminergic agonist or agonist precursor in large doses, which in turn results in a secondary down-regulation of dopamine post-synaptic receptors, and a net reduction in dopaminergic activity that occurs when the agonist or precursor is withdrawn.

Alpert et al. (1978) administered very high doses of L-dopa for 6 – 7 weeks to a small group of schizophrenics, some of whom were also suffering from tardive dyskinesia. These investigators observed a worsening of symptomatology at the beginning of therapy, followed by a clear-cut improvement in both dyskinesia and psychotic symptoms, which persisted after withdrawal of the drug. In a second study, Beramendi et al. (1980) treated 12 patients with L-dopa carbidopa, 9 with haloperidol and 10 with placebo. Approximately 50% of the L-dopa carbidopa group showed clinically significant improvement 4 weeks after termination of treatment, although overall the haloperidol group fared better.

This approach definitely represents a novel means of pharmacological treatment, the desired therapeutic effect occurring when the treatment is stopped, and persisting for some time after that, however, more study in this area is needed to verify the efficacy of this approach (Friedhoff and Miller, 1983).

LITHIUM

The use of lithium in the treatment of schizophrenia was first reported by Cade (1949). In the initial trial he treated six patients with dementia praecox, and stated that 'although there was no fundamental improvement in any of them, three who were usually restless, noisy and shouting nonsensical abuse . . . lost their excitement and restlessness and became quiet and amenable for the first time in years . . . they reverted to their previous state upon cessation of lithium medication'. Since then over 20 clinical studies evaluating the use of lithium in schizophrenia have been published (Delva and Letemendia, 1982). However, interpretation of the result has been limited either by inadequate sample size or by the scarcity of adequately controlled study (Prien, 1979).

There are very few studies which report the efficacy of lithium in schizophrenics whose symptomatology does not include an affective component. Shopsin et al. (1971) published the first controlled study of lithium versus chlorpromazine in 21 acute newly admitted schizophrenics. Chlorpromazine treatment was clearly superior to lithium within a 3-week period of active medication. Although this study shows that chlorpromazine may well be superior to lithium in the treatment of acute schizophrenia, as it is in acute manic patients who are highly active (Prien et al., 1972), it cannot be concluded that lithium has no value in the long-term treatment of schizophrenia. However, it does indicate the limited value of lithium as an antipsychotic.

Alexander et al. (1979) reported a double-blind controlled study comparing lithium with placebo in five schizophrenic and eight schizoaffective patients. He reported a favorable improvement in two schizophrenics and relapse in one patient after lithium withdrawal. Obviously the sample is too small to draw any general conclusion.

Two studies (Small et al., 1975; Growe et al., 1979) do suggest that adding lithium to conventional antipsychotics may be of some modest benefit to some 'core' schizophrenics. Small et al. (1975) stabilized 22 long-term hospitalized chronic schizophrenics on the optimum dosage of the antipsychotic known to give maximal improvement and/or best tolerance, and added lithium or placebo to their regimen in a crossover design. Patients were exposed to each treatment twice, each time for 4 weeks (four periods and three crossovers in random sequence). A variety of scale ratings showed the significant superiority of lithium over placebo. Growe et al. (1979) published a controlled double-blind study on eight patients with the same design as Small et al. but using one rating scale. The conclusion of both studies was that a trial of lithium combined with antipsychotics is warranted in schizophrenics who are refractory to antipsychotics alone.

The pre-clinical studies of the lithium effects on neurotransmitter synthesis and function have reported an inhibitory effect on dopamine turnover (Gerbino et al., 1978) which might explain the antipsychotic property, if any, of lithium.

In sum, although some studies have seemed to indicate a therapeutic value for lithium in schizophrenia, other studies have reported conflicting results. All of the studies have methodological difficulties based on small sample size or insufficient controls. Van Kammen and DeFraites (1979) emphasize that even studies that reported antipsychotic action with lithium do not claim that lithium is more effective than established antipsychotics. Clearly, antipsychotic neuroleptic drugs remain the medication of choice for schizophrenia, although a combination of lithium and antipsychotics could be useful in some refractory or schizoaffective patients. More research is needed and the question of lithium efficacy in psychosis remains unresolved.

CONCLUSION

In the last 10 years we have seen the introduction of several new compounds for treatment of psychosis. As we have indicated in the preceding text the pharmacologic agents span both a wide variety of transmitter systems and chemical classes. In addition to the knowledge gained from the clinical trials with this impressive array of new and diverse drugs we have also expanded our basic understanding of the many pharmacologic actions these compounds have. New techniques have been developed and have been applied not only in the laboratory but also in the clinic (e.g. radioreceptor assay).

Despite this flurry of activity and expansion of knowledge in the field of psychopharmacology, the question of primary significance must remain: what clinical benefits have derived from these endeavors? Unhappily, progress in the area of patient treatment has been elusive. Most of the antipsychotic drugs currently available today have what could be regarded as a less than satisfactory spectrum of action. They treat some symptoms well while having little or no effect on others. Additionally, the side effects associated with this class of drugs can be very difficult to manage acutely and one of the most significant long-term risks – tardive dyskinesia – has yet to be successfully addressed.

In sum, our progress in the more basic areas of psychopharmacology has not been accompanied by similar strides in the clinic.

REFERENCES

Alexander, P. E., Van Kammen, D. P. and Bunney, W. E. (1979) Antipsychotic effects of lithium in schizophrenia. Am. J. Psychiatry 135, 283 – 287.

Alpert, M., Friedhoff, A. J., Marcos, L. R. and Diamond, F. (1978) Paradoxical reaction to L-dopa in schizophrenic patients. Am. J. Psychiatry 135, 1329 – 1332.

Amakura, T. and Majima, T. (1973) Comparison of therapeutic effects of FK-880 and perphenazine in schizophrenia by a double-blind study. Jentgens Med. J. 19, 239 – 249.

Anderson, K., D'Elia, G., Hallberg, B., Perris, G., Rapp, W. and Roman, G. (1971) The treatment of chronic schizophrenia. Preliminary results of a controlled comparison of pimozide (oral) with trifluoperazine. Clin. Trials J. 8 (Suppl. II), 72.

Asada, S., Ishimaru, T., Kubo, S., Kodama, H., Masuda, K., Kawamura, T., Nomura, S., Miyake, Y., Tsukue, I., Ishakawa, H., Sasaki, T., Jitsuiki, S., Kimura, N. and Shimonaga, K. (1976) Etude des effects cliniques du sulpiride et de la perphenazine chez 82 schizophrenics par la methode du double aveugle. L'Encephale. II. 73 – 83.

Atsmon, A., Blum, I., Wijsenbeck, H., Maoz, P., Steiner, M. and Ziegelman, A. (1971) The short-term effects of adrenergic-blocking agents in a small group of psychotic patients. Psychiatr. Neurol. Neurochir. 74, 251 – 258.

Atsmon, A., Blum, I., Steiner, M., Latz, A. and Wijsenbeek, H. (1972) Further studies with propranolol in psychotic patients. Psychopharmacologia 27, 249 – 254.

Bankier, R. G. (1973) A comparison of fluspiriline and trifluoperazine in the treatment of acute schizophrenic psychosis. J. Clin. Pharmacol. 13, 44 – 47.

Bellomo, L. E. and Fernandez, H. (1972) Investigacion a doble ensayo ciego de la sulprida en pacientes psicoticas. Minerva Psiquiatrica Argentina, 29 – 50.

Belmaker, R. H., Ebstein, R. P., Dasberg, H., Levy, A., Sedvall, G. and Van Praag, H. M. (1979) The effect of propranolol treatment in schizophrenia on CSF amine metabolites and prolactin. Psychopharmacologia 63, 293 – 296.

Beramendi, V., Alpert, M., Guimon, J., Friedhoff, A. J. and Gutierrez, M. (1980) Estudio controlado de la L-dopa enesquizofrenia con referencia a la teroria de la hipersesibilidad de los receptores dopaminergicos. Arch. Neurobiol. 43, 107 – 124.

Blanco, J. M., Sanchez, J. C., Diaz, J. A. and Zubia, B. Z. 1972) Ensayo clinico con dogmatily placebo ensquizofrenicas cronicos estuido de 89 enfermes con application de la escala de Harris, Letemendia y Willems. Arch. Neurobiol. 35, 3 – 22.

Boban, J., Melon, J., Marmont, C., Dufrasne, M. and Pinchard, A. (1970) Neuroleptiques a longue duree d'action. Etude pilote du penfluridol (R-16341). Acta Psychiatr. Neurol. Scand. 70, 523 – 551.

Borenstein, P. and Bles, G. (1965) Effects cliniques electroencephalographiques en de metoclopramide. Psychiatr. Ther. 20, 975 – 995.

Borgen, L. A. (1979) Trebenzomine: a new psychotropic agent with potential as an antipsychotic and an antidepressant. Psychopharmacol. Bull. 15, 92 – 94.

Bratfos, O. and Haug, J. O. (1979) Comparison of sulpiride and chlorpromazine in psychosis: a double-blind multicenter study. Acta Psychiatr. Scand. 60, 1 – 9.

Bremmer, R. M., Greengrass, P. M., Morville, M. and Blackburn, K. J. (1978) Effect of tolamolol and other beta-adrenoceptor blocking drugs on [^{3}H]haloperidol binding to rat striatal membrane preparations. J. Pharm. Pharmacol. 30, 388 – 390.

Bunney, Jr., W. E., Van Kammen, D. P., Post, R. M. and Garland, B. A. (1984) A possible role for dopamine in schizophrenia and manic depressive illness (a review of evidence). In: E. Usdin, I. J. Kopin and J. Barchas (Eds), Catecholamines: Basic and Clinical Frontiers, Vol. 2. Pergamon Press, New York, 1807 – 1819.

Cade, J. F. J. (1949) Lithium salts in treatment of psychotic excitement. Med. J. Aus. 36, 349 – 352.

Cassano, G. B., Castrogiovanni, P. and Conti, L. (1975) Sulpiride versus haloperidol in schizophrenia: a double-blind comparative trial. Curr. Ther. Res. 17, 189 – 201.

Chouinard, G., Lehmann, H. E. and Ban, T. A. (1970) Pimozide in the treatment of chronic schizophrenic patients. Curr. Ther. Res. 12, 598.

Clark, M. L., Huber, W. K., Sakata, K., Fowles, D. C. and Searfctinides, E. A. (1970) Molindone in chronic schizophrenia. Clin. Pharmacol. Ther. 11, 668 – 688.

Corism, A. U., DelZompo, M., Manconi, S., Cianchetti, G., Magoni, A. and Gessa, G. L. (1977) Sedative hypnotic and antipsychotic effects of low doses of apomorphine in man. Adv. Biochem. Psychopharmacol. 16, 645 – 648.

Culler, N. R., Jeste, D. V., Karoum, F. and Wyatt, R. J. (1982) Low-dose apomorphine reduces serum homovanillic acid concentration in schizophrenic patients. Life Sci. 30, 753 – 756.

Darondel, A. and Fengler, B. (1981) Open study of haldol decanoate in psychotic syndromes. Proc. III World Congress of Biological Psychiatry, June 1981.

Delva, N. J. and Letemendia, F. J. J. (1982) Lithium treatment in schizophrenia and schizoaffective disorder. Br. J. Psychiatry 141, 387 – 400.

Denber, H. C. (1973) AHR-2277 – a new major neuroleptic with minimal side effects. Ann. Med. Psychol. (Paris) 1, 131 – 138.

Edwards, J., Alexander, J. R., Alexander, M. S., Gordon, A. and Zutch, T. (1980) Controlled trial of sulpiride in chronic schizophrenic patients. Br. J. Psychiatry 137, 522 – 529.

Elizur, A., Segal, Z., Yeret, A., Davidson, S. and Atsmon, A. (1979) Antipsychotic effect of propranolol on chronic schizophrenics: study of gradual treatment regimen. Psychopharmacologia 60, 189 – 194.

Falloon, I., Watt, D. C. and Shepherd, M. (1978) A comparative controlled trial of pimozide and fluphenazine decanoate in the continuation therapy of schizophrenia. Psychol. Med. 8, 59 – 60.

Frederiksen, P. K. (1975) Baclofen in the treatment of schizophrenia. Lancet 1, 702 – 703.

Freeman, H. and Frederick, A. N. S. (1969) Comparison of trifluperazine and molindone in chronic schizophrenic patients. Curr. Ther. Res. 11, 670 – 676.

Friedhoff, A. J. and Miller, J. C. (1983) Clinical implication of receptor sensitivity modification. Ann. Rev. Neurosci. 6, 121 – 148.

Gallant, D. M. and Bishop, M. P. (1968) Molindone: a controlled evaluation in chronic schizophrenic patients. Curr. Ther. Res. 10, 441 – 447.

Gallant, D. M., Bishop, M. P., Steel, C. A., Bishop, G. and Guerrero-Figueroa, R. (1973) Molindone: a cross-over evaluation of capsule and tablet formulations in severely ill schizophrenic patients. Curr. Ther. Res. 15, 915 – 918.

Gallant, D. M., Mielke, D. H., Spirtes, M. A., Swanson, W. C. and Bost, R. (1974) Penfluridol: an efficacious long-acting oral antipsychotic compound. Am. J. Psychiatry 131, 699 – 702.

Gallant, D. M., Mielke, D. H., Oelsner, T., Kessler, C. M., Tomlinson, W. K. and Cohen, G. H. (1975) Butaclamol hydrochloride (AY-23,208): an early evaluation in severely ill schizophrenics. Dis. Nerv. Syst. 36, 7 – 8.

Gardos, A. and Cole, J. O. (1977) Weight reduction in schizophrenics by molindone. Am. J. Psychiatry 134, 302 – 304.

Gardos, A., Cole, J. O., Volicer, L., Orzack, M. H. and Oliff, A. C. (1973) A dose-response study of propranolol in chronic schizophrenics. Curr. Ther. Res. 15, 314 – 323.

Georgotas, A., Gerbino, L., Jordan, B., McCarthy, M., Gershon, S., Kleinberg, D., Lautin, A., Stanley, M. and Rotrosen, J. (1981) A double-blind comparison of trebenzomine and thioridazine in the treatment of schizophrenia. Psychopharmacology 73, 292 – 294.

Gerbino, L., Oleshansky, M. and Gershon, S. (1978) Clinical use and mode of action of lithium. In: M. A. Lipton, A. DiMascio and K. F. Killam (Eds), Psychopharmacology: A Generation of Progress. Raven Press, New York., pp. 1261 – 1276.

Gordon, H. L., Law, A., Hohman, K. E. and Groth, C. (1960) The problem of overweight in hospitalized psychiatric patients. Psychiatr. Q. 34, 69 – 82.

Gottfries, C. (1971) Flupenthixol and trifluoperazine: a double-blind investigation in the treatment of schizophrenias. Br. J. Psychiatry 119, 547 – 548.

Growe, G. A., Crayton, J. W., Klass, D. B., Evans, H. and Strizich, M. (1979) Lithium in chronic schizophrenia. Am. J. Psychiatry 136, 454 – 455.

Hanssen, T., Heyden, T., Sundberg, I., Alfredsson, G., Nyback, H. and Wetterberg, L. (1980) Propranolol in schizophrenia. Arch. Gen. Psychiatry 37, 685 – 690.

Hollister, L. E., Davis, K. L. and Berger, P. A. (1975) Butaclamol hydrochloride in newly admitted schizophrenics. Psychopharmacol. Comm. 1, 493 – 500.

Hollister, L. E., Davis, K. L., Wermuth, B., Berger, P. A. and Stunkard, A. J. (1976) The use of baclofen in schizophrenia. New Clinical Drug Evaluation Unit Intercom 8.

Jimerson, D. C., Van Kammen, D. P., Post, R. M., Docherty, J. P. and Bunney, Jr., W. E. (1982) Diazepam in schizophrenia: a preliminary double-blind trial. Am. J. Psychiatry 139, 489 – 491.

Karson, C. N., Weinberger, D. R., Bigelow, L. and Wyatt, R. J. (1982) Clonazepam treatment of chronic schizophrenia: negative results in a double-blind, placebo-controlled trial. Am. J. Psychiatry 139, 1627 – 1628.

King, D. J., Turkson, S. N. A., Liddle, J. and Kinney, C. D. (1980) Some clinical and metabolic aspects of propranolol in chronic schizophrenia. Br. J. Psychiatry 137, 458 – 468.

Lautin, A., Angrist, B., Stanley, M., Gershon, S., Heckl, K. and Karobath, M. (1980) Sodium valproate in schizophrenia: some biochemical correlates. Br. J. Psychiatry 137, 240 – 244.

Lindstrom, L. H. and Persson, E. (1980) Propranolol in chronic schizophrenia: a controlled study in neuroleptic-treated patients. Am. J. Psychiatry 137, 126 – 130.

Lingjaerde, O. (1982) Effects of the benzodiazepine derivative estazolam in patients with auditory hallucination: a multi-centre double-blind, cross-over study. Acta Psychiatr. Scand. 65, 339 – 354.

Linnoila, M., Viukari, M. and Hietala, O. (1976) Effect of sodium valproate on tardive dyskinesia. Br. J. Psychiatry 129, 114 – 119.

McCreadie, R. G., Heykants, J. J. P., Chalmers, A. and Anderson, A. M. (1979) Plasma pimozide profiles in chronic schizophrenics. Br. J. Clin. Pharmacol. 7, 533 – 534.

McCreadie, R. G., Dingwall, J. M., Wiles, D. H. and Heykants, J. J. P. (1980) Intermittent pimozide versus fluphenazine decanoate as maintenance therapy in chronic schizophrenia. Br. J. Psychiatry 137, 510 – 517.

McCreadie, R. G., Mackie, M., Morrison, D. and Kidd, J. (1982) Once weekly pimozide versus fluphenazine decanoate as maintenance therapy in chronic schizophrenia. Br. J. Psychiatry 140, 280 – 286.

Meco, G., Casacchia, M., Attenni, M., Iafrate, I., Ecari, U. and Argenta, G. (1981) Haloperidol decanoate: an open study in acute and chronic schizophrenic outpatients. Proc. III World Congress of Biological Psychiatry p. 300.

Meltzer, H. Y. (1982) Dopamine autoreceptor stimulation: clinical significance. Pharm. Biochem. Behav. (Suppl. 1) 17, 1 – 10.

Meltzer, H. Y., Goode, D. J., Young, M., Strahilevitz, M., Creese, I. and Snyder, S. H. (1978) Serum prolactin and clinical response. In: Scientific Proceedings of the 131st Annual Meeting of the American Psychiatric Association (APA), Atlanta, Georgia, U.S.A., 1978. Published by APA, p. 209.

Mielke, D. H., Gallant, D. M., Kessler, C. and Roniger, J. J. (1975) Lenperone: a controlled evaluation in chronic schizophrenic patients. Curr. Ther. Res. 18, 636 – 640.

Nagao, T., Ohshimo, T., Mitsunobu, K., Sato, M. and Otsuki, S. (1979) Cerebrospinal fluid monoamine metabolites and cyclic nucleotides in chronic schizophrenic patients with tardive dyskinesia or drug induced tremor. Biol. Psychiatry 14, 509 – 523.

Nestoros, J. N., Suranyi-Cadotti, B. E., Spees, R. C., Schwartz, G. and Nair, N. P. (1982) Prog. Neuropsychopharmacol. Biol. Psychiatry 6, 513 – 516.

Oritz, A., Dabbagh, M. and Gershon, S. (1984) Lithium: clinical use, toxicology, and mode of action. In: J. G. Bernstein (Ed.), Clinical Psychopharmacology. John Wright, PSG Inc., Boston, pp. 111 – 144.

Peet, M., Middlemiss, D. N. and Yates, R. A. (1980) Pharmacokinetic interaction between propranolol and chlorpromazine in schizophrenic patients. Lancet ii, 978.

Peet, M., Middlemiss, D. N. and Yates, R. A. (1981a) Propranolol in schizophrenia. II. Clinical and biochemical aspects of combining propranolol with chlorpromazine. Br. J. Psychiatry 138, 112 – 117.

Peet, M., Bethell, M. S., Coates, A., Khammee, A. K., Hall, P., Cooper, S. J., King, D. J. and Yates, R. A. (1981b) Propranolol in schizophrenia. I. Comparison of propranolol, chlorpromazine, and placebo. Br. J. Psychiatry 139, 105 – 111.

Peselow, E. D. and Stanley, M. (1982) Clinical trial of benzamides in psychiatry. In: J. Rotrosen and M. Stanley (Eds), The Benzamides: Pharmacology, Neurobiology, and Clinical Aspects. Raven Press, New York. pp. 163 – 194.

Prien, R. F. (1972) Comparison of lithium carbonate and chlorpromazine in the treatment of mania. Arch. Gen. Psychiatry 31, 189 – 192.

Prien, R. J. (1979) Lithium in the treatment of schizophrenia and schizoaffective disorder. Arch. Gen. Psychiatry 36, 852 – 853.

Quitkin, F., Rifkin, A., Kane, J., Ramos-Loren, J. R. and Klein, D. F. (1978) Long-acting oral vs. injectable antipsychotic drugs in schizophrenia. Arch. Gen. Psychiatry 35, 889.

Ridges, A. P., Lawton, K., Harper, P., Ghosh, G. and Hindson, N. (1977) Propranolol in schizophrenia. Lancet ii, 986.

Robert, E. (1972) An hypothesis suggesting that there is a defect in GABA system in schizophrenia. Neurosci. Res. Prog. Bull. 10, 468 – 481.

Roose, K. (1981) Monthly haloperidol decanoate as a replacement for maintenance therapy. Proceedings from III World Congress of Biological Psychiatry, p. 410.

Sheppard, G. P. (1979) High-dose propranolol in schizophrenia. Br. J. Psychiatry 134, 470 – 476.

Shopsin, B., Kim, S. S. and Gershon, S. (1971a) A controlled study of lithium vs. chlorpromazine in acute schizophrenics. Br. J. Psychiatry 119, 435 – 440.

Simpson, G. M. and Lee, J. H. (1978) A ten-year review of antipsychotics. In: M. A. Lipton, A.

DiMascio and K. F. Killam (Eds), Psychopharmacology: A Generation of Progress. Raven Press, New York, pp. 1131 – 1137.

Simpson, G. M., Amin, M. and Edwards, J. G. (1971) A double-blind comparison of molindone and trifluoperazine in the treatment of acute schizophrenia. J. Clin. Pharmacol. 11, 228 – 236.

Simpson, G. M., Branchey, M. H. and Shrivastava, R. K. (1976) Baclofen in schizophrenia. Lancet i, 966.

Small, J. G., Kellams, J. J., Milstein, V. and Moore, J. (1975) A placebo controlled study of lithium combined with neuroleptics in chronic schizophrenia patients. Am. J. Psychiatry 132, 1315 – 1317.

Smith, R. C., Tamminga, G. and Davis, J. M. (1977) Effect of apomorphine on schizophrenia symptoms. J. Neural. Transm. 40, 171 – 176.

Snyder, S. H. (1980) Dopamine receptors, neuroleptics and schizophrenia. Am. J. Psychiatry 138, 460.

Stanley, M., Rotrosen, J., Sculerati, N., Gershon, S., Kuhn, C. and Cohen, B. M. (1979a) Atypical antidopaminergic properties of CI-686: a potential antipsychotic agent. Psychopharmacologia 66, 23 – 27.

Stanley, M., Lautin, A., Rotrosen, J. and Gershon, S. (1979b) Antipsychotic efficacy of metoclopramide. Do DA/neuroleptic receptors mediate the action of antipsychotic drugs. IRCS Med. Sci. 7, 322.

Stam, F. C. (1971) Enkele ervaringen met propranolol-behandelingen van schizophrenen. Ned. Tydschr. Psychiatr. 13, 422 – 426.

Sterkmans, P., Brugmans, J. and Gevers, F. (1968) The clinical efficacy of pimozide in chronic psychotic patients. Clin. Trials J. 5, 1107 – 1112.

Sterkmans, P., Brugmans, J. and Gevers, F. (1969) Clinical evaluation of fluspirilene, a long-acting injectible neuroleptic drug. Clin. Trials J. 6, 19 – 25.

Tamminga, G. A., Schaffer, M. H., Smith, J. M. and Davis, J. M. (1978) Schizophrenic symptoms improved with apomorphine. Science 200, 567 – 568.

Taverna, P., Ghisoni, T. and Pogg, E. (1972) Controlled study of the antipsychotic efficacy of sulpiride. Psychol. Med. 4, 811 – 818.

Toru, M., Shimazono, Y., Miyaska, M., Kakubo, T., Mori, Y. and Nasu, T. (1972) A double-blind comparison of sulpiride with chlorpromazine in chronic schizophrenia. J. Clin. Pharmacol. 12, 221 – 229.

Van Kammen, D. P. and DeFraites, E. G. (1979) Lithium treatment in schizophrenia: a review of treatment and prophylaxis in schizophrenia, schizo-affective disorders, and periodic catatonia. In: T. B. Cooper, S. Gershon, N. S. Kline and M. Schou (Eds), Lithium, Controversies and Unresolved Issues. Excerpta Medica, Amsterdam, pp. 85 – 97.

Van Praag, H. M., Schut, T., Dols, L. and Van Schilfgaarden, R. (1971) Controlled trial of penfluridol in acute psychosis. Br. Med. J. 4, 710 – 713.

Von Zerssen, D. (1976) Beta-adrenergic blocking agents in the treatment of psychosis. A report on 17 patients. Adv. Clin. Pharmacol. 12, 105 – 114.

Wazer, D. E., Rotrosen, J. and Stanley, M (1982) The benzamides: evidence for action of dopamine receptors – shortcomings of current models. In: J. Rotrosen and M. Stanley (Eds), The Benzamides: Pharmacology, Neurobiology and Clinical Aspects. Raven Press, New York, pp. 83 – 95.

Yorkston, N. J., Zaki, S. A., Malik, M. K. U., Morrison, R. C. and Havard, C. W. H. (1974) Propranolol in the control of schizophrenic symptoms. Br. Med. J. 4, 633 – 635.

Yorkston, N. J., Themen, J. F. and Havard, C. W. H. (1976) Propranolol to control schizophrenic symptoms: 55 patients. Adv. Clin. Pharmacol. 12, 91 – 94.

Yorkston, N. J., Pitcher, D. R., Gruzelier, J. H., Hollander, D. and Sargeant, H. G. S. (1977) Propranolol as an adjunct to the treatment of schizophrenia. Lancet ii, 575 – 578.

Yorkston, N. J., Zaki, S. A., Weller, M. P., Gruzelier, J. H. and Hirsch, S. R. (1981) DL-Propranolol and chlorpromazine following admission for schizophrenia. Acta Psychiatr. Scand. 63, 13 – 27.

Young, J. P. R., Hughes, W. C. and Lader, M. H. (1976) Br. Med. J. 1, 1116 – 1118.

Burrows/Norman/Davies (eds) Antipsychotics

Chapter 13

Antipsychotic effect of the benzodiazepines

ODD LINGJÆRDE

Section of Clinical Psychiatry, University of Tromsø, and Åsgård Sykehus, 9010 Åsgård, Norway

INTRODUCTION

Psychotic patients may be given benzodiazepines for different purposes: for insomnia, for anxiety and tension, for neuroleptic-induced side effects like akathisia and tardive dyskinesia, and, finally, for psychotic symptoms proper, such as hallucinations, delusions, thought disturbances, and psychotic excitement and aggression. It is the possible antipsychotic effect that is to be addressed in this survey.

Do benzodiazepines really have an effect on psychotic symptoms – an effect that is not only secondary to the anxiolytic and sedating effects? It is probably fair to say that many psychiatrists doubt it, and it is commonly agreed that the benzodiazepines, at least generally speaking, are inferior to the neuroleptics in this respect. However, besides many negative reports, the literature reveals a number of uncontrolled and controlled trials that seem to indicate that benzodiazepines may, at least under certain circumstances, exert a true antipsychotic effect, and that they may enhance the antipsychotic effect of the neuroleptics. If so, the benzodiazepines may have a more important role to play in the treatment of psychoses than they have been given until now, especially in patients who do not respond satisfactorily to neuroleptics alone, or who are bothered by side effects like tardive dyskinesia.

Many of the studies on benzodiazepines in psychoses were reported in the 1960's, and several of them do not stand up to present-day standards of clinical trials.

However, there are also some more recent trials, and there has been a renewed interest in the possible antipsychotic effect of benzodiazepines since it has been shown that high-dose diazepam treatment may be remarkably effective in some schizophrenic patients.

In the following, the pertinent literature will be briefly surveyed, with special emphasis on controlled trials. Since almost all trials on the possible antipsychotic effect of the benzodiazepines have been carried out on schizophrenic patients (often without further specification), the results to be presented are relevant mainly for this diagnostic category.

This survey does not intend to be totally comprehensive. Other surveys of the antipsychotic/antischizophrenic effects of benzodiazepines can be found in Nestoros (1980) and Lingjaerde (1983).

In the following, dosage is always given as total daily dose.

SOME EARLY, UNCONTROLLED TRIALS

In the early 1960's there appeared several reports claiming that diazepam had an excellent therapeutic effect in many schizophrenic patients, notably on auditory hallucinations (e.g. Pöldinger, 1963; Vinar and Taussigova, 1966), whereas at least as many reports were quite negative (e.g. Deberdt et al., 1962; Lehmann and Ban, 1964; see Lingjaerde, 1983, for further references). There were also negative reports on chlordiazepoxide (Deberdt et al., 1962). On the other hand, there were reports that chlordiazepoxide enhanced the antipsychotic effect of neuroleptics (Dye, 1961; Monroe and Wise, 1965). Thus, these early reports on uncontrolled trials seemed promising to some extent, but as a whole they were rather inconsistent and unconvincing.

At about the same time controlled trials also began to appear. However, as we shall see shortly, these trials have also given equivocal results.

We shall have a look first at controlled trials of benzodiazepines against placebo, next at controlled trials of benzodiazepines against neuroleptics, and then at controlled trials of benzodiazepines against placebo in addition to neuroleptics. Finally, some recent – mainly uncontrolled – promising studies with very high dosage of diazepam will be mentioned.

BENZODIAZEPINES VERSUS PLACEBO

Hankoff et al. (1962) compared meprobamate, chlorpromazine, chlordiazepoxide (mostly 30 mg), and placebo, with each drug being given for 2 weeks, in 134 mostly schizophrenic outpatients. The improvement on chlorpromazine and chlordiazepoxide was better than on placebo with regard to global change, and especially with regard to reducing manifest anxiety. Unfortunately, the effect is not specified for schizophrenic and non-schizophrenic patients.

In a controlled cross-over trial of chlordiazepoxide (1 mg/kg) against thioridazine

(5 mg/kg) and placebo in 24 schizophrenic men, Holden et al. (1968) found that chlordiazepoxide was inferior to thioridazine, but significantly better than placebo on several single symptoms: negativism, euphoria, disturbance of life drive, confusion, and appetite increase. Azima et al. (1962), on the other hand, found that chlordiazepoxide (20 – 200 mg) had no better effect than placebo.

Turning now to diazepam, some early studies concluded that this drug was not markedly superior to placebo in hospitalized schizophrenics, and inferior to neuroleptics (Merlis et al., 1982; Hollister et al., 1963). Gundlach et al. (1966), in a 6-week trial with diazepam (maximum 40 mg) vs. placebo in 100 outpatients, 63 of whom were schizophernics, also found no significant difference in favor of diazepam, neither overall nor in the schizophrenic subgroup. On the contrary, patients on diazepam more often developed suicidal or paranoid thoughts, prompting the authors to conclude that diazepam (alone) may be contraindicated in psychotic patients. A better effect of diazepam than placebo in schizophrenic patients was, however, reported by Venkoba Rao (1964).

In another trial by Nishikawa et al. (1982), the prophylactic effect of diazepam (15 mg), imipramine (50 mg), chlorpromazine (75 mg), haloperidol (3 mg), and placebo was compared in a total of 55 schizophrenics in remission. Fifty per cent relapse was seen within 16 days with placebo, 88 days with diazepam, 30 days with imipramine, 165 days with chlorpromazine, and 74 days with haloperidol. However, only chlorpromazine and haloperidol had significantly prolonged the mean remission period at the end of the 3-year trial period. It may be objected that all drugs were probably given in suboptimal dosage in this trial.

Summing up, the controlled trials of benzodiazepines (chlordiazepoxide and diazepam, mostly in conventional dosage) against placebo that have been mentioned so far, have not shown a convincing antipsychotic effect. A more promising trial of high-dose diazepam vs. placebo will, however, be mentioned later (Nestoros et al., 1982).

BENZODIAZEPINES VERSUS NEUROLEPTICS

From the mostly negative results of the placebo-controlled trials, one would not expect benzodiazepines to stand up in direct comparison against the neuroleptics in psychotic patients. Nevertheless, there have appeared several controlled studies in which benzodiazepines seem to have about the same effect as standard neuroleptics, or even better. However, in interpreting the results of such trials, that have often been performed on a limited number of patients, one always has to be aware of the risk of drawing the false conclusion that there is no difference, when in reality there is one – probably in favor of the neuroleptics.

Maculans (1964) compared diazepam (maximum 60 mg), chlorpromazine (maximum 600 mg), and chlorprothixene (maximum 600 mg), each drug given for 3 weeks, in a cross-over trial with one-week placebo intervals between the active drugs, in 37 chronic schizophrenics. An overall improvement was noted in 53% on chlorprothixene, 46% on chlorpromazine, and 59% on diazepam. The symptoms that seemed to respond best to diazepam, were anxiety-tension, depression, somatization, emotional apathy, seclusiveness, and confused behavior. It was concluded that the trial had yielded definite evidence of diazepam's antipsychotic activity, comparable to and even surpassing that of the two neuroleptics. However, the weight of the evidence in the report does not seem to warrant this optimistic conclusion.

As mentioned in the previous section, Holden et al. (1968) found chlordiazepoxide (1 mg/kg) to be inferior to thioridazine (5 mg/kg) in a cross-over trial in chronic schizophrenic men, whereas Hankoff et al. (1962) found both chlordiazepoxide and chlorpromazine to be better than placebo, and chlordiazepoxide in fact to be better than chlorpromazine in certain respects. Smith (1961) also reported chlordiazepoxide, in the high dosage of 150 – 700 mg, to be better than chlorpromazine (150 – 600 mg). Merlis et al. (1962) compared chlordiazepoxide (75 mg), diazepam (30 mg), chlorpromazine (150 mg), and placebo, but found no difference between the four compounds.

In a trial by Lerner et al. (1979), 40 acute psychotic patients, including schizophrenics, were randomized to receive intravenous haloperidol (20 – 35 mg) or diazepam (30 – 40 mg). Both groups showed marked and rapid improvement, with no significant difference between them. No placebo group was included, but considering the proven effectiveness of haloperidol in acute psychosis, the trial strongly indicates that diazepam may have a true therapeutic effect in such patients.

Summing up, controlled trials of benzodiazepines vs. neuroleptics in psychotic patients are, on a whole, rather inconclusive, some trials indicating an inferior effect of the benzodiazepine, some equal effectiveness, and some even a superior effect of the benzodiazepine.

BENZODIAZEPINES VERSUS PLACEBO IN ADDITION TO NEUROLEPTICS

So far we have seen that benzodiazepines alone – some positive controlled trials notwithstanding – have not been convincingly demonstrated to have a true antipsychotic effect. In this section, however, several trials will be mentioned that show very convincingly that benzodiazepines may enhance the antipsychotic effect of neuroleptics, in patients where neuroleptics alone have had unsatisfactory effect. Even in this area, though, there are some negative findings.

The negative studies are primarily the three large and thoroughly analyzed trials carried out by Kurland, Hanlon, Michaux and collaborators (Michaux et al., 1966; Hanlon et al., 1969, 1970, 1975; Kurland and Hanlon, 1971). In these trials, acutely disturbed, predominantly schizophrenic patients were treated with chlorpromazine, thioridazine, or fluphenazine, either alone or in combination with chlordiazepoxide

(30 or 40 mg), imipramine (not to be discussed here), or placebo. In all three studies, an attenuating effect of chlordiazepoxide on the antipsychotic effect of the phenothiazines was observed. On the average, patients receiving chlordiazepoxide in addition to their phenothiazine medication showed less overall improvement than patients receiving phenothiazine alone, a result that was found to be due principally to decreased effectiveness in the alleviation of symptoms of psychosis such as perceptual and thought disorders (Kurland and Hanlon, 1971). Some of the inferior effect of the chlordiazepoxide-phenothiazine combination, at least in the chlorpromazine trial, may have been due to a lower dose of the phenothiazine in patients receiving the combination compared to patients on phenothiazine alone, but this does not explain the overall results. An interesting aspect of the chlorpromazine trial, however, is that the chlorpromazine-chlordiazepoxide combination was significantly better than chlorpromazine alone in the most disturbed 20% of the patients, and also in the high-agitated and the high-retarded patients. In evaluating the results of these trials, it should also be considered that a fixed, low dosage of chlordiazepoxide was given (30 mg in two trials and 40 mg in the third), and that the patient groups are not very well-defined.

More favorable effects of chlordiazepoxide in addition to neuroleptics have been reported by Ulett et al. (1964) and Kellner et al. (1975). In the former study, chlordiazepoxide (40 mg) in addition to thioridazine, tetrabenazine, or fluphenazine was followed by a noticeable behavioral improvement, when compared with the addition of placebo, in a group of 21 chronic psychotic (mainly schizophrenic) women. The latter study was a multiple cross-over trial on six anxious schizophrenic patients who had not responded to neuroleptics alone. In three patients, chlordiazepoxide, in a dosage of up to 300 mg in addition to individually optimized neuroleptic medication, was superior to placebo, not only on anxiety, tension and somatic symptoms, but also on typically schizophrenic symptoms like hallucinations, delusions, and thought disturbances. Two patients showed no significant difference between chlordiazepoxide and placebo, whereas one patient seemed to be more depressed on chlordiazepoxide.

Surprisingly, there seems to have been carried out only one controlled trial comparing diazepam and placebo in addition to neuroleptics in psychotic patients. In this trial (Lingjærde et al., 1979), 23 chronic psychotic patients (19 schizophrenics) were maintained on their previous neuroleptic medication, that was not quite effective, and were given in addition diazepam (15 mg) or placebo, 3 weeks each, in a randomized cross-over design. Although no dramatic changes were seen, diazepam was significantly better than placebo in improving the total score on the Brief Psychiatric Rating Scale, and on the symptoms suspiciousness and unusual thought content – the difference was nearly significant also for anxiety and hallucinatory behavior.

Lorazepam (6 mg) was compared with placebo in 60 haloperidol-treated acutely psychotic patients in a 4-week study by Guz et al. (1972). A significant difference in favor of lorazepam was found for the symptoms anxious mood, delusions-hallucinations, and behavior, whereas the difference in global improvement was of only marginal significance (depending on type and time of evaluation).

Camazepam (40 mg) has also been tested against placebo in haloperidol-treated schizophrenic patients (Marneros, 1979). No significant difference was seen with regard to typically psychotic symptoms like delusions and hallucinations, whereas camazepam was significantly superior to placebo on affective symptoms like anxiety, tension, irritability, aggressivity, and psychomotor unrest.

Another recently introduced benzodiazepine, estazolam (a triazolobenzodiazepine), that seemed to have a remarkable antihallucinatory effect in an uncontrolled trial (Lingjærde and Astrup, 1978), was compared with placebo in a double-blind, double cross-over trial on 58 patients with auditory hallucinations (Lingjærde, 1982). Forty-nine of the patients were schizophrenic, and all except five patients were continued on previous neuroleptic medication throughout the trial period, which consisted of three 3-week periods. Estazolam (6 mg) was given either in the first and third period, or in the second period, and placebo in the remaining periods. Estazolam was found to have a significantly better effect than placebo on the global clinical state, on frequency and attitude toward the auditory hallucinations, as well as on compulsive thoughts and visual hallucinations.

Summing up, there is rather convincing evidence that various benzodiazepines may enhance the antipsychotic effect of neuroleptics, in patients showing an unsatisfactory response to neuroleptics alone. This effect may be seen even with ordinary dosage of benzodiazepines. As will appear from the next section, however, more dramatic improvement may be seen by giving diazepam – alone or in combination with neuroleptics – in substantially higher dosage.

HIGH-DOSE DIAZEPAM TREATMENT IN SCHIZOPHRENIA

Chlordiazepoxide in high dosage has been given to schizophrenic patients in several earlier studies (e.g. Smith, 1961; Kellner et al., 1975), with promising results (see above). Perhaps these studies deserve some more interest. During recent years, however, studies with high-dose diazepam treatment in schizophrenia have attracted more interest, and some of these studies are therefore to be mentioned in some detail.

Beckmann and Haas (1980), in an uncontrolled study, treated nine schizophrenics of the paranoid-hallucinatory type, and six of the schizoaffective type with diazepam alone in rapidly increasing dosage, up to 400 mg; most patients were given a maximum of 200 mg. The paranoid-hallucinatory patients showed marked improvement of symptoms like anxiety, hallucinations, conceptual disorganization, unusual thoughts, and uncooperativeness. Five of the schizoaffective patients, on the other hand, had to be withdrawn from the trial because of unmanageable hyperactivity, excitation, and insomnia. In the total group, there was remarkably little sedation except after the first 50 mg dose. Above ca. 60 mg, a rather marked stimulating and euphoriant effect was seen, and in several patients a loss of social and sexual inhibitions. Initially, some muscular weakness, dysarthria, and ataxia were observed, mostly in older patients.

Nestoros et al. (1983), also in an open trial, gave up to 200 mg diazepam to 10 hospitalized chronic schizophrenic patients who were resistant to standard neuroleptics, in addition to previous neuroleptic treatment. The diazepam dose was adjusted daily to avoid oversedation, with maximum dose varying from 35 to 200 mg. The addition of diazepam produced marked improvement in 3, moderate in 4, mild in 1, and no change in 2 patients. Marked improvement was seen in symptoms such as anxiety, emotional withdrawal, conceptual disorganization, tension, mannerism-posturing, suspiciousness, hostility, and hallucinatory behavior. All improved patients were of the paranoid type, whereas the unresponsive were of the undifferentiated type. All patients initially tolerated a high dosage of diazepam without sedation. However, later on all patients experienced sedation, necessitating dose reduction. Two patients exhibited a loss of inhibition of aggressive behavior, but this was controlled by temporarily increasing the dosage to sedating levels.

Nestoros et al. (1982) have also carried out a controlled trial in which 12 paranoid schizophrenic patients were randomly assigned to receive diazepam or placebo for one week, followed by a 6-week period during which patients not responding during the first week were given 30 mg haloperidol in addition to previous medication. During the first week, the dosage was increased as quickly as possible, provided that little or no side effects were present, to a maximum dose of diazepam ranging from 70 to 400 mg. Within a few hours to a few days from the onset of diazepam treatment, both positive symptoms like auditory hallucinations and persecutory delusions, and negative symptoms like emotional withdrawal and blunted affect, were dramatically eliminated in 5 out of 6 patients. Placebo failed to produce any improvement in 5 out of 6 patients. Diazepam seemed to act more rapidly than haloperidol. All patients tolerated high doses of diazepam without sedation as long as they were actively psychotic, whereas sedation appeared when schizophrenic symptoms were no longer present.

Less positive results were obtained by Jimerson et al. (1982) in a preliminary trial on five schizophrenic and one schizoaffective patient. After at least 2 weeks on placebo, diazepam was given in increasing dosage, according to tolerance, to a maximum of 300 mg. Three patients, who obtained a maximum dose of less than 120 mg, did not show any certain improvement, whereas the other three showed only a limited decrease in psychosis rating.

Summing up, high-dose diazepam seems to be well-tolerated by most manifestly psychotic patients, and to have a remarkable anxiolytic as well as antipsychotic effect in some schizophrenics, especially of the paranoid subgroup. However, further studies are needed in order to gain more knowledge about the optimal dosages and indications in such patients.

A NOTE ON THE MECHANISM OF ACTION

It is now well-established that benzodiazepines act mainly – perhaps exclusively – by enhancing GABA-ergic transmission in the brain (see Haefely et al., 1983, for survey). A functional deficiency in the GABA-ergic systems in the brain has been implicated in schizophrenia. However, according to a comprehensive survey, neither biochemical nor pharmacological studies have been able to demonstrate a clear and reproducible GABA disturbance in schizophrenia (Garbutt and van Kammen, 1983). But these authors also state that, in their view, the complexity of the GABA system and the heterogeneity of schizophrenia suggest that GABA may still play a role in the disorder.

It is more likely, though, that the antipsychotic effect of the benzodiazepines is mediated by a GABA-ergic inhibition of dopaminergic systems in the brain. As discussed in more detail in other chapters in this volume, neuroleptics seem to exert their antipsychotic effect by blocking certain dopamine receptors in the brain, and it has been shown that benzodiazepines potentiate several behavioral and biochemical effects of neuroleptics (Keller et al., 1976; Singhal et al., 1983).

There are no indications that the enhancing effect of benzodiazepines on the antipsychotic effect of neuroleptics is due to a pharmacokinetic interaction. Such a mechanism also could not explain the presumed antipsychotic effect of high doses of diazepam given alone.

CONCLUSIONS

The total picture of clinical trials with benzodiazepines in psychotic patients is still somewhat confusing. The reported results vary from 'worse than placebo' to 'better than standard neuroleptics'. Obviously, further studies are required to clarify the picture. Until then, however, some tentative conclusions may be drawn:

1) Benzodiazepines alone, in conventional doses (as given in neurotic states), have no convincing antipsychotic effect, although they may reduce anxiety and insomnia in psychotic patients.
2) In high dosage (e.g. 10 times higher than usually given in neurotic states, or even higher), benzodiazepines like chlordiazepoxide and diazepam, given alone, seem to have a therapeutic effect in psychotic patients, especially in paranoid-hallucinatory schizophrenics. This effect includes improvement of anxiety and tension, but also of typically psychotic symptoms such as hallucinations, delusions, and disturbed thought. Some patients may react with loss of social and sexual inhibition on this high-dose treatment (at least with diazepam).
3) Benzodiazepines, in ordinary dosage, may enhance the antipsychotic effect of neuroleptics. This effect seems to be most marked in patients with auditory hallucinations, in whom neuroleptics alone have had little or no effect. Effect may

also be seen on several other symptoms, such as visual hallucinations, delusions, suspiciousness, and compulsive thoughts, as well as on anxiety and tension.
4) The benzodiazepines may differ in their ability to enhance the antipsychotic effect of neuroleptics, but there are no comparative trials directly addressing this question. The author, from his personal experience, is inclined to believe that the triazolobenzodiazepine estazolam is superior to several other benzodiazepines, e.g. diazepam, in this respect. It remains to be seen whether this is a general characteristic of this subclass of benzodiazepines.

REFERENCES

Azima, A., Arthurs, D. and Silver, A. (1962) The effects of chlordiazepoxide (librium) in anxiety states: a multi-blind study. Can. Psychiatr. Assoc. J. 7, 44 – 50.

Beckmann, H. and Haas, S. (1980) High dose diazepam in schizophrenia. Psychopharmacology 71, 79 – 82.

Deberdt, R, Gross, H., Kaltenbäck, E. and Mühlau, M. (1962) Klinische Erfahrungen mit Benzodiazepinderivaten. Paper presented at the III CINP Congress, Munich, Sept. 2 – 5.

Dye, E. N. (1961) Dual pharmacotherapy in grossly disturbed psychotic patients. Am. J. Psychiatry 118, 548 – 549.

Garbutt, J. C. and van Kammen, D. P. (1983) The interaction between GABA and dopamine: implications for schizophrenia. Schizophr. Bull. 9, 336 – 353.

Gundlach, R., Engelhardt, D. M., Hankoff, L., Paley, H., Rudorfer, L. and Bird, E. (1966) A double-blind outpatient study of diazepam (Valium) and placebo. Psychopharmacologia 9, 81 – 92.

Guz, I., Moraes, R. and Sartoretto, J. N. (1972) The therapeutic effects of lorazepam in psychotic patients treated with haloperidol: a double-blind study. Curr. Ther. Res. 14, 767 – 774.

Haefely, W., Polc, P., Pieri, L., Schaffner, R. and Laurent, J.-P. (1983) Neuropharmacology of benzodiazepines: synaptic mechanisms and neural basis of action. In: E. Costa (Ed.), The Benzodiazepines: From Molecular Biology to Clinical Practice. Raven Press, New York, pp. 21 – 66.

Hankoff, L. D., Rudorfer, L. and Paley, H. M. (1962) A reference study of ataraxics. A two-week double blind outpatient evaluation. J. New Drugs 2, 173 – 178.

Hanlon, T. E., Ota, K. Y., Agallianos, D. D., Berman, S. A., Bethon, G. D., Kobler, F. and Kurland, A. A. (1969) Combined drug treatment of newly hospitalized, acutely ill psychiatric patients. Dis. Nerv. Syst. 30, 104 – 116.

Hanlon, T. E., Ota, K. Y. and Kurland, A. A. (1970) Comparative effects of fluphenazine, fluphenazine-chlordiazepoxide and fluphenazine-imipramine. Dis. Nerv. Syst. 31, 171 – 176.

Hanlon, T. E., Blatchley, R. J. and Kurland, A. A. (1975) Effects of control techniques in a controlled clinical trial. Int. Pharmakopsychiatry 10, 169 – 176.

Holden, J. M. C., Itil, T. M., Keskiner, A. and Fink, M. (1968) Thioridazine and chlordiazepoxide, alone and combined, in the treatment of chronic schizophrenia. Compr. Psychiatry 9, 633 – 643.

Hollister, L. E., Bennett, J. L., Kimbell, Jr., I., Savage, C. and Overall, J. E. (1963) Diazepam in newly admitted schizophrenics. Dis. Nerv. Syst. 24, 746 – 749.

Jimerson, D. C., van Kammen, D. P., Post, R. M., Docherty, J. P. and Bunney, Jr., W. E. (1982) Diazepam in schizophrenia: a preliminary double-blind trial. Am. J. Psychiatry 139, 489 – 491.

Keller, H. H., Schaffner, R. and Haefely, W. (1976) Interaction of benzodiazepines with neuroleptics at central dopamine neurons. Naunyn-Schmiedeberg's Arch. Pharmacol. 294, 1 – 7.

Kellner, R., Wilson, R. M., Muldawer, M. D. and Pathak, D. (1975) Anxiety in schizophrenia. The response to chlordiazepoxide in an intensive design study. Arch. Gen. Psychiatry 32, 1246 – 1254.

Kurland, A. A. and Hanlon, T. E. (1971) The use of psychotropic drug combinations. Comments and observations. Pharmakopsychiatr. Neuropsychopharmacol. 4, 297 – 307.

Lehmann, H. E. and Ban, T. A. (1964) Notes from the log-book of a psychopharmacological research unit. II. Can. Psychiatr. Assoc. J. 9, 111 – 113.

Lerner, Y., Lwow, E., Levitin, A. and Belmaker, R. H. (1979) Acute high-dose parenteral haloperidol treatment of psychosis. Am. J. Psychiatry 136, 1061 – 1064.

Lingjærde, O. (1982) Effect of the benzodiazepine derivative estazolam in patients with auditory hallucinations. A multicentre double-blind, cross-over study. Acta Psychiatr. Scand. 65, 339 – 354.

Lingjærde, O. (1983) Benzodiazepines in the treatment of schizophrenia. In: E. Costa (Ed.), The Benzodiazepines: From Molecular Biology to Clinical Practice. Raven Press, New York, pp. 369 – 381.

Lingjærde, O. and Astrup, C. (1978) Mulig antipsykotisk virkning av benzodiazepiner, med saerlig henblikk på estazolam (Domnamid). Nord. Psykiatr. Tidsskr. 32, 421 – 424.

Lingjærde, O., Engstrand, E., Ellingsen, P., Stylo, D. A. and Robak, O. H. (1979) Antipsychotic effect of diazepam when given in addition to neuroleptics in chronic psychotic patients: a double-blind clinical trial. Curr. Ther. Res. 26, 505 – 514.

Maculans, G. A. (1964) Comparison of diazepam, chlorprothixene and chlorpromazine in chronic schizophrenic patients. Dis. Nerv. Syst. 25, 164 – 168.

Marneros, A. (1979) Anxiolytische Zusatzbehandlung bei den affektbetonten Schizophrenien. Therapiewoche 29, 7533 – 7538.

Merlis, S., Turner, W. J. and Krumholz, W. (1962) A double blind comparison of diazepam, chlordiazepoxide, and chlorpromazine in psychotic patients. J. Neuropsychiatry 3 (Suppl. 11), 133 – 138.

Michaux, M. H., Kurland, A. A. and Agallianos, D. D. (1966) Chlorpromazine-chlordiazepoxide and chlorpromazine-imipramine treatment of newly hospitalized, acutely ill psychiatric patients. Curr. Ther. Res. 8 (Suppl.), 117 – 152.

Monroe, R. R. and Wise, III, S. P. (1965) Combined phenothiazine, chlordiazepoxide and primidone therapy for uncontrolled psychotic patients. Am. J. Psychiatry 122, 694 – 698.

Nestoros, J. N. (1980) Benzodiazepines in schizophrenia: a need for reassessment. Int. Pharmacopsychiatry 15, 171 – 179.

Nestoros, J. N., Suranyi-Cadotte, B. E., Spees, R. C., Schwartz, G. and Nair, N. P. V. (1982) Diazepam in high doses is effective in schizophrenia. Prog. Neuro-Psychopharmacol. Biol. Psychiat. 6, 513 – 516.

Nestoros, J. N., Nair, N. P. V., Pulman, J. R., Schwartz, G. and Bloom, D. (1983) High doses of diazepam improve neuroleptic-resistant chronic schizophrenic patients. Psychopharmacology 81, 42 – 47.

Nishikawa, T., Tsuda, A., Tanaka, M., Koga, I. and Uchida, Y. (1982) Prophylactic effect of neuroleptics in symptom-free schizophrenics. Psychopharmacology 77, 301 – 304.

Pöldinger, W. (1963) Klinische Erfahrungen mit dem Benzodiazepinderivat Valium, einem neuen Psychopharmakon. Schweiz. Med. Wochenschr. 93, 797 – 801.

Singhal, R. L., Rastogi, R. B. and Lapierre, Y. D. (1983) Diazepam potentiates the effect of neuroleptics on behavioral activity as well as dopamine and norepinephrine turnover: do benzodiazepines have antipsychotic potency? J. Neural Transm. 56, 127 – 138.

Smith, M. E. (1961) A clinical study of chlorpromazine and chlordiazepoxide. Conn. Med. 25, 153 – 157.

Ulett, G. A., Bowers, C. A., Heusler, A. F., Quick, R., Word, T. and Word, V. (1964) A study of behavior and EEG patterns of patients receiving tranquilizers with and without the addition of chlordiazepoxide. J. Neuropsychiatry 5, 558 – 565.

Venkoba Rao, A. (1964) A controlled trial with 'Valium' in some psychiatric disorders. Indian J. Psychiatry 6, 188 – 192.

Vinar, O. and Taussigova, D. (1966) Therapeutic effects of diazepam in psychotics. Act. Nerv. Super. 8, 441 – 444.

Burrows/Norman/Davies (eds) Antipsychotics

Chapter 14

The long-acting neuroleptic drugs and their treatment systems

P. F. MARRIOTT, T. R. NORMAN
and
G. D. BURROWS

Department of Psychiatry, University of Melbourne, The Austin Hospital, Heidelberg, Victoria 3084, Australia

INTRODUCTION

By definition, the long-acting neuroleptics are drugs which provide antipsychotic activity for a duration of one or more weeks following a single dose. They can be orally administered but usually are injectable. It has long been obvious that any oral medication can result in poor patient compliance with a defaulting rate of 30 – 60%. The most common indication for long-acting neuroleptics is as maintenance therapy for chronic schizophrenia. They have also been used in mania, schizoaffective disorders, adolescent schizophrenia, mentally-retarded disorders if psychotic or displaying disturbed behaviour, elderly patients with late onset schizophrenia, mild to moderate dementia with paranoid features, and epilepsy with schizophrenia. Other important indications are for chronic schizophrenia with concomitant medical conditions which may become life-threatening, as when the diabetic patient, or the patient with renal disease or hypertension, may reject his necessary medication under the influence of his schizophrenic delusions.

CLASSIFICATION AND PHARMACOLOGY OF LONG-ACTING NEUROLEPTICS

The most commonly available long-acting neuroleptics are classified according to their chemical structure in Table 1. An alternative classification divides the drugs into two types according to the mechanism of their prolonged duration of action (Ban and Ceskova, 1980). Most long-acting neuroleptics are esters of long-chain fatty acids with an oily vehicle, e.g. sesame oil, for the vehicle medium. These are Type 1 drugs. In Type 2 drugs, the active agent itself has a high intrinsic lipophilicity. With both types this high lipophilicity results in slow release from injection site, slow tissue distribution, and prolonged biotransformation to less lipophilic, more polar and finally water-soluble compounds that are excreted. For example, the ester fluphenazine decanoate has an elimination half-life of 21 days, compared with 18 hours for fluphenazine hydrochloride. Penfluridol, a Type 2 drug, is the only oral preparation currently available with a duration of antipsychotic action of one week. In some patients the interval between doses can be increased by daily increments, as far as 14 days. However, careful patient selection is necessary. Penfluridol is strongly absorbed by the brain, and shows markedly delayed elimination without metabolism, from the brain (Floru, 1975). Fluspirilene, which is injected intramuscularly as microcrystals in an aqueous suspension, also has a duration of action of approximately one week (Lingjaerde, 1973).

TABLE 1

Types of long-acting neuroleptics.

Group	Subgroup	Name
Phenothiazine	Piperazine	Fluphenazine decanoate Fluphenazine enanthate Perphenazine enanthate Pipothiazine undecylenate Pipothiazine palmitate
Thioxanthene		Flupenthixol decanoate Clopenthixol decanoate
Butyrophenone		Haloperidol decanoate
Diphenylbutylpiperidine		Fluspiriline Penfluridol*
Dibenzothiepine		Oxyprothepine decanoate

* Oral preparation.

TABLE 2

Therapeutic dosage range.

Name	Dose range (mg)	Duration (wks)
Fluphenazine decanoate	12.5 – 75	3 – 6
Fluphenazine enanthate	12.5 – 75	1 – 3
Perphenazine enanthate	12.5 – 75	1 – 3
Pipothiazine undecylenate	50 – 450	1 – 3
Pipothiazine palmitate	50 – 600	3 – 6
Flupenthixol decanoate	10 – 80	2 – 4
Clopenthixol decanoate	–	2 – 4
Haloperidol decanoate	200 – 800	2 – 4
Fluspirilene	2 – 20	1
Penfluridol*	30 – 150	1
Oxyprothepine decanoate	–	1 – 3

* Oral preparation.

Therapeutic dosage ranges and duration of action of long-acting neuroleptics are summarized in Table 2.

USE OF LONG-ACTING NEUROLEPTICS

One of the main indications for long-acting neuroleptics is schizophrenia. There is no 'cure'; like a number of other medical conditions, e.g. diabetes, arthritis or hypertension, it pursues a long course over many years with intermittent relapse. The clinician will need to follow a treatment plan which assesses the individual's response to a specific drug and use other types of neuroleptic if progress is slow or unsatisfactory. A random sample of 50 outpatients of a clinic population of 400 attending an Australian Depot Neuroleptic Clinic gave results as follows: patients had been on fluphenazine decanoate 1 – 4 years; 22.5% were employed; 36% were unemployed; 22% (all women) were engaged in home duties; 18% were receiving invalid pensions (Marriott et al., 1982). The family must become involved in the treatment plan. A discussion with the family should cover these areas: 1) the diagnosis; 2) the potential long-term problem; 3) the drugs – dose, side effects and how to treat them; 4) drug defaulting and possible relapse; 5) support and supervision; 6) drug interactions, including alcohol; 7) expectations from treatment. A booklet on the subject is often helpful.

Follow-up and management in the first year of treatment

Choice of the treatment centre should occur following recovery from the acute phase of the illness, taking into account such factors as location.

FORMATION OF A SPECIALIZED CLINIC

a) An initial enquiry into local needs, selection of treatment area.
b) Team selected and trained. A team approach with individual case manager.
c) Standardized procedures adopted.
d) An automatic follow-up system.
e) Rational approach in psychopharmacology, with teaching programme.
f) Accurate records for regular evaluation; regular team meetings.
g) Flexibility with dosage and treatment intervals of injections.
h) Co-ordination with other local services.
i) Psychosocial treatment for the individual and family.
j) Long-term psychological support.

Fig. 1. Some requirements for formation of the Depot Neuroleptic Clinic.

Initial appointment should be made within 2 weeks of leaving hospital. At each visit a plan should be followed (see Appendix). Drug changes include reduction of oral neuroleptics, and of other oral medication including antiparkinson drugs. The dose of long-acting medication can be varied, depending on clinical assessment, and can later be stabilized. Then the interval between injections can be tentatively increased. Evaluation for side effects occurs, with possible dosage manipulation and antiparkinson medication. During this phase depression needs evaluation and treatment.

Outpatient treatment in the second and third year of treatment

By this time the dose of the long-acting neuroleptic has been stabilized at the lowest possible level to maintain remission. The widest interval between injections can be attempted. Side effects are likely to be minimal but should be treated. Other treatments include the non-drug needs of the patient and the family, e.g. a retraining programme. Early signs of relapse need detection, including drug defaulting or refusal of injections, insomnia, or new stresses in the family. Prompt treatment via an effective follow-up system is essential (see Fig. 2).

Outpatient treatment in year four and subsequent years

Dose and treatment interval have become standardized. Observation and treatment for tardive dyskinesia is imperative. This important topic is covered in Chapter 15. Other special problem areas include the question of whether the patient should cease drug treatment. If this decision is made by the patient, relative or doctor, a high chance of relapse is likely (e.g. 80%, see Johnson et al., 1983). Therefore, careful follow-up for one year is mandatory following cessation of long-acting drugs. Many patients remain on maintenance injections of a suitable long-acting neuroleptic for life.

THE FOLLOW-UP SYSTEM

1) Automatic recall system with standardized procedures
2) *System* known to team and hospital
3) *Explanation* of follow-up to
   a) patient
   b) relatives
   c) local doctor
   d) other services
4) *Specific steps*
   a) telephone
   b) letter
   c) home visits nurse/occupational therapist/social worker/doctor
   d) visit relative or friend/neighbour
   e) visit at work site
   f) communicate to team at hospital if emergency
   g) team meeting regarding results of visit and further management
   h) involve local doctor if relapsing
5) *Community nursing service* – service provided
   a) support family
   b) crisis assessment
   c) assess problem, e.g. side effects
   d) routine injection at home
   e) non-attendance
   f) evening visits
6) *Concept of long-term support via team approach*

Fig. 2. Details of the follow-up system to assist patient compliance.

The Depot Neuroleptic Clinic

Once the patient's treatment involves the use of an injectable long-acting neuroleptic, it is important to refer such a patient to a specialized clinic with staff having considerable experience in this area. Often a teaching programme is needed to train staff in the use of injectable neuroleptics and associated procedures. A number of rules can be formulated. These include the following of the standard procedures in the use of depot neuroleptics and associated drugs. In the active phase of the illness, the use of oral neuroleptics; short intervals between injections; constant evaluation for side effects and their prompt treatment; the treatment of depression. In the residual or chronic phase the oral medication is reduced; then the dose of depot neuroleptic fixed, and later the interval between injections increased. Education for patient and family is essential to enable the system to work smoothly. It is possible to give each patient a book. Co-ordination with the parent hospital or other community agencies should also occur. It should also be possible for team members to provide psychosocial treatment for the individual and the family.

Contraindications to long-acting neuroleptics

There are few absolute contraindications other than a history of serious hypersensitivity to drugs, drug allergies or past drug reactions or side effects. Some relative contraindications include: a) severe brain damage, idiopathic parkinsonism and severe epilepsy; b) previous adverse drug reactions to other forms of neuroleptics, e.g. severe akathisia. However, in most cases an individual assessment is warranted. A low test-dose can be given in hospital with careful monitoring and prompt treatment of side effects or any other problems.

Severe renal, cardiac or hepatic disease patients with schizophrenia may require lower doses of the drug, due to impairment of biotransformation or excretion.

The presence of severe affective disorder as well as schizophrenia has, in the past, been considered a contraindication (Ayd, 1974) but more recent work (Knights et al., 1979; Johnson et al., 1983) indicates that severe depression is part of the schizophrenic process and should be treated as such (see also Möller and von Zerssen, in preparation). Indeed, some 25 – 50% of patients with chronic schizophrenia may become depressed in the post-psychotic phase (or in the 6 months following an acute schizophrenic episode or relapse) (Mandel et al., 1982). The recognition of depressive symptoms may reflect the more careful follow-up given to patients on depot preparations.

Quitkin et al. (1975) suggest that depression can occasionally result from too high a dose of neuroleptic. There is anecdotal evidence that some patients who appear to respond to long-acting neuroleptics with depression, may benefit from smaller injections at more frequent intervals. This maintains a sufficient mean plasma level of drug for antipsychotic effect, while reducing the peak plasma level that may cause the adverse response.

Adverse side effects

In the first year or two of treatment, some of the most common side effects will cease with time or reduce in severity due to dose reduction of the long-acting neuroleptic, cessation of oral medication and increase in the interval between injections, among other causes. Hypotension and anticholinergic effects appear to be a problem only in the first few months of treatment. Weight gain can be monitored by dose and interval adjustment and diet (Marriott et al., 1981a). Menstrual disturbance occurs with these preparations, loss of libido is less common. Liver disease and blood dyscrasias are rare. There have been rare reports of epileptic seizures. Minor ECG changes have been reported.

Extrapyramidal side effects (EPS) are the most common. The incidence appears to be 80% in the first 2 years of treatment (Knights et al., 1979). However, at active Depot Neuroleptic Clinics rather than research trials, these side effects could be reduced to 20% (Johnson et al., 1981; Marriott et al., 1981b).

Long-term problems are still being evaluated. The contribution of the long-acting preparations to tardive dyskinesia remains unclear. Our study of 400 outpatients showed an incidence of 10% with a 2.1 ratio of females to males (Marriott et al., 1978). See also Chapter 15, this volume.

To minimize long-term hazards of long-acting neuroleptics, the clinician must aim to reduce and stabilize the dose, then later try to increase the interval between injections. The Australian experience is limited to fluphenazine decanoate (Marriott et al., 1973) and we believe it is possible to increase the interval from 3 to 6 weeks. The choice of the final interval is determined by clinical assessment, in that patients remain in remission.

Treatment of extrapyramidal side effects

This requires a standardized treatment plan. A brief sheet on side effects and how to treat them should be available to outpatients and family. There should be prompt treatment, with emotional support and explanation of what is happening. Tremor, rigidity and bradykinesia and the dystonias respond best to anticholinergic agents such as benztropine. Akathisia or motor restlessness, may take some time to respond to treatment. Later dosage reduction will enable cessation of such oral medication. The antiparkinson drugs should *not* be given prophylactically as they may cause further problems and may contribute to tardive dyskinesia.

Marriott and Hiep (1978) in a retrospective study with two groups of patients (total 69 females) found no difference between the group given antiparkinson drugs prophylactically and those given antiparkinson drugs only when the symptoms justified them.

Relapse rates

Of concern is the reported relapse rate of 20 – 60%, despite medication and intensive psychosocial therapy or support (Hogarty et al., 1979). Marriott et al. (1978, 1981b) found a relapse rate of 19.2% (28 out of 146 outpatients), 53.6% of those readmitted had unofficially increased the intervals between injections. Johnson and colleagues (1983) reported on a stabilized group of 56 chronic schizophrenics on fluphenazine decanoate or flupenthixol decanoate. The relapse rate at the end of an 18 months follow-up was 23.2%. Wiles and colleagues (Wiles and Gelder, 1979; Wistedt et al., 1982) suggest that there may be a critical plasma level of fluphenazine required; the suggestion needs further evaluation.

Pregnancy and long-acting neuroleptics

Most female patients receiving long-acting neuroleptics are in the child-bearing age range. These preparations pass through the placenta, but there have been no indications of harmful effects to the foetus.

The clinician can minimize problems during pregnancy and the puerperium by careful planning. The pregnant woman should be on the lowest possible dose, with maximum intervals between injections, and no additional psychotropic drugs. The psychiatric history will provide information as to whether previous pregnancies have resulted in relapses. Most likely times for relapse are in the last trimester and in the 3 months following the delivery. The majority of patients will relapse if neuroleptics are discontinued. However, the drug will usually be present in the first 3 months of pregnancy since even on cessation of fluphenazine decanoate, the active drug can be detected in the plasma for many weeks in some patients (Wistedt et al., 1982). Of special importance is the woman on high doses of neuroleptic, which will be retained by the neonate from the foetal circulation. The baby should therefore be carefully examined for clinical signs of sedation or side effects such as hyperactivity and hypertonia, which have been reported with chlorpromazine (Hill et al., 1966). Extrapyramidal features require treatment with low doses of antihistamines (e.g. diphenhydramine) or antiparkinsonian drugs.

A specific method was developed for management of women with schizophrenia, mostly chronic, who had become pregnant (Marriott, 1978). Of 203 females attending the clinic, there were 25 pregnancies. Seven (28%) were terminated, there were 8 (32%) spontaneous abortions and 10 (40%) delivered normal infants. Because of a history of previous relapses, all pregnant women continued to receive their injections of fluphenazine decanoate. Of the 10 who had babies, two relapsed in the last month of pregnancy and three within 3 months of the delivery. Only one infant was breast fed, the clinic's policy being to discourage breast feeding under these conditions. Only one baby had side effects, these were hypertonia, irritability and arching of the neck and back. These signs resolved spontaneously within a few days of delivery without the need for further drug treatment.

In summary, the management of the pregnant woman on a long-acting neuroleptic requires continuation of the drug, support and close observation for relapse or not managing the new baby or household duties. If the baby is breast fed, it should be observed for signs of sedation or side effects. Counselling for further contraception is also advised.

SUMMARY AND SOME UNRESOLVED QUESTIONS

Long-acting neuroleptics can reduce the problem of relapse by overcoming, to a large extent, the problem of non-compliance, in patients who suffer from chronic schizophrenia. However, some research groups have questioned whether these preparations and the associated specialized delivery systems have indeed reduced the relapse rate, as compared to oral neuroleptics and the more conventional outpatient therapies.

Some indications for the management of patients have been outlined. Special reference has been made to the pregnant woman who suffers from chronic schizophrenia, since a large proportion of female patients are in the child-bearing age range.

Preliminary work by Wiles and his associates (Wistedt et al., 1982) has suggested critical plasma levels, below which the individual patient relapses.

Two final questions are often asked by patients and relatives. Firstly, how long does one stay on the injections? The current response seems to be at least 3 – 5 years or perhaps for life. The last question relates to the need to identify the patient who can do well without medication.

APPENDIX

THE INTERVIEW PROCEDURE

1. *Before seeing* patient please ensure you have the following: case notes and various treatment cards.
   (a) Please read up these areas in particular to gain information on:
      (i) the diagnosis
      (ii) the treatment plan
      (iii) the drugs last prescribed
      (iv) the time interval since last appointment
      (v) the past medical and psychiatric history
   (b) Focus in particular on the details of the last appointment:
      (i) the treatment given: dose and intervals of fluphenazine decanoate
      (ii) have available the results of investigations ordered
      (iii) is an interpreter needed.
2. At each visit assess the person as an individual and be complete in the evaluation, explaining to the person the aim is to assess their response to treatment. Include these areas:
   (a) present history since last appointment
   (b) changes in life style; change in job; appearance of new stresses or a flare-up of chronic stresses that would lead to the individual being at risk; changes in the family behavioural patterns
   (c) briefly ask about specific systems such as sleep, appetite, bowels, menses, libido, CNS, alcohol and drugs
   (d) at what stage is the illness and what is the change: towards relapse or improvement
   (e) check mental state examination
   (f) evaluation of side effects from information provided by patient, relative or staff
   (g) assessment of the physical state e.g. CNS examination which will aid in evaluation of side effects, e.g. extrapyramidal
   (h) any tests required
   (i) oral medication – whether taken, any side effect problem.
3. Based on the foregoing, formulate a treatment plan and explain it to the patient, and if required, the relatives. Please use these headings:
   (a) Decide whether the person is:
      (1) in remission/relapsing/has chronic features
      (2) has side effects
      (3) is depressed
      (4) has social problems and needs retraining
      (5) needs group or individual supporting therapy

   (6) requires evaluation for other medical problems
  (b) Decide on:
   (1) dose of fluphenazine decanoate/interval between injections/oral medication
   (2) treatment of side effects
   (3) aims of the supportive session
   (4) requires other services in hospital/community
   (5) co-ordination with other medical units/referral.
4. Treatment plan is briefly recorded.
5. Next appointment.

REFERENCES

Ayd, F. J. (1974) Side effects of depot fluphenazines. Compr. Psychiatry 15, 277 – 284.

Ban, T. and Ceskova, E. (1980) Long-acting antipsychotic drugs. Psychopharmacol. Bull. 16, (4), 6 – 13.

Floru, L. (1975) Aspects of long-term treatment with neuroleptics. J. Int. Med. Res. 3, 114 – 123.

Hill, R., Desmond, M. and Kay, T. (1966) Extrapyramidal dysfunction in an infant of a schizophrenic mother. J. Pediatrics 69, 589.

Hogarty, G., Schooler, N., Ulrich, R. et al. (1979) Fluphenazine and social therapy in the aftercare of schizophrenic patients. Arch. Gen. Psychiatry 36, 1283 – 1294.

Johnson, D. A. W., Pasterski, G., Ludlow, J., Street, K. and Taylor, R. (1983) The discontinuance of maintenance neuroleptic therapy in chronic schizophrenic patients: drug and social consequences. Acta Psychiatr. Scand. 67, 339 – 352.

Knights, A., Okasha, M., Salih, M. and Hirsch, S. (1979) Depressive and extrapyramidal symptoms and clinical effects. A trial of fluphenazine versus flupenthixol in maintenance of schizophrenic outpatients. Br. J. Psychiatry 135, 515 – 523.

Lingjaerde, O. (1973) Symposium on depot neuroleptics. Acta Psychiatr. Scand. 246, 9 – 14.

Mandel, M., Severe, M., Schooler, N. et al. (1982) Development and prediction of post-psychotic depression in neuroleptic-treated schizophrenics. Arch. Gen. Psychiatry 39, 197 – 203.

Marriott, P. (1978) A five-year follow-up at a depot phenothiazine clinic. In: F. J. Ayd (Ed.), Depot Fluphenazines: Twelve Years Experience. Ayd Medical Communications, Baltimore. pp. 46 – 71.

Marriott, P. and Hiep, A. (1978) Drug monitoring at an Australian depot phenothiazine clinic. J. Clin. Psychiatry 39, 206 – 212.

Marriott, P., Grigor, J. and Hiep, A. et al. (1973) A psychiatric clinic for depot phenothiazines. Med. J. Aust. 2, 957 – 960.

Marriott, P., Pansa, M. and Hiep, A. (1978) The effect of treatment variables on outcome in schizophrenics receiving depot neuroleptics over two years. Presented at the 11th CINP Congress, Vienna, Austria.

Marriott, P., Pansa, M. and Hiep, A. (1981a) Depot fluphenazine maintenance treatment and associated weight changes. Compr. Psychiatry 22, 320 – 325.

Marriott, P., Pansa, M. and Hiep, A. (1981b) Who likes injections: outcome with depot neuroleptic outpatients: a two-year follow-up. Presented at the Royal Australian and New Zealand College of Psychiatrists' Annual Congress, October 1981, Hong Kong.

Marriott, P., Hiep, A. and Martin, R. (1982) A four-year evaluation of an Australian Depot Neuroleptic Clinic. Br. J. Clin. Soc. Psychiatry 1, 55 – 57.

Möller, H.-J. and von Zerssen, D. (1984) Depression and schizophrenia. In: G. D. Burrows, T. R. Norman and G. Rubinstein (Eds), Handbook of Studies on Schizophrenia. Elsevier Biomedical Press, Amsterdam (in preparation).

Quitkin, F., Rifkin, A. and Klein, D. (1975) Very high dosage vs standard dosage. Fluphenazine in schizophrenics. Arch. Gen. Psychiatry 32, 1276 – 1281.

Wiles, D. and Gelder, M (1979) Plasma fluphenazine levels by radioimmunoassay in schizophrenic patients treated with injections of fluphenazine decanoate. Br. J. Clin. Pharmacol. 8, 565 – 570.
Wistedt, B., Jorgensen, A. and Wiles, D. (1982) A depot neuroleptic withdrawal study. Plasma concentration of fluphenazine and flupenthixol and relapse frequency. Psychopharmacology 78, 301 – 304.

Burrows/Norman/Davies (eds) Antipsychotics

Chapter 15

Tardive dyskinesia: The major problem with antipsychotic maintenance therapy

PHILIP A. BERGER

and

MEREDITH J. DUNN

Norris Mental Health Clinical Research Center, Stanford University School of Medicine, Stanford, CA 94305, U.S.A.

INTRODUCTION

Tardive dyskinesia is the major problem which limits the use of antipsychotic medications as maintenance treatment for patients with psychopathology. The introduction of the first effective antipsychotics in the early 1950's caused a revolution in psychiatric treatment and greatly improved the prognosis for patients with chronic psychotic disorders. Not only do antipsychotic drugs rapidly control acute psychotic symptoms and behavior in a wide variety of psychotic disorders, but the antipsychotics have long-term preventative or ameliorative effects on patients with chronic schizophrenia. However, the antipsychotics are not effective for every patient and can cause the sometimes irreversible disorder of involuntary movement known as tardive dyskinesia (Berger, 1978).

Tardive dyskinesia was first described in the late 1950's and was associated with the prolonged use of antipsychotics in psychiatric patients (Schonecker, 1957; Sigwald et al., 1959). The syndrome was designated 'tardive dyskinesia' to distinguish it from the early-onset extrapyramidal reactions of antipsychotics, and to signify a movement disorder that could manifest itself and persist for years, even after treatment with the precipitating agent had been discontinued (Faurbye et al., 1964; ACNP – FDA Task Force, 1973).

Tardive dyskinesia is a complex neurological syndrome of involuntary hyperkinetic movements. It most often affects the mouth, lips, tongue and jaw (the bucco-linguo-masticatory triad) causing smacking and pursing of the lips, tongue writhing and thrusting, sucking, chewing movements, and tic-like motions of the lips, eyes, eyebrows, and muscles of facial expression. The movements may also involve the limbs or trunk, with axial dystonias, finger and toe movements, shoulder shrugging, pelvic rotations, rocking and swaying, lordosis, or other involuntary choreoathetoid movements. Grunting, difficulty swallowing, and respiratory arrhythmias, have also been reported (Paulson, 1975; Kobayashi, 1976; Baldessarini and Tarsy, 1978; Craig and Richardson, 1982; Faheem et al., 1982).

Anxiety or volitional motor activity usually increases the movements of tardive dyskinesia. Attempts to voluntarily control the dyskinesia often result in increased movements, particularly in muscle groups on which the patient's attention is not focused. The movements of tardive dyskinesia tend to lessen with relaxation or sedation, and disappear in sleep (Berger and Rexroth, 1980a).

Tardive dyskinesia is of increasing concern to psychiatrists, physicians in other specialities, and to the public. In the United States, a one million dollar malpractice award given to a patient with tardive dyskinesia has further alarmed physicians (Fieger, 1983). The syndrome is therefore posing complex ethical and legal dilemmas for physicians and patients. More important than the legal dilemmas posed by tardive dyskinesia is the handicap for individual patients caused by this disorder.

The symptoms of tardive dyskinesia can be socially embarrassing. They can also cause significant disability, sometimes interfering with speech, eating, dexterity, and respiration. Aspiration pneumonitis is a rare complication (Kobayashi, 1977). Tardive dyskinesia may reduce life expectancy (Mehta et al., 1978). Because of its resistance to the available treatments, non-remitting tardive dyskinesia has made physicians re-evaluate the use of antipsychotic treatment in psychiatric patients. Several recent comprehensive reviews have discussed the clinical phenomenology, prevalence, pathophysiology, and experimental treatment of this disorder (Baldessarini et al., 1980; Berger and Rexroth, 1980b; Crane and Smith, 1980; Gardos and Cole, 1980; Klawans et al., 1980; Kane and Smith, 1982).

SUBTYPES OF TARDIVE DYSKINESIA

There are several suggestions in the literature for possible ways to subtype tardive dyskinesia. Tardive dyskinesia which is obvious while the patient is being treated with antipsychotics is called 'overt' tardive dyskinesia. Patient whose symptoms only appear when antipsychotics are withdrawn are said to have 'covert' tardive dyskinesia.

An important division can be made between tardive dyskinesia which persists after antipsychotic medications have been discontinued and tardive dyskinesia which spontaneously remits. These categories have been called 'irreversible' and 'reversible' tardive dyskinesia but these terms are misleading. Since there are no effective treatments for tardive dyskinesia, the syndrome is not reversed. Thus, a division into 'persistent' or 'non-remitting' tardive dyskinesia and 'remitting' tardive dyskinesia is probably more appropriate. When tardive dyskinesia spontaneously remits, the remission usually takes place during the first 3 months after antipsychotic medications are withdrawn. Thus, patients whose tardive dyskinesia continues beyond 3 months after antipsychotics are discontinued are thought to have the non-remitting type of this disorder.

For the majority of patients with tardive dyskinesia the distinction between remitting and non-remitting forms of the disorder is a useful one. However, there are exceptions. Longitudinal studies of patients with remitting tardive dyskinesia have demonstrated that some patients have a recurrence of symptoms from 3 to 7 years after antipsychotic discontinuation (Wegner and Kane, 1982). Most of these patients have a recurrence while being treated with antipsychotics. In addition, some patients with non-remitting tardive dyskinesia may become symptom-free at a later time whether on or off antipsychotics (Berger and Rexroth, 1980b). Despite these occasional unusual cases, the distinction between remitting and non-remitting tardive dyskinesia has proved to be a useful one for both the clinician and researcher (Berger and Rexroth, 1980a).

A third method for subtyping tardive dyskinesia is based on its response to pharmacological agents which alter brain dopamine and acetylcholine activity. Classical tardive dyskinesia is the pharmacological mirror-image of Parkinson's disease and of the extrapyramidal reactions caused by antipsychotics. Parkinson's disease is improved by dopamine agonists and by anticholinergics, and exacerbated by dopamine antagonists and cholinomimetics. Classical tardive dyskinesia is suppressed by dopamine antagonists and by cholinomimetics and generally worsened by dopamine agonists and anticholinergic agents (Moore and Bowers, 1980).

However, some patients with tardive dyskinesia have atypical responses to these drugs and may exhibit improvement with dopamine agonists or anticholinergics as do patients with Parkinson's disease (Casey and Denny, 1977). Some investigators have proposed that these different pharmacological responses should be considered two pharmacological subtypes of tardive dyskinesia. Other investigators suggest that only patients who improve with cholinomimetics and dopamine antagonists should be classified as having tardive dyskinesia, while patients with the opposite pharmacological response are more appropriately considered to have a variant of parkinsonian or extrapyramidal symptoms. Perhaps a compromise would be to consider tardive dyskinesia patients whose pharmacological response is the mirror-image of Parkinson's disease to have classical tardive dyskinesia, while those whose responses are parallel to Parkinson's disease have atypical tardive dyskinesia (Berger and Rexroth, 1980b).

PREVALENCE AND RISK FACTORS

An accurate determination of the prevalence of tardive dyskinesia is difficult because of differences in the methods of diagnosis and assessment used by various investigators. A review of the literature yields reports of prevalence ranging from 0.5 to 56%, with an average reported prevalence of 15 – 20% in institutionalized patients (Berger and Rexroth, 1980b; Kane and Smith, 1982). A study by Smith et al. (1979) undertook a systematic investigation of the distribution of tardive dyskinesia in 293 psychiatric inpatients using the Abnormal Involuntary Movement Scale (AIMS) developed by the Psychopharmacology Research Branch of the NIMH. Thirty percent of the patients examined in the study had symptoms of tardive dyskinesia which could be rated as at least moderate ($\geqslant 3$) on the AIMS. Among children given neuroleptics for childhood schizophrenia, autism, and behavioral disorders in the mentally retarded, prevalence of tardive dyskinesia has been suggested to range from 20 to 40% (Caine et al., 1978).

The prevalence of tardive dyskinesia seems to be increasing. Baldessarini (1974) obtained a mean prevalence of 15% from 25 publications covering 28,000 patients. Kane and Smith (1982) reviewed 56 studies from 1959 to 1979 involving a total of 34,555 patients. They report a mean prevalence of 20%. The average prevalence for the 23 studies reported between 1960 and 1969 was 14.6%, while the prevalence for the 33 studies reported between 1970 and 1979 was 23.9%. Jeste and Wyatt (1981) also conclude that the prevalence of tardive dyskinesia is increasing. They report that 11 studies published between 1976 and 1980 report a prevalence of 25.7%.

The apparent increase in the prevalence of tardive dyskinesia has several possible explanations. Some of the increase could be due to increased awareness of the condition. In earlier years, tardive dyskinesia may have been underdiagnosed, while it may be overdiagnosed now as a result of the increased publicity that the syndrome has recently received. A true increase in prevalence could be due to persistent or non-remitting cases of tardive dyskinesia. If the incidence of the disorder remained stable, the prevalence would increase since an increasing number of patients has been exposed to antipsychotics each year since they were introduced. Higher doses of medication may have been used in recent years and new classes of antipsychotics have been introduced, some of which have higher potency and are more selective at blocking dopamine receptors. The clinically equivalent doses of these newer antipsychotics are not well-established and a trend towards greater exposure to antipsychotic medication is more likely with agents of increasing potency (Kane and Smith, 1982).

There are two important qualifications to this apparent increase in the prevalence of tardive dyskinesia that should be considered. First, the prevalence of tardive dyskinesia is not synonymous with the prevalence of non-remitting tardive dyskinesia. Many patients with tardive dyskinesia spontaneously recover during the first 6 weeks to 3 months after antipsychotic medications are withdrawn. Clearly, this remitting form of tardive dyskinesia is less of a public health problem. The important question is whether the prevalence of non-remitting tardive dyskinesia is increasing. This question cannot be answered from available data.

Second, the prevalence of tardive dyskinesia reported in recent reviews has not been corrected for the prevalence of spontaneous orofacial dyskinesia. This syndrome is indistinguishable from tardive dyskinesia but occurs in patients who have not taken antipsychotics (Altrocchi, 1972). Some studies indicate that 1 – 2% of tardive dyskinesia is actually spontaneous dyskinesia; other studies suggest that as many as 10 – 20% of all patients in mental institutions, nursing home residents, and the elderly may suffer from spontaneous dyskinesia (Greenblatt et al., 1968; Degwitz, 1969). Spontaneous dyskinesia may be even more common among schizophrenic patients. In a survey of 411 hospitalized patients with chronic schizophrenia, spontaneous involuntary movement disorders were found in 47 patients who had never been exposed to antipsychotic medication (Cunningham Owens et al., 1982). Kane and Smith (1982) summarizing 19 investigations involving 11,000 psychiatric patients who had not been treated with antipsychotics, reported the prevalence of spontaneous orofacial dyskinesia to be 5%. Assuming that the uncorrected prevalence for tardive dyskinesia is approximately 20%, a prevalence figure corrected for spontaneous dyskinesia would be 15%.

Spontaneous orofacial dyskinesia may be the correct diagnosis for those patients presenting with the symptoms of tardive dyskinesia, but who are without any history of drug exposure or who only have a history of having taken tricyclic antidepressants, antihistamines, anticholinergics, and other non-antipsychotic medications (Berger and Rexroth, 1980b).

The identification of patients at high risk for developing tardive dyskinesia would be of tremendous benefit in the determination of the appropriate pharmacological approach to patients with schizophrenia. However, the search for specific factors that might cause only certain patients receiving antipsychotics to develop tardive dyskinesia has proven to be difficult. It is even difficult to demonstrate that the risk of tardive dyskinesia increases with increasing exposure to antipsychotic drugs. Attempts to identify a dose-response curve for tardive dyskinesia are complicated by the relative infrequency of the disorder, the retrospective nature of the available data, and the inherent methodological problems in evaluating the pharmacological data. A retrospective evaluation of varying compliance rates as well as possible individual differences in absorption and metabolism of antipsychotics is almost impossible.

Kane and Smith (1982), in a review of the literature of 18 studies exploring the relationship between the prevalence of tardive dyskinesia and cumulative drug dose, find only four studies that report a significant positive relationship. The four studies that did report a positive relationship involved samples of patients with relatively low cumulative drug exposure. Thus, for those patients vulnerable to tardive dyskinesia, a dose-response relationship may occur at a relatively low cumulative dose, while for patients without the underlying vulnerability, cumulative dosage beyond this range may not lead to increases in the risk for tardive dyskinesia.

The relationship between length of exposure to antipsychotics and prevalence of tardive dyskinesia has the same intuitive appeal as the relationship between cumulative dose and prevalence but is also as difficult to demonstrate. Of 21 investigations, only six found increasing length of exposure to be a significant risk factor for tardive dyskinesia (Kane and Smith, 1982). Two of these investigations involve samples with only relatively brief exposure. Several investigations suggest that a substantial percentage of patients who develop tardive dyskinesia have their first symptoms within 3 years of their first exposure to antipsychotics. While it is always assumed that tardive dyskinesia will become more severe or persistent with continued exposure to antipsychotics, this assumption has not been proven and there are reports which suggest that tardive dyskinesia can remit even when a stable dose of antipsychotics is continued (Berger and Rexroth, 1980a). Thus, there may be a period of maximum risk for development of tardive dyskinesia that occurs with relatively brief exposure in patients who are vulnerable. Patients without this vulnerability may be able to receive antipsychotics for extended periods without increasing their risk of developing tardive dyskinesia.

The association between the prevalence of tardive dyskinesia and age is more firmly established (Baldessarini et al., 1980). Of 20 studies with adequate age distributions, 13 reports found a statistically significant relationship between the prevalence of tardive dyskinesia and age (Kane and Smith, 1982). This increase in prevalence with age might reflect the non-remitting character of tardive dyskinesia among older individuals. The recent investigation by Smith and Baldessarini (1980) reports a strong correlation between age and severity of tardive dyskinesia and a strong inverse correlation between age and the rate of spontaneous remission of tardive dyskinesia. Both of these factors could contribute to the higher prevalence rates of tardive dyskinesia in groups of elderly patients even if incidence was not affected by age.

Kane and Smith (1982) summarize the relative prevalence of tardive dyskinesia in men and women. These data from 31 publications include 33 groups comprising a total of more than 15,000 patients. In 29 of the 33 samples, the prevalence of tardive dyskinesia was higher in the female sample than in the male sample. The average unweighted ratio of female-to-male prevalence for the 31 samples in which this value could be computed was 1.68 to 1. Another general trend in this investigation was for the ratio of female to male prevalence to increase as the criterion used to define tardive dyskinesia became more severe. Thus, it appears that women have a somewhat higher overall prevalence of tardive dyskinesia than men, and that the more severe forms of the disorder are more likely to develop in women.

The search for a correlation between drug type and tardive dyskinesia has met with mixed success. Tardive dyskinesia usually occurs after several years of antipsychotic treatment, although onset within the first 6 months of treatment has been reported. The phenothiazines and butyrophenones have most often been associated with tardive dyskinesia and long-acting fluphenazine has been reported to be both less liable (Ayd, 1973) and more liable (Gardos et al., 1977) to cause tardive dyskinesia; but all classes of antipsychotics seem to be capable of producing the movement disorder. Cases of tardive dyskinesia have also occasionally been reported following the use of anticholinergics (Birket-Smith, 1974), antihistamines (Davis, 1976), large doses of tricyclic antidepressants (Fann et al., 1976), amphetamines (Mattson and Calverley, 1968), and the anticonvulsant phenytoin (Chadwick et al., 1976). However, as described above, tardive dyskinesia-like syndromes unrelated to the use of antipsychotics may represent spontaneous orofacial dyskinesia and there is no convincing evidence that medications other than the antipsychotics can cause tardive dyskinesia (Berger and Rexroth, 1980a).

All antipsychotic drugs currently marketed in the United States and the antidepressant amoxapine which has antipsychotic activity have been reported to cause tardive dyskinesia. The effort to relate the relative risk of tardive dyskinesia to a specific antipsychotic is encumbered by the unreliability of drug histories and the fact that most chronically ill psychiatric patients have received more than one antipsychotic agent. Thus, there is little evidence to implicate specific drugs or drug classes in the development of tardive dyskinesia. Clearly, if one drug was associated with an increased risk it would be difficult to determine this fact even if the effect was large because of the inherent methodological difficulties. A related question is the relative risk of specific drugs or drug classes in their likelihood of worsening or converting a remitting tardive dyskinesia to a non-remitting condition. Unfortunately, there are no well-designed studies which have been able to answer this question (Berger and Rexroth, 1980b; Kane and Smith, 1982).

Another intuitively appealing hypothesis which relates to a possible risk factor in tardive dyskinesia is the suggestion that drug holidays or intermittent treatment with antipsychotics would decrease the risk for tardive dyskinesia. Jeste et al. (1979) took 21 hospitalized tardive dyskinesia patients and discontinued their antipsychotic medication. After 3 months without medication, 12 patients were found to have no dyskinetic movements. The dyskinetic symptoms persisted in the other nine patients. The patients with non-remitting tardive dyskinesia were then compared to those with remitting tardive dyskinesia in an attempt to find discriminating factors between the two groups. An analysis of variance showed no significant differences in age, sex, diagnosis, localization of dyskinetic symptoms, amount or type of antipsychotics given, EEG abnormalities, severity of psychopathology, severity of dyskinesia, or presence of parkinsonian symptoms. The group of patients with non-remitting dyskinesia were found to have a history of significantly longer antipsychotic treatment as well as a significantly greater number of drug-free intervals of at least 2 months duration. Significant differences were also found in the total percent of drug-free time since initiation of antipsychotic therapy, in the duration of the tardive dyskinesia, and in the duration of psychiatric illness. A step-wise discriminant function analysis showed clear separation of the two patient groups, with the best discriminating factor being the number of drug-free intervals; this variable alone correctly separated 76% of the dyskinetic cases into non-remitting or remitting (Jeste et al., 1979).

Crane (1974) examined the relationship between continuity of treatment and ratings for tardive dyskinesia. He measured continuity of treatment as the percentage of time exposed to drug from the beginning of treatment to the time of the investigation. Continuity of treatment did not correlate with ratings for tardive dyskinesia. However, continuity of treatment was significantly correlated with maximum dose, prescribed for at least 6 months, and the duration of antipsychotic treatment.

Thus, at the present time, there is insufficient evidence to either recommend drug holidays or continuous drug treatment. On the one hand, drug-free intervals may be helpful in identifying patients whose tardive dyskinesia is masked by antipsychotics. On the other hand, the drug-free intervals may increase or decrease the risk of tardive dyskinesia and may increase or decrease the risk of a non-remitting form of tardive dyskinesia. Obviously this is an area which urgently requires investigation because it has practical implications for how patients should be treated with antipsychotics.

There are a number of other factors which have been suggested to increase or decrease the risk of tardive dyskinesia based on plausible hypotheses. Unfortunately, the literature is confusing and contradictory and there is not enough evidence to evaluate the effect of these variables on the risk of developing tardive dyskinesia. Electroconvulsive therapy has been suggested to put patients at greater risk for tardive dyskinesia (Gardos et al., 1977). However, a review of the literature shows little controlled evidence to support this conclusion. A number of investigators have suggested that patients with organic brain disease are more likely to develop tardive dyskinesia if treated with antipsychotics. However, this assumption has been challenged by other investigators (Smith et al., 1979). At present, organic brain dysfunction or disease cannot be considered an established risk factor for tardive dyskinesia.

Several investigators have suggested that patients with a greater sensitivity to extrapyramidal side effects early in their treatment with antipsychotics are more likely to develop tardive dyskinesia. Despite this frequent suggestion, there is only one study in the literature which investigates this question. In a sample of more than 300 patients, previous history of antipsychotic-induced extrapyramidal reactions was the same in patients with and without tardive dyskinesia (Jus et al., 1976). Thus, one cannot conclude that patients with a greater sensitivity to extrapyramidal reactions are more likely to develop tardive dyskinesia.

Several investigators have speculated that the use of anticholinergic antiparkinsonian medications might increase the risk of tardive dyskinesia. This speculation may be based on the reciprocal pharmacological relationship between Parkinson's disease and tardive dyskinesia. Unfortunately, there is little evidence to substantiate the proposed relationship between anticholinergic drug use and tardive dyskinesia. In 13 of 18 investigations, use of antiparkinsonian anticholinergic drugs was not significantly related to the development of tardive dyskinesia (Kane and Smith, 1982).

The use of multiple antipsychotic agents known as 'polypharmacy' in the same patient has been suggested to be a risk factor for tardive dyskinesia. The four controlled investigations which have examined the possible role of polypharmacy in tardive dyskinesia have been unable to demonstrate an association between antipsychotic polypharmacy and an increased risk for tardive dyskinesia (Kane and Smith, 1982). Several anecdotal reports have suggested that patients with affective illness may be more likely to develop tardive dyskinesia than patients with schizophrenia. However, since no controlled investigations have been carried out, one cannot conclude that patients with affective disorders are more likely to develop tardive dyskinesia if treated with antipsychotics (Berger and Rexroth, 1980a).

Using a different approach to the investigation of risk factors for tardive dyskinesia, Wegner and colleagues (1977) found an unusually high prevalence of the rare B-mitten EEG dysrhythmia; 10 of the 11 patients with tardive dyskinesia studied exhibited the B-mitten pattern. A subsequent study compared 21 tardive dyskinesia patients with controls matched for age, sex, diagnosis, cumulative antipsychotic exposure, and maximum antipsychotic dose; 92.5% of the tardive dyskinesia patients were found to have the B-mitten EEG dysrhythmia, as compared to 33.3% of the controls (Wegner et al., 1979). Wegner et al. (1979) suggest that the subcortical B-mitten dysrhythmia may indicate a pre-existing structural or functional vulnerability of the nigrostriatal system to antipsychotic-induced dysregulation; the dysregulation is then sufficient to cause the symptoms of tardive dyskinesia. This provocative hypothesis will obviously require further study.

DIFFERENTIAL DIAGNOSIS OF TARDIVE DYSKINESIA

Tardive dyskinesia must be differentiated from other similar involuntary movement disorders. Spontaneous orofacial dyskinesia as described earlier is clinically indistinguishable from antipsychotic-induced tardive dyskinesia (Altrocchi, 1972). Spontaneous orofacial dyskinesia is common among psychiatric patients and other elderly institutional or nursing home residents who have no history of antipsychotic drug use. The prevalence of spontaneous orofacial dyskinesia increases with age, is more common among patients with dementia or other significant neurological findings, but occasionally occurs in elderly subjects without neurological or psychological disorders. In a recent review of epidemiological studies of untreated psychiatric patients, the mean prevalence in 11,000 patients was reported to be 5% (Kane and Smith, 1982). In samples of patients treated with antipsychotics, the presence of tardive dyskinesia includes the sum of patients with spontaneous orofacial dyskinesia and patients with antipsychotic-induced tardive dyskinesia.

Another movement disorder which frequently affects the oral musculature and which can cause tremor, chorea, and torticollis is orofaciocervical dystonia (OFCD), or the Meige syndrome (Glazer et al., 1983). The syndrome was first described in 1910 by Henri Meige (1910) and more recently was given the eponym Brueghel's syndrome by Marsden (1976). The Meige syndrome is currently considered a variant of idiopathic, adult onset torsion dystonia. The syndrome is distinguished from other facial spasms or tics by an unusual bilateral symmetric distribution of spasms with a predominantly median focus.

Meige symptoms can occur without a specific cause, in combination with a well-defined neurological disorder, and in patients with levodopa- and antipsychotic-induced dyskinesias (Tolosa, 1979). More recent reports suggest that the Meige syndrome and other dystonias can be produced or at least precipitated by antipsychotics (Burke et al., 1982). Some physicians use the term Meige syndrome as a synonym for spontaneous orofacial dyskinesia. Others suggest that the movements of tardive dyskinesia or spontaneous orofacial dyskinesia are more rapid and therefore are more appropriately called choreiform movements or dyskinesias rather than dystonias. For most patients with tardive dyskinesia, the individual movements last much less than 5 seconds. Patients with Meige syndrome or other idiopathic dystonias usually have movements that are sustained for 5 seconds or longer (Glazer et al., 1983). Since both tardive dyskinesia and Meige syndrome can occur following antipsychotic treatment or spontaneously, differentiating tardive dyskinesia, spontaneous orofacial dyskinesia and idiopathic Meige syndrome from antipsychotic-induced Meige syndrome is virtually impossible in patients who have received antipsychotics.

Other dystonias can often be more easily distinguished from tardive dyskinesia or tardive dystonia. The dystonias are a diverse group of neurological states with sustained involuntary twisting movements affecting muscle groups in the limbs, trunk, neck or face. Dystonia musculorum deformans is frequently hereditary and can be distinguished from tardive dyskinesia by a careful history. Secondary dystonias can be produced by numerous neurological disorders, several classes of medications, and certain toxins. These disorders are not likely to be confused with tardive dyskinesia because of the history of the primary precipitating factor.

Patients with Parkinson's disease who are being treated with high doses of levodopa may develop symptoms exactly like those of tardive dyskinesia. Levodopa dyskinesia tends to show increased oral preponderance with age, while tardive dyskinesia gets worse with age without any change in symptom distribution (Gerlach, 1977). The clear association with levodopa therapy obviates any problems in differential diagnosis, but the close similarity between tardive dyskinesia and levodopa dyskinesia is interesting and may be helpful in understanding the pathophysiology of tardive dyskinesia.

Mixed syndromes of parkinsonian side effects or extrapyramidal reactions and tardive dyskinesia can occur in schizophrenic patients who are taking antipsychotics. In a single case report, a patient with such a mixed presentation was given the cholinomimetic physostigmine; his tardive dyskinesia improved and his parkinsonian symptoms increased. The patient was then given anticholinergic agents; these had the opposite effect, improving his extrapyramidal reactions while exacerbating his tardive dyskinesia (DeFraites et al., 1977).

An investigation by Wolf et al. (1983) suggests that patients with tardive dyskinesia who continue to receive antipsychotics have more extrapyramidal reactions than patients without tardive dyskinesia. In this study, a positive correlation was reported between the severity of tardive dyskinesia ratings and the severity of ratings of extrapyramidal reactions. This suggests that patients with tardive dyskinesia should also be evaluated for extrapyramidal reactions.

Some elderly patients have an acute dystonic reaction to antipsychotic treatment; this may be combined with the classical signs of tardive dyskinesia. This so-called Pisa syndrome is characterized by rotation and flexion of the upper trunk, neck, and head to one side. It is improved with anticholinergic treatment and reversible with discontinuation of antipsychotic therapy. Both the clinical manifestations of the Pisa syndrome and its pharmacological response make it easily distinguishable from tardive dyskinesia (Ekbom et al., 1972).

In pure form, Huntington's chorea can be distinguished from tardive dyskinesia on the basis of family history and by noting progressive dementia with no neuroleptic history. Many patients with Huntington's disease are taking antipsychotics, however, and there are many cases for which no reliable family history is available. In such situations, the differential diagnosis of Huntington's chorea from tardive dyskinesia can be difficult to make with certainty (Buxton, 1976).

A more easily distinguishable movement disorder is the 'rabbit syndrome'. This is a late-onset antipsychotic-induced extrapyramidal syndrome which is characterized by rhythmic involuntary movements (5.0 – 5.5/sec) of the masticatory musculature, resembling the chewing movements of a rabbit (Weiss et al., 1980). Unlike tardive dyskinesia, the rabbit syndrome responds to anticholinergic medications and readily reverses when antipsychotics are discontinued (Souner and DiMascio, 1977). The rabbit syndrome is also differentiated by its persistence in Stage I NREM sleep (Villeneuve et al., 1973); tardive dyskinesia disappears in sleep.

The symptoms of tardive dyskinesia must also be distinguished from the abnormal, repetitive movements which are part of the schizophrenic syndrome. In 1907, Kraepelin observed a 'type of convulsive movement, involving the muscles of the eye and speech, which is both characteristic and of frequent occurrence in dementia praecox . . . There may be associated with them smacking of the lips, clucking the tongue, sudden grunting, sniffing, and coughing. Furthermore, in the lips we observe very rapid rhythmical movements. More often there exists a peculiar choreiform movement of the mouth which may be described as an athetoid ataxia' (Kraepelin, 1907).

In a 1911 description of schizophrenia, Bleuler noted 'grimaces of all kinds, peculiar ways of shrugging the shoulder, extraordinary movements of the tongue and lips' (Bleuler, 1950). These early reports of unmedicated schizophrenics show that the movement disorders or 'stereotypies' of schizophrenia itself can closely resemble antipsychotic-induced tardive dyskinesia.

Choreas and choreoathetoses have multiple causes and can sometimes have symptoms which overlap with the symptoms of tardive dyskinesia. Hereditary choreas, drug-induced choreas from oral contraceptives, and phenytoin, and choreas due to CNS toxicity have been reported with choreiform symptoms of the trunk and limbs which are similar to the movements of some patients with tardive dyskinesia. Chorea gravidarum occurs in 1 of every 2,000 to 3,000 pregnancies and can occasionally resemble the movements of tardive dyskinesia. Endocrine and infectious choreas have also been reported to have symptoms similar to those observed in both Huntington's disease and tardive dyskinesia (Granacher, 1981).

Finally, any standard textbook of neurology includes a long list of other conditions which can be associated with choreoathetoid movement disorders. Certain infectious, vascular, neoplastic, toxic (heavy metals), degenerative, and metabolic disorders can all present with choreiform movements. These conditions are distinguished from tardive dyskinesia by the presence of the other symptoms of the primary disorder.

THE PATHOPHYSIOLOGY OF TARDIVE DYSKINESIA

Tardive dyskinesia is hypothesized to result from an increased responsiveness or supersensitivity of dopamine receptor sites induced by long-term antipsychotic blockade (Klawans, 1973). Antipsychotics are proposed to improve schizophrenic symptoms by blocking certain dopamine receptors in the mesolimbic-mesocortical pathway in the central nervous system (Carlsson and Lindquist, 1963). It is possible that the antipsychotic dopamine receptor blockade produces a 'chemical denervation' of the dopamine receptors in the nigrostriatal pathway; prolonged chemical denervation may in turn produce a denervation supersensitivity of striatal dopamine receptors, such that any dopamine reaching the receptors causes an abnormal and increased response from the dopamine neurons. This functional dopaminergic overactivity leads to an imbalance between dopamine and acetylcholine in the nigrostriatum, which manifests itself in the symptoms of tardive dyskinesia (Klawans, 1973; Davis and Berger, 1978; Gerlach et al., 1974).

A balance of dopaminergic and cholinergic influence on the striatum has been demonstrated to be necessary for the normal functioning of the striatum and for the maintenance of normal movement and behavior (Klawans, 1973). While Parkinson's disease is thought to result from an abnormal cholinergic dominance in the striatum, hyperkinetic, stereotyped movements like those of tardive dyskinesia have generally been related to relative dopaminergic dominance, based upon either dopaminergic hyperfunction or cholinergic hypofunction. The general exacerbation of tardive dyskinesia by anticholinergic antiparkinsonian medications and the dopamine precursor levodopa leading respectively to decreased cholinergic and increased dopaminergic activity, provides evidence for a state of dopaminergic dominance in tardive dyskinesia (Klawans, 1973; Davis and Berger, 1978).

The hypothesis of denervation supersensitivity in the nigrostriatal dopamine tracts stems from a well-documented analogous phenomenon in peripheral receptor sites and receives support from a number of animal studies (Klawans, 1973). Several studies find that the chronic administration of antipsychotics to animals, followed by discontinuation of the medication, produced enhanced behavioral sensitivity to dopamine agonists such as apomorphine or methylphenidate (Tarsy and Baldessarini, 1973; Davis et al., 1978). In another study, rats with unilateral striatal lesions, when treated with haloperidol for 6 days, showed an increased turning response to apomorphine (Sayers and Burki, 1976). Chronic exposure of animals to antipsychotics is reported to lead to a prolonged requirement for increased doses of the same agent or another, dissimilar antipsychotic agent to block the behavioral effects of the dopamine agonist apomorphine (Asper et al., 1973). These findings are consistent with the development of dopamine receptor supersensitivity.

An increase in striatal dopamine receptor sites or affinity, as demonstrated by enhanced binding of tritiated spiroperidol, has also been observed following chronic administration of antipsychotics to animals (Burt et al., 1977). The increase in striatal binding affinity correlates well with the degree of behavioral supersensitivity to apomorphine observed in the same animals (Snyder et al., 1977).

A study presents animal data indicating that the initial behavioral and biochemical evidence for striatal dopamine receptor blockade by trifluoperazine disappears within a few weeks of initiating drug administration (Clow et al., 1979). Apomorphine-induced stereotypy is initially antagonized by trifluoperazine, but returns to control levels within 3 months of antipsychotic treatment; within 6 months of treatment, the antipsychotic-treated animals show an enhanced response to apomorphine. Changes in receptor affinity parallel the behavioral changes. There is a reduction in affinity after one month of antipsychotic treatment, followed by a tendency for increased receptor affinity with no obvious change in the number of binding sites appearing within 6 months of antipsychotic administration.

Another study found that chronic treatment with haloperidol, chlorpromazine, and loxapine, but not with clozapine, potentiated apomorphine-induced stereotypies in rats (Burki et al., 1976). Clozapine also did not produce the increased striatal levels of the dopamine metabolite homovanillic acid that had been noted after treatment with the other neuroleptics. These interesting results led to the suggestion that clozapine, an antipsychotic with high affinity for brain muscarinic cholinergic receptors, may not cause tardive dyskinesia (Burki et al., 1976).

Antipsychotics increase spinal fluid homovanillic acid presumably because they block dopamine receptors and increase dopamine turnover (Carlsson and Lindquist,

1963). The investigation of possible abnormalities in the dopamine metabolism of tardive dyskinesia patients also includes measurements of cerebrospinal fluid (CSF) levels of homovanillic acid in tardive dyskinesia, but with variable results (Gerlach et al., 1975a). One study reports reduced dopamine turnover in tardive dyskinesia (Chase, 1974). Still another preliminary study reported elevated homovanillic acid concentrations in tardive dyskinesia patients (Tarsy and Baldessarini, 1976). Nagao et al. (1979) measured CSF levels of homovanillic acid, 3-methoxy-4-hydroxyphenylglycol, and 5-hydroxyindoleacetic acid, the major metabolites of dopamine, norepinephrine, and 5-hydroxytryptamine (serotonin), as well as cyclic 3′,5′-adenosine monophosphate (cyclic AMP) and cyclic 3′,5′-guanosine monophosphate (cyclic GMP); they found no differences between tardive dyskinesia patients and a control group. They suggest that their inability to find differences may be due to the use of older, chronic schizophrenics with long antipsychotic histories as a control group; they report that homovanillic acid levels in both tardive dyskinesia patients and chronic antipsychotic-treated schizophrenics are higher than in normal volunteers, and suggest that the high levels of homovanillic acid in the schizophrenic controls may be related to some kind of pre-tardive dyskinesia state.

It has been suggested that the prolonged and often irreversible course of tardive dyskinesia is more consistent with permanent structural alterations of the brain than with the purely pharmacological state of chemical denervation supersensitivity. However, neuropathological studies in laboratory animals following antipsychotic administration and post-mortem studies of tardive dyskinesia patients have been unable to demonstrate consistent pathological changes in the brain (Baldessarini and Tarsy, 1976). Christensen and colleagues (1970) reported cell degeneration in 27 of 28 brains from dyskinetic patients as compared to only 7 of 28 controls matched for sex, age, and diagnosis; however, other investigators have not been able to confirm these findings. Computerized axial tomography (CAT) scans were made of the brains of tardive dyskinesia patients; essentially normal results were seen, with no caudate atrophy (Gelenberg, 1976).

Thus, a supersensitivity of dopamine receptors in the striatum in an attempt to compensate for post-synaptic blockade by antipsychotics is a plausible hypothesis for the neurochemical basis of tardive dyskinesia. The evidence for this hypothesis comes from the pharmacological responses of patients with tardive dyskinesia and from animal investigations of dopamine and acetylcholine interactions after antipsychotic administration. While the evidence is suggestive, the dopamine supersensitivity hypothesis of tardive dyskinesia does not explain the differential vulnerability of patients to the disorder, nor does it explain paradoxical pharmacological responses to dopaminergic and anticholinergic medications seen in patients with atypical tardive dyskinesia.

Furthermore, the dopamine supersensitivity hypothesis has not yet been confirmed by direct examination of dopamine receptor activity in patients with tardive dyskinesia and normal controls. Whilst such investigations may have been unthinkable in the past, they may now be possible using positron emission transaxial tomography (PETT). Spiperone which binds to dopamine receptors has been used in preliminary PETT scans of normal controls and patients with Parkinson's disease. These preliminary scans suggest that receptor differences in striatal dopamine receptors can be visualized using this technique and that tardive dyskinesia patients should be studied. PETT scan studies may provide evidence that cortical dopamine neurons are involved in tardive dyskinesia.

A recent case report describes a patient with a cerebral infarct in the region of the left motor cortex. This patient subsequently developed unilateral tardive dyskinesia suggesting that his infarct in the left motor cortex provided unilateral immunity to the involuntary movements of tardive dyskinesia. This single case suggests that in addition to striatal neurons, cortical neurons may also be involved in the pathophysiology of tardive dyskinesia (Mcentee and Newman, 1981).

THE PHARMACOLOGY AND EXPERIMENTAL TREATMENT OF TARDIVE DYSKINESIA

The literature on tardive dyskinesia is filled with reports of effective treatments which have not been confirmed by subsequent investigations. Methodological problems abound in the assessment of pharmacological treatments for this disorder. The spontaneous improvement seen in many tardive dyskinesia patients is often not taken into account in study designs (Berger and Rexroth, 1980a). Tardive dyskinesia patients who have been antipsychotic-free for years occasionally show a slow improvement in their symptoms; early signs of tardive dyskinesia often completely remit. Thus, positive effects attributed to the experimental treatment may actually be manifestations of the natural progression of the disorder. In order to control for the possibility of a slow improvement process, protocols should be designed with a placebo period following as well as preceding the period of drug administration. Protocols which compare movement frequency at the end of investigational drug treatment with a preceding baseline or placebo period, and not a subsequent placebo period, bias toward finding a positive drug effect (Davis et al., 1979).

Other methodological problems in the evaluation of treatments for tardive dyskinesia include the difficulty in making an initial diagnosis. Since there are no laboratory tests to validate or refute the diagnosis of tardive dyskinesia, the clinical history and physical examination must be reliable. Another problem comes from the initial enthusiasm for any new treatment. When a new treatment is introduced, initial reports are usually highly encouraging. Gradually unfavorable results are reported. Unfortunately, there is a general tendency for the scientific literature to report initial positive results more frequently than subsequent studies which fail to replicate the initial findings (Jeste and Wyatt, 1982).

As described earlier in this chapter, classical tardive dyskinesia is the pharmacological mirror-image of Parkinson's disease. Patients with tardive dyskinesia have their symptoms suppressed by antipsychotics and by cholinomimetics. This pattern of pharmacological response has led to the suggestion that tardive dyskinesia reflects a relative dopaminergic predominance over cholinergic activity in nigrostriatal dopamine neurons. Nigrostriatal dopamine neurons can be inhibited by cholinomimetics and by agents which increase the activity of the neurotransmitter gamma-aminobutyric acid (GABA) in the CNS. Thus, three important strategies for the experimental treatment of tardive dyskinesia reflect this general pharmacological characterization of the disorder. Experimental treatments for tardive dyskinesia include dopamine antagonists, cholinomimetics, and putative GABA-ergic drugs. In addition, because there is currently no satisfactory treatment for non-remitting tardive dyskinesia, a wide variety of pharmacological agents have been used as experimental treatments without a specific theoretical rationale (Berger and Rexroth, 1980a; Jeste and Wyatt, 1982).

The most effective and most controversial treatments for tardive dyskinesia are the antipsychotic drugs themselves (Jeste and Wyatt, 1982). Every antipsychotic available in the United States seems capable of suppressing the symptoms of tardive dyskinesia. The atypical antipsychotic clozapine may be an exception to this rule since clozapine is not only less effective at suppressing the symptoms of tardive dyskinesia but can sometimes exacerbate the existing tardive dyskinesia.

Jeste and Wyatt (1982) summarize 19 double-blind investigations using typical antipsychotics to treat tardive dyskinesia. Most of these investigations find antipsychotics significantly more effective than placebo in suppressing the symptoms of tardive dyskinesia. While antipsychotics vary in their sedative properties, they do not appear to differ in their ability to decrease the symptoms of tardive dyskinesia. This suggests that antipsychotics have a specific dyskinesia-suppressing effect independent of their sedative action. The obvious problem with the use of antipsychotics for the treatment of tardive dyskinesia is the fact that these agents cause the disorder in the first place. It is intuitively reasonable to expect that continued treatment with antipsychotics should worsen the underlying cause of tardive dyskinesia even while suppressing the symptoms. Antipsychotics might also be expected to convert remitting tardive dyskinesia to non-remitting tardive dyskinesia. However, neither of these assumptions has been adequately tested. The possibility that continued administration of antipsychotics to patients with tardive dyskinesia may exacerbate the tardive dyskinesia has neither been confirmed nor refuted by any investigation. Clearly, such an investigation is extremely important since the question of whether or not to continue antipsychotics in a patient with tardive dyskinesia is currently one of the most important dilemmas for those who treat chronic schizophrenics.

Reserpine and tetrabenazine deplete dopamine by preventing dopamine storage thus reducing dopaminergic activity. Several uncontrolled or brief, placebo-controlled trials of reserpine and tetrabenazine report some improvement in dyskinetic symptoms (Kobayashi, 1976). Not all patients responded to treatment;

those who did respond to tetrabenazine showed a gradual loss of benefit when the treatment was continued for 18 months (Kazamatsuri et al., 1973). A recent report suggests that reserpine can improve tardive dyskinesia initially but aggravate the syndrome when discontinued (Donatelli et al., 1983).

Alpha-methyl-*p*-tyrosine, which reduces dopamine synthesis by inhibition of tyrosine hydroxylase, has been reported to have some positive effects in tardive dyskinesia (Gerlach and Thorsen, 1976). Alpha-methyldopa, another blocker of dopamine synthesis, has shown inconsistent results in clinical trials (Viukari and Linnoila, 1975). Oxypertine, which may deplete dopamine, has been shown to have positive effects in at least one study (Chien et al., 1978). Papaverine, a smooth muscle relaxant, which may antagonize dopamine, has also been reported to improve tardive dyskinesia (Gardos et al., 1976). It must be kept in mind however, that like antipsychotics, dopamine antagonists, dopamine-depleting agents, and blockers of dopamine synthesis could theoretically exacerbate the underlying defect of tardive dyskinesia with long-term use.

The dopamine agonist apomorphine and the dopamine precursor levodopa would be expected to increase dopaminergic predominance and so exacerbate the symptoms of tardive dyskinesia. However, several investigators have suggested that there may be a biphasic response to these drugs, with low doses actually producing a reduction in the movements of tardive dyskinesia (Smith et al., 1977). It has been suggested that both levodopa and apomorphine, in low doses, stimulate inhibitory presynaptic dopamine receptors, thereby decreasing dopamine release (Carroll et al., 1977). Again, this reduced dopamine release might eventually be expected to increase dopamine receptor supersensitivity and exacerbate tardive dyskinesia. Tarsy and colleagues (1979) gave low doses of apomorphine and three doses of levodopa (50, 100 and 250 mg) to 10 tardive dyskinesia patients and obtained inconsistent results. Three patients were reported to show a biphasic response to the levodopa, with improvement of symptoms at low doses and exacerbation at the highest dose. However, when two of these three patients were put on a maintenance low-dose treatment of levodopa, they showed an initial decrease and then an increase in the severity of their tardive dyskinesia.

A different approach to the treatment of tardive dyskinesia has been used by Alpert and Friedhoff (1980). These investigators propose to reduce nigrostriatal dopamine receptor supersensitivity by temporarily increasing dopamine concentrations with levodopa. Animal experiments suggest that levodopa can reverse the behavioral manifestation of haloperidol-induced supersensitivity to dopamine agonists. While this hypothesis is attractive and the preliminary results are encouraging, the levodopa 'desensitization' treatment temporarily worsens both the tardive dyskinesia and the psychosis, making the treatment difficult to use practically.

Although the cholinergic pharmacology of tardive dyskinesia is not completely clear, the general exacerbation of symptoms with anticholinergics leads to the suggestion that treatment with cholinomimetics might improve the syndrome (Davis and Berger, 1978). Cholinomimetics which have been used as experimental treatments for tardive dyskinesia include physostigmine, deanol, choline, lecithin, and tetrahydroaminoacridine (THA, tacrine). In a review of 13 studies using physostigmine as a treatment for tardive dyskinesia, 52% of 71 patients improved (Jeste and Wyatt, 1982). Physostigmine is not a practical treatment for tardive dyskinesia because it is currently administered intravenously and is too short-acting and has too many side effects. Oral physostigmine as a possible treatment of tardive dyskinesia should be explored (Berger and Rexroth, 1980b).

Deanol may be the most extensively studied treatment for tardive dyskinesia. The drug is generally considered a cholinomimetic, but there is no clear evidence that it is a true precursor of acetylcholine. Early studies with deanol were uncontrolled and reported high rates of success. More recent investigations with more careful study designs have failed to confirm this initial optimism (Berger and Rexroth, 1980b; Jeste and Wyatt, 1982).

Choline is the natural precursor of acetylcholine. There are now six published reports of choline chloride treatment for tardive dyskinesia (Berger and Rexroth, 1980b; Jeste and Wyatt, 1982). Of 36 patients treated with choline chloride, 44% were reported to be improved. Unfortunately, the drug has cholinomimetic side effects and produces a body odor similar to 'dead fish', presumably due to the oxidation of choline to trimethylamine by bacteria in the gastrointestinal tract. Thus, the use of choline on a routine clinical basis would be inconvenient and unpleasant and its status in the treatment of tardive dyskinesia will require further testing.

Lecithin, phosphatidylcholine, is metabolized to choline in the gastrointestinal tract and liver. It raises plasma choline concentrations and does not produce the body odor caused by the ingestion of choline. In seven published investigations, the overall improvement rate was 48% (Jeste and Wyatt, 1982). Lecithin can also cause cholinomimetic side effects and weight gain due to its high caloric content. Thus, like choline chloride, lecithin remains a research tool rather than a practical treatment for tardive dyskinesia (Berger and Rexroth, 1980b).

The most recent cholinomimetic used for the treatment of tardive dyskinesia is tetrahydroaminoacridine (tacrine). In a preliminary study with eight patients, tacrine was reported to cause a reduction in tardive dyskinesia movements of about 40% (Ingram and Newgreen, 1983).

Thus, the use of cholinomimetics as experimental treatments for tardive dyskinesia has not produced a practical treatment. Even if cholinomimetics improve tardive dyskinesia, it is not clear that they act by increasing cholinergic activity. If increased cholinergic activity is the mechanism of action, it is possible that the cholinergic activity decreases dopamine release from dopamine neurons in the striatum. Once again, there is a possibility that the decreased dopamine release could further exacerbate the post-synaptic dopamine supersensitivity thought to cause tardive dyskinesia. Cholinomimetics may therefore only cause temporary improvement and may eventually worsen tardive dyskinesia. Further investigations are clearly needed using less toxic and more potent cholinomimetics.

The relationship between gamma-aminobutyric acid (GABA) and other neurotransmitters in the nigrostriatum has been the subject of considerable controversy in neurochemistry. One suggestion is that GABA, like acetylcholine, exerts an inhibitory influence on dopaminergic neurotransmission (Groves et al., 1975). According to this hypothesis, GABA agonists, as well as cholinomimetics, would act to decrease dopamine hyperactivity in nigrostriatal dopamine neurons. Some investigators suggest that GABA or GABA agonists also affect motor function independent of the state of the dopamine system (Tamminga et al., 1979). Antipsychotic drugs produce changes in the metabolism and release of GABA, possibly diminishing GABA neuronal activity within extrapyramidal nuclei and so leading to tardive dyskinesia. CSF levels of GABA were reported to be significantly decreased in drug-free tardive dyskinesia patients; however, this finding is not specific to tardive dyskinesia and may indicate an alteration in GABA-mediated neuronal transmission in a group of neurological syndromes. In an animal study, decreased brain glutamate decarboxylase activity was found in the substantia nigra of rats and monkeys who were dyskinetic after receiving an antipsychotic diet (Gunne, 1983). While this finding suggests a primary role for GABA in animal dyskinesia, it has not yet been determined whether this GABA-synthesizing enzyme is also deficient in human patients with tardive dyskinesia.

The benzodiazepines facilitate brain GABA activity. Several investigators have reported positive effects of benzodiazepines on tardive dyskinesia (Sedman, 1976). However, none of the investigations has involved prolonged administration in a placebo-controlled double-blind design. There has also been little systematic attempt in these studies to separate an antidyskinetic effect of benzodiazepines from their sedative and muscle relaxant actions (Berger and Rexroth, 1980b).

Other putative GABA agonists which have been used as experimental treatments for tardive dyskinesia include baclofen (*p*-chlorophenyl-GABA), sodium valproate, muscimol (3-hydroxy-5-aminomethylisoxazole), gamma-acetylenic GABA, and gamma-vinyl-GABA. Baclofen is probably not a GABA agonist but may act on substance P or as a phenylethylamine analogue (Davis et al., 1976); it was reported to be effective in several short-term double-blind studies (Jeste and Wyatt, 1979). Sodium valproate is a GABA-transaminase inhibitor and has had positive effects in several uncontrolled, short-term double-blind studies (Linnoila et al., 1976). Muscimol, a structural analogue of GABA, potently mimics GABA activity in a number of biochemical, neurophysiological, and pharmacological characteristics (Tamminga et al., 1979). Muscimol is reported to have caused a significant diminution in the movements of tardive dyskinesia; it has also been used as an experimental treatment for schizophrenia however, and has been found to exacerbate psychosis in some cases (Tamminga et al., 1979). Gamma-acetylenic GABA has been reported to be useful in treating patients with tardive dyskinesia who were also receiving antipsychotics in a single trial (Casey et al., 1979). Gamma-vinyl-GABA may be even more effective than gamma-acetylenic GABA in preliminary trials but more carefully controlled investigations are needed with both compounds.

Thus, there is only preliminary evidence that putative GABA agonists have a specific antidyskinetic effect. No GABA agonist can yet be recommended as a practical treatment for tardive dyskinesia. Further therapeutic trials are underway and should help delineate the role, if any, of GABA agonists in the treatment of tardive dyskinesia.

The possible roles of serotonin and norepinephrine in tardive dyskinesia have been explored with a number of pharmacological agents. Tryptophan was administered to tardive dyskinesia patients in order to increase brain serotonin concentrations; a transient reduction in symptoms was seen in one study, but a subsequent double-blind study showed no significant effects (Jeste and Wyatt, 1982). Cyproheptadine, a serotonin receptor blocker, was found to have positive results in one study (Goldman, 1976) and both positive and negative results in another (Nagao et al., 1979).

In preliminary trials, tardive dyskinesia and levodopa-induced dyskinesia have been reported to be improved by the dopamine-beta-hydroxylase-inhibitors, fusaric acid (Viukari and Linnoila, 1977) and disulfiram (Birket-Smith and Vang Andersen, 1973). Both of these agents reduce the synthesis of norepinephrine; the positive results of the studies suggest that norepinephrine, as well as dopamine, may play a role in the etiology of tardive dyskinesia. However, the efficacy of fusaric acid and disulfiram needs to be confirmed before serious consideration can be given to the role of norepinephrine in tardive dyskinesia.

The effects of lithium carbonate treatment have also been studied in tardive dyskinesia, with conflicting results. Lithium may have a weak antipsychotic-like effect on dopamine activity (Beitman, 1978). Four of five tardive dyskinesia patients treated with lithium showed decreased CSF concentrations of homovanillic acid (Gerlach et al., 1975b); this is consistent with a postulated lithium-induced reduction of dopamine activity. The antipsychotic-like activity of lithium might explain the short-term amelioration of tardive dyskinesia seen in several studies; it would also explain the appearance of dyskinetic symptoms later in some patients receiving lithium (Beitman, 1978).

A possible prophylactic effect of lithium carbonate has been been reported by two groups of investigators (Klawans et al., 1977; Pert et al., 1978). Using the animal model of tardive dyskinesia and tritiated spiroperidol binding, these investigators demonstrated that in at least one experimental condition, pretreatment and concomitant treatment with lithium prevented the development of dopamine supersensitivity (Pert et al., 1978). The clinical implications of this study are extremely important but there is little clinical evidence yet to support the prophylactic use of lithium for tardive dyskinesia.

Other pharmacological agents have been used as experimental treatments for tardive dyskinesia. There is little theoretical basis for the use of most of these compounds, and none have as yet been demonstrated to be of practical value. These compounds include manganese, niacinamide, phenytoin, melanocyte-stimulating hormone-release inhibiting factor 1, morphine sulfate, barbiturates, naloxone, an enkephalin analogue, FK 33-824, pyridoxine hydrochloride, propranolol, clonidine, and estrogens (Berger and Rexroth, 1980b; Jeste and Wyatt, 1982).

Non-pharmacological treatments have also been used in an attempt to improve tardive dyskinesia. The most successful non-pharmacological treatment may be the prescription of well-fitting dentures. Dental or denture problems can cause abnormal movements of the tongue, jaw, and lips and make tardive dyskinesia movements worse. Other non-pharmacological treatments include stereotaxic surgery (Nashold, 1969), and cerebellar stimulation through an implanted cerebellar pacemaker (Heath, 1977). Electroconvulsive therapy (ECT) was reported to be effective in improving dyskinesia in two reports (Price and Levin, 1978), while another group of investigators found no significant change in tardive dyskinesia symptoms following ECT (Asnis and Leopold, 1978). Both biofeedback (Albanese and Gaarder, 1977) and transcutaneous nerve stimulation (Betts et al., 1979) have been used in patients with tardive dyskinesia but the results are too preliminary to yield definite conclusions.

DIRECTIONS FOR FUTURE RESEARCH IN TARDIVE DYSKINESIA

The etiology, pathophysiology, possible modes of prevention, treatment, or cure of tardive dyskinesia have yet to be determined. Given the continuing rise in prevalence figures, it is imperative that vigorous, well-designed clinical and preclinical studies be continued in order to understand and to control this serious disorder.

To facilitate both epidemiological and experimental pharmacological studies, strict standards for diagnosis and assessment of tardive dyskinesia must be used. A comprehensive epidemiological study can then examine the possible association of tardive dyskinesia with such factors as: specific antipsychotics; high- or low-dose antipsychotic treatment; depot or oral antipsychotic preparations; antipsychotic drug holidays; extrapyramidal reactions; the use of anticholinergic antiparkinsonian agents, lithium carbonate, or tricyclic antidepressants in combination with antipsychotics; ECT; and organic brain disease. The possibility of a correlation between tardive dyskinesia and plasma neuroleptic concentrations or plasma neuroleptic activity should be examined. Clinical studies should also be conducted to determine biochemical or physiological correlates of tardive dyskinesia. A multicenter prospective study could then rigorously test the possible associations suggested by the epidemiological study.

The possible use of antipsychotic medications as a treatment for tardive dyskinesia should be vigorously explored in carefully controlled studies. The untested assumption that antipsychotics temporarily suppress the symptoms but eventually worsen the disorder has greatly modified the treatment practices of physicians and may be depriving patients of continued treatment for their psychosis and possibly for their tardive dyskinesia. On the other hand, prolonged antipsychotic treatment in patients with tardive dyskinesia may exacerbate the underlying pathology of this disorder and may therefore worsen the symptoms or convert a remitting tardive dyskinesia to a non-remitting type. In this case, the risk of continued maintenance treatment for chronic schizophrenic patients would be greater than is currently appreciated.

The actions of cholinomimetics and GABA agonists in the treatment of tardive dyskinesia should be further examined in basic and animal neuropharmacological studies. It is possible that these agents improve tardive dyskinesia by decreasing dopamine release; like antipsychotics these agents would provide the receptor with less dopamine. With such a mode of action, both cholinomimetics and GABA agonists might ultimately cause or increase dopamine receptor supersensitivity. The improvement seen in the symptoms of tardive dyskinesia might then be only temporary, and continued use of these agents might eventually exacerbate the movement disorder. However, as is the case with antipsychotics, the predicted exacerbation is based on a primitive understanding of pathophysiology of tardive dyskinesia which may be invalid. It is also possible that cholinomimetics and GABA agonists may improve tardive dyskinesia by mechanisms unrelated to the dopamine system.

The development and testing of new pharmacological agents for the treatment of tardive dyskinesia should continue. Clinical tests of experimental drug treatments must be carefully designed; the protocols should be double-blind and include both pre- and post-experimental drug-placebo periods to avoid confounding the results of the treatment with the natural course of the disorder.

The development and testing of antipsychotic agents that may not cause tardive dyskinesia deserve high priority. Clozapine-like drugs currently offer the most promise for effective antipsychotic activity without the production of tardive dyskinesia. High-dose diazepam, high-dose propranolol, thyrotropin-releasing hormone, beta-endorphin, and des-tyrosine-gamma-endorphin have been suggested to be effective treatments for schizophrenia which may not cause tardive dyskinesia. Unfortunately, the initial positive claims for these treatments as antipsychotic agents are now controversial (Berger and Rexroth, 1980b).

Recently, the question of a possible mesolimbic equivalent to tardive dyskinesia has been raised. As previously described, numerous animal studies give support to the hypothesis of antipsychotic-induced dopamine receptor supersensitivity in the nigrostriatal dopamine tract. It has been suggested that the mesolimbic dopamine tract, proposed as the neuroanatomical substrate of schizophrenia, might also develop supersensitivity. Evidence from animal studies indicates the possibility of mesolimbic supersensitivity, but the data are clearly preliminary and may not be applicable to human patients (Davis and Rosenberg, 1979).

Three groups of investigators recently discussed the possible existence of a mesolimbic equivalent of tardive dyskinesia in humans treated with antipsychotics. Davis and Rosenberg (1979) call the syndrome 'the limbic system equivalent of tardive dyskinesia'. They suggest that the symptoms might include anxiety, sleeplessness, and agitation; such symptoms were reported in many studies of 'antipsychotic withdrawal symptoms'. A more serious consequence of the hypothetical syndrome of mesolimbic supersensitivity might be exacerbation of schizophrenic symptoms in some patients who initially showed an improvement with these medications. Long-term antipsychotic treatment in a non-psychotic patient might also eventually lead to psychosis; there is one report of a patient who developed psychosis for the first time when antipsychotics were withdrawn (Sale and Kristall, 1978). Chouinard and Jones (1980) called the hypothetical syndrome 'supersensitivity psychosis'. They report a subpopulation of schizophrenic patients who require increasing doses of fluphenazine for symptom control who relapse rapidly on drug withdrawal and exhibit a high incidence of tardive dyskinesia. Wilson et al. (1983) use the term 'tardive dysmentia' to describe the hypothesized antipsychotic-induced limbic system dopamine supersensitivity syndrome. These investigators found a high correlation between tardive dyskinesia ratings and a syndrome including unstable mood and loquaciousness. They suggest that tardive dysmentia may include a hypomanic state characterized by euphoria, but also by explosive changes in affect and rapid swings between social withdrawal and intrusive behavior.

The speculative existence of a mesolimbic equivalent of tardive dyskinesia is an alarming possibility. Further clinical and preclinical studies are urgently needed to determine whether prolonged antipsychotic treatment does produce mesolimbic dopamine receptor supersensitivity and what the clinical consequences of such supersensitivity might be.

ACKNOWLEDGEMENT

The research reported in this manuscript is supported by the National Institute of Mental Health Specialized Research Center Grant MH 30854, and by the Veterans Administration through the Palo Alto Veterans Administration Medical Center Schizophrenia Biologic Research Center.

REFERENCES

Albanese, H. and Gaarder, K. (1977) Biofeedback treatment of tardive dyskinesia. Two case reports. Am. J. Psychiatry 134, 1149 – 1150.

Alpert, M. and Friedhoff, A. J. (1980) Clinical application of receptor modification. In: W. E. Fann, R. C. Smith and J. M. Davis (Eds), Tardive Dyskinesia: Research and Treatment. SP Medical and Scientific Books, New York, pp. 471 – 473.

Altrocchi, P. H. (1972) Spontaneous oral-facial dyskinesia. Arch. Neurol. 26, 506 – 512.

American College of Neuropsychopharmacology – FDA Task Force (1973) Neurological syndromes associated with antipsychotic drug use. Arch. Gen. Psychiatry 28, 463 – 467.

Asnis, G. M. and Leopold, M. A. (1978) A single-blind study of ECT in patients with tardive dyskinesia. Am. J. Psychiatry 135, 1235 – 1237.

Asper, H., Baggiolini, M. and Burki, H. R. (1973) Tolerance phenomena with neuroleptics. Eur. J. Pharmacol. 22, 287 – 294.

Ayd, Jr., F. J., (1973) Neuroleptic-induced extrapyramidal reactions: incidence, manifestations and management. In: F. J. Ayd, Jr. (Ed.), The Future of Pharmacotherapy New Drug Delivery System. Baltimore International Drug Therapy Newsletter, pp 77 – 88.

Baldessarini, R. J. (1974) Tardive dyskinesia: an evaluation of the etiologic association with neuroleptic therapy. Can. Psychiatr. Assoc. J. 19, 551 – 554.

Baldessarini, R. J. and Tarsy, D. (1976) Mechanisms underlying tardive dyskinesia. In: M. Yahr (Ed.), Proceedings of the Association of Research in Nervous and Mental Disorders. Raven Press, New York, pp. 443 – 446.

Baldessarini, R. J. and Tarsy, D. (1978) Tardive dyskinesia. In: M. A. Lipton, A. DiMascio and K. F. Killam (Eds), Psychopharmacology: A Generation of Progress. Raven Press, New York, pp. 993 – 1004.

Baldessarini, R. J., Cole, J. O. and Davis, J. M. (1980) Task Force Report of the American Psychiatric Association on Late Neurological Effects of Antipsychotic Drugs. American Psychiatric Association, Washington, D. C.

Beitman, B. D. (1978) Tardive dyskinesia reinduced by lithium carbonate. Am. J. Psychiatry 135, 1229 – 1230.

Berger, P. A. (1978) Medical treatment of mental illness. Science 200, 974 – 981.

Berger, P. A. and Rexroth, K. (1980a) Tardive dyskinesia: clinical, biological, and pharmacological perspectives. Schiz. Bull. 6, 102 – 116.

Berger, P. A. and Rexroth, K. (1980b) Tardive dyskinesia. In: F. J. Ayd, Jr. (Ed.), Haloperidol Update: 1958 – 1980. Ayd Medical Communications, Baltimore, pp. 174 – 196.

Betts, W. C., Johnstone, F. S. and Pratt, M. J. (1979) An effective palliative treatment for phenothiazine-induced tardive dyskinesia. N. C. Med. J. 40, 286.

Birket-Smith, E. (1974) Abnormal involuntary movements induced by anticholinergic therapy. Acta Neurol. Scand. 50, 801 – 811.

Birket-Smith, E. and Vang Andersen, J. (1973) Treatment of side-effects of levodopa. Lancet i, 431.

Bleuler, E. (1950) Dementia Praecox or the Group of Schizophrenics. Translated by J. Zinkin, 1911 German Edition. International University Press, New York.

Burke, R. E., Fahn, S., Ilson, J., Gollomp, S. and Jankovic, J. (1982) Tardive dystonia. Abstract from the Annual Meeting of the American Academy of Neurology, Toronto, Canada.

Burki, H. R., Sayers, A. C. and Ruch, W. (1976) Einfluss von Anticholinergika sowie Clozapin auf die durch Haloperidol induzierte Aktivierung des dopaminergen Systems im Striatum der Ratte: Neurochemische Ergebuisse. Arzneim. Forsch. (Drug Res.) 26, 1094 – 1096.

Burt, D. R., Creese, J. and Snyder, S. H. (1977) Antischizophrenic drugs: chronic treatment elevates dopamine receptor binding in brain. Science 196, 326 – 328.

Buxton, M. (1976) Diagnostic problems in Huntington's chorea and tardive dyskinesia. Compr. Psychiatry 17, 325 – 333.

Caine, E. D., Margolin, D. I. and Brown, G. L. (1978) Gilles de la Tourette's Syndrome, tardive dyskinesia and psychosis in an adolescent. Am. J. Psychiatry 135, 241 – 243.

Carlsson, A. and Lindquist, M. (1963) Effect of chlorpromazine or haloperidol on formation of 3-methoxytyramine and normetanephrine in mouse brain. Acta Pharmacol. Toxicol. 20, 140 – 144.

Carroll, B. J., Curtis, G. C. and Kokmen, E. (1977) Paradoxical response to dopamine agonists in tardive dyskinesia. Am. J. Psychiatry 134, 785 – 789.

Casey, D. E. and Denney, P. (1977) Pharmacological characterization of tardive dyskinesia. Psychopharmacologia 54, 1 – 8.

Casey, D. E., Gerlach, J. and Magelund, G. (1979) Gamma-acetylenic GABA in tardive dyskinesia. Arch. Gen. Psychiatry 37, 1376 – 1379.

Chadwick, D., Reynolds, E. H. and Marsden, C. D. (1976) Anticonvulsant-induced dyskinesias: a comparison with dyskinesias induced by neuroleptics. J. Neurol. Neurosurg. Psychiatry 39, 1210 – 1218.

Chase, T. N. (1974) Catecholamine metabolism and neurologic disease. In: E. Usdin and S. M. Snyder (Eds), Frontiers in Catecholamine Research. Pergamon Press, New York, pp. 941 – 945.

Chien, C., Jung, K. and Ross-Townsend, A. (1978) Efficacies of agents related to GABA, dopamine and acetylcholine in the treatment of tardive dyskinesia. Psychopharmacol. Bull. 14, 20 – 22.

Chouinard, G. and Jones, B. D. (1980) Neuroleptic-induced supersensitivity psychosis: clinical and pharmacologic characteristics. Am. J. Psychiatry 137, 16 – 21.

Christensen, E., Moller, J. E. and Faurbye, A. (1970) Neurological investigation of 28 brains from patients with dyskinesia. Acta Psychiatr. Scand. 46, 14 – 23.

Clow, A., Jenner, P. and Theodorou, A. (1979) Striatal dopamine receptors become supersensitive while rats are given trifluoperazine for 6 months. Nature (London) 278, 59 – 61.

Craig, T. J. and Richardson, M. A. (1982) Swallowing, tardive dyskinesia, and anticholinergics. Am. J. Psychiatry 139, 1083.

Crane, G. E. (1974) Factors predisposing to drug-induced neurologic effects. In: I. S. Forrest, C. J. Carr, and E. Usdin (Eds), The Phenothiazines and Structurally Related Drugs. Raven Press, New York, pp. 269 – 279.

Crane, G. E. and Smith, R. C. (1980) The prevalence of tardive dyskinesia. In: W. E. Fann, R. C. Smith and J. M. Davis (Eds), Tardive Dyskinesia: Research and Treatment. Spectrum Publications, New York, pp. 269 – 279.

Cunningham Owens, D. G., Johnstone, E. C. and Frith, C. D. (1982) Spontaneous involuntary disorders of movement – their prevalence, severity, and distribution in chronic schizophrenics with and without treatment with neuroleptics. Arch. Gen. Psychiatry 39, 452 – 461.

Davis, K. L. and Berger, P. A. (1978) Pharmacological investigations of the cholinergic imbalance hypotheses of movement disorders and psychosis. Biol. Psychiatry 13, 23 – 49.

Davis, K. L. and Rosenberg, G. (1979) Is there a limbic system equivalent of tardive dyskinesia? Biol. Psychiatry 14, 699 – 703.

Davis, K. L., Hollister, L. E. and Berger, P. A. (1976) Baclofen in schizophrenia. Lancet i, 1245.

Davis, K. L., Hollister, L. E. and Vento, A. L. (1978) Choline chloride in methylphenidate- and apomorphine-induced stereotypy. Life Sci. 22, 2171 – 2178.

Davis, K. L., Berger, P. A. and Hollister, L. E. (1979) Clinical and preclinical experience with choline chloride in Huntington's disease and tardive dyskinesia: unanswered questions. In: A. Barbeau, J. H. Growdon and R. J. Wurtman (Eds), Nutrition and The Brain. Raven Press, New York, pp. 305 – 315.

Davis, W. A. (1976) Dyskinesia associated with chronic antihistamine use. N. Engl. J. Med. 294, 113.

De Fraites, E. G., Davis, K. L. and Berger, P. A. (1977) Coexisting tardive dyskinesia and Parkinsonism: a case report. Biol. Psychiatry 12, 267 – 272.

Degwitz, R. (1969) Extrapyramidal motor disorders following longterm treatment with neuroleptic drugs. In: G. E. Crane and R. Gardiner (Eds), Psychotropic Drugs and Dysfunctions of The Basal Ganglia. Washington Public Health Service Publication No. 1938, pp. 22 – 32.

Donatelli, A., Geisen, L. and Feuer, E. (1983) A case report of adverse effects of reserpine on tardive dyskinesia. Am. J. Psychiatry 140, 239 – 240.

Ekbom, K., Lindholm, H. and Ljungberg, L. (1972) New dystonic syndrome associated with butyrophenone therapy. Z. Neurol. 202, 94 – 103.

Faheem, A. D., Brightwell, D. R., Burton, G. C. and Struss, A. (1982) Respiratory dyskinesia and dysarthria from prolonged neuroleptic use: tardive dyskinesia Am. J. Psychiatry 139, 517 – 518.

Fann, W. E., Sullivan, J. L. and Richman, B. W. (1976) Dyskinesias associated with tricyclic antidepressants. Br. J. Psychiatry 128, 490 – 493.

Faurbye, A., Rasch, P. J. and Peterson, P. B. (1964) Neurological symptoms in pharmacotherapy of psychoses. Acta Psychiatr. Scand. 40, 10 – 27.

Fieger, G. N. (1983) After the flood: the progeny of Faigenbaum versus Oakland Medical Center. Abstract from the Annual Meeting of the American College of Neuropsychopharmacology, San Juan, Puerto Rico.

Gardos, G. and Cole, J. O. (1980) Overview: public health issues in tardive dyskinesia. Am. J. Psychiatry 137, 776 – 781.

Gardos, G., Cole, J. O. and Sniffin, C. (1976) An evaluation of papaverine in tardive dyskinesia. J. Clin. Pharmacol. 16, 304 – 310.

Gardos, G., Cole, J. O. and La Brie, R. A. (1977) Drug variables in the etiology of tardive dyskinesia: application of discriminant function analysis. Prog. Neuro-Psychopharmacol. 1, 147 – 154.

Gelenberg, A. J. (1976) Computerized tomography in patients with tardive dyskinesia. Am. J. Psychiatry 133, 578 – 579.

Gerlach, J. (1977) Relationship between tardive dyskinesia, L-dopa-induced hyperkinesia and Parkinsonism. Psychopharmacologia 51, 259 – 263.

Gerlach, J. and Thorsen, K. (1976) The movement pattern of oral tardive dyskinesia in relation to anticholinergic and antidopaminergic treatment. Int. Pharmacopsychiatry 11, 1 – 7.

Gerlach, J., Reisby, N. and Randrup, A. (1974) Dopaminergic hypersensitivity and cholinergic hypofunction in the pathophysiology of tardive dyskinesia. Psychopharmacologia 34, 21 – 35.

Gerlach, J., Thorsen, K. and Fog, R. (1975a) Extrapyramidal reactions and amine metabolites in cerebrospinal fluid during haloperidol and clozapine treatment of schizophrenic patients. Psychopharmacologia 40, 341 – 350.

Gerlach, J., Thorsen, K. and Munkvad, I. (1975b) Effect of lithium in neuroleptic-induced tardive dyskinesia compared with placebo in a double-blind cross-over trial. Pharmakopsychiatr. Neuro-psychopharmakol. 8, 51 – 56.

Glazer, W. M., Moore, D. C., Hansen, T. C. and Brenner, L. M. (1983) Meige syndrome and tardive dyskinesia. Am. J. Psychiatry 140, 798 – 799.

Goldman, D. (1976) Treatment of phenothiazine-induced dyskinesia. Psychopharmacologia 47, 271 – 272.

Granacher, R. P. (1981) Differential diagnosis of tardive dyskinesia: an overview. Am. J. Psychiatry 138, 1288 – 1297.

Greenblatt, D. L., Dominick, J. R. and Stotsky, B. A. (1968) Phenothiazine-induced dyskinesia in nursing home patients. J. Am. Geriatr. Soc. 16, 27 – 34.

Groves, P. M., Wilson, C. J. and Young, S. J. (1975) Self inhibition by dopaminergic neurons: an alternative to the ‘normal feed-back loop’ hypothesis for the mode of action of certain psychotropic drugs. Science 190, 522 – 529.

Gunne, L. (1983) The pathophysiology and biochemistry of tardive dyskinesia. Abstract from the Annual Meeting of the American College of Neuropsychopharmacology, San Juan, Puerto Rico.

Heath, R. G. (1977) Modulation of emotion with a brain pacemaker. J. Nerv. Ment. Dis. 165, 300 – 317.

Ingram, N. A. W. and Newgreen, D. B. (1983) The use of tacrine for tardive dyskinesia. Am. J. Psychiatary 140, 1629 – 1631.

Jeste, D. V. and Wyatt, R. J. (1979) In search of treatment for tardive dyskinesia: review of the literature. Schiz. Bull. 5, 251 – 293.

Jeste, D. V. and Wyatt, R. J. (1981) Changing epidemiology of tardive dyskinesia: an overview. Am. J. Psychiatry 138, 297 – 309.

Jeste, D. V. and Wyatt, R. J. (1982) Therapeutic strategies against tardive dyskinesia – two decades of experience. Arch. Gen. Psychiatry 39, 803 – 816.

Jeste, D. V., Potkin, S. G. and Sinha, S. (1979) Tardive dyskinesia – reversible and persistent. Arch. Gen. Psychiatry 36, 585 – 590.

Jus, A., Pineau, R. and Lachance, R. (1976) Epidemiology of tardive dyskinesia, I and II. Dis. Nerv. Syst. 37, 210 – 214; 257 – 261.

Kane, J. M. and Smith, J. M. (1982) Tardive dyskinesia: prevalance and risk factors, 1959 to 1979. Arch. Gen. Psychiatry 39, 473 – 481.

Kazamatsuri, H., Chien, C. and Cole, J. O. (1973) Long-term treatment of tardive dyskinesia with haloperidol and tetrabenazine. Am. J. Psychiatry 130, 479 – 483.

Klawans, Jr., H. L., (1973) The pharmacology of tardive dyskinesias. Am. J. Psychiatry 130, 82 – 86.

Klawans, H. L., Weiner, W. J. and Nausieda, P. A. (1977) The effect of lithium on an animal model of tardive dyskinesia. Prog. Neuropsychopharmacol. 1, 53 – 60.

Klawans, H. L., Goetz, C. G. and Perlik, S. (1980) Tardive dyskinesia: review and update. Am. J. Psychiatry 137, 900 – 908.

Kobayashi, R. M. (1976) Orofacial dyskinesia – clinical features, mechanisms and drug therapy. West J. Med. 125, 277 – 288.

Kobayashi, R. M. (1977) Drug therapy of tardive dyskinesia. N. Engl. J. Med. 296, 257 – 260.

Kraepelin, E, (1907) Clinical Psychiatry. Translated by A. Diefendorf Ross. Macmillan Company, New York, p. 229.

Linnoila, M., Viukari, M. and Hietala, O. (1976) Effect of sodium valproate on tardive dyskinesia. Br. J. Psychiatry 129, 114 – 119.

Marsden, C. D. (1976) Blepharospasm-oromandibular dystonia syndrome. J. Neurol. Neurosurg. Psychiatry 39, 1204 – 1209.

Mattson, R. H. and Calverley, J. (1968) Dextroamphetamine-sulfate-induced dyskinesias. J. Am. Med. Assoc. 204, 108 – 110.

Mcentee, W. J. and Newman, G. C. (1981) A case report of tardive hemidyskinesia. Am. J. Psychiatry 138, 1380 – 1381.

Mehta, D., Mallya, A. and Volavka, J. (1978) Mortality of patients with tardive dyskinesia. Am. J. Psychiatry 135, 371 – 372.

Meige, H. (1910) Les convulsions de la face: une forme clinique de convulsion faciale bilaterale et mediane. Rev. Neurol. 21, 437 – 443.

Moore, D. C. and Bowers, M. B. (1980) Identification of a subgroup of tardive dyskinesia patients by pharmacologic probes. Am. J. Psychiatry 137, 1202 – 1205.

Nagao, T., Ohshimo, T. and Mitsunobu, K. (1979) Cerebrospinal fluid monoamine metabolites and cyclic nucleotides in chronic schizophrenic patients with tardive dyskinesia or drug-induced tremor. Biol. Psychiatry 14, 509 – 523.

Nashold, B. S. (1969) The effects of central tegmental lesions on tardive dyskinesia. In: G. E. Crane and R. Gardner (Eds), Psychotropic Drugs and Dysfunctions of the Basal Ganglia. Public Health Service publication, 1938. National Institute of Mental Health, pp. 111 – 119.

Paulson, G. W. (1975) Tardive dyskinesia. Ann. Rev. Med. 26, 75 – 81.

Pert, A., Rosenblatt, J. E. and Sevel, C. (1978) Long-term treatment with lithium prevents the development of dopamine receptor supersensitivity. Science 201, 171 – 173.

Price, T. R. P. and Levin, R. (1978) The effects of electroconvulsive therapy on tardive dyskinesia. Am. J. Psychiatry 112, 983 – 987.

Sale, I. and Kristall, H. (1978) Schizophrenia following withdrawal from chronic phenothiazine administration: a case report. Aust. N. Z. J. Psychiatry 12, 73 – 75.

Sayers, A. C. and Burki, H. R. (1976) Einfluss von Anticholinergika sowie Clozapin auf die durch Haloperidol induzierte Aktivierung des dopaminergen Systems im Striatum der Ratte: Pharmakologische Ergebnisse. Arzneim. Forsch. (Drug Res.) 26, 1092 – 1093.

Schonecker, M. (1957) Ein eigentumliches Syndrom in oralen Bereich bei Megaphenapplikation. Nervenartz 28, 35.

Sedman, G. (1976) Clonazepam in the treatment of tardive oral dyskinesia. Br. Med. J. 2, 583.

Sigwald, T., Bouttier, D. and Raymondeaud, C. (1959) Quatre cas de dyskinisie facio-bucco-linguo-masticatrice a evolution prolongee secondaire a un traitement par les neuroleptiques. Rev. Neurol. 100, 751 – 755.

Smith, J. M. and Baldessarini, R. J. (1980) Changes in prevalence, severity, and recovery in tardive dyskinesia with age. Arch. Gen. Psychiatry 37, 1368 – 1373.

Smith, J. M., Kucharski, L. T. and Oswald, W. T. (1979) A systematic investigation of tardive dyskinesia in inpatients. Am. J. Psychiatry 136, 918 – 922.

Smith, R. C., Tamminga, C. A. and Haraszti, J. (1977) Effect of dopamine agonists in tardive dyskinesia. Am. J. Psychiatry 134, 763 – 768.

Snyder, S. H., Creese, I. and Burt, D. R. (1977) Dopamine receptor binding in mammalian brain: relevance to psychiatry. In: E. Usdin, J. Barchas and D. Hamburg (Eds), Neuroregulators and Psychiatric Disorders. Oxford University Press, New York, pp. 526 – 537.

Souner, R. and DiMascio, A. (1977) The effect of benztropine mesylate in the rabbit syndrome and tardive dyskinesia. Am. J. Psychiatry 139, 1301 – 1302.

Tamminga, C. A., Crayton, J. W. and Chase, T. N. (1979) Improvement in tardive dyskinesia after muscimol therapy. Arch. Gen. Psychiatry 36, 595 – 598.

Tarsy, D. and Baldessarini, R. J. (1973) Pharmacologically-induced behavioral supersensitivity to apomorphine. Nature (London) 245, 262 – 263.

Tarsy, D. and Baldessarini, R. J. (1976) The pathophysiologic basis of tardive dyskinesia. Presented at the Symposium on Biochemical Basis of Drug Side Effects in Psychiatry, Society of Biological Psychiatry, San Francisco, California.

Tarsy, D., Gardos, G. and Cole, J. O. (1979) The effect of dopamine agonists in tardive dyskinesia. Neurology 29, 606.

Tolosa, E. S. (1979) Meige disease (idiopathic orofaciocervical dystonia): a clinical study of 16 patients. Neurology 29, 605.

Viukari, M. and Linnoila, M. (1975) Effect of methyldopa on tardive dyskinesia in psychogeriatric patients. Curr. Ther. Res. 18, 417 – 424.

Viukari, M. and Linnoila, M. (1977) Effect of fusaric acid on tardive dyskinesia and mental state in psychogeriatric patients. Acta Psychiatr. Scand. 56, 57 – 61.

Villeneuve, A., Jus, K. and Jus, A. (1973) Polygraphic studies of tardive dyskinesia and of the rabbit syndrome during different stages of sleep. Biol. Psychiatry 6, 259 – 275.

Wegner, J. T. and Kane, J. M. (1982) Follow-up study of the reversibility of tardive dyskinesia. Am. J. Psychiatry 139, 368 – 369.

Wegner, J. T., Struve, F. A. and Kane, J. M. (1977) The B-mitten EEG pattern and tardive dyskinesia: a possible association. Am. J. Psychiatry 134, 1143 – 1145.

Wegner, J. T., Struve, F. A. and Kantor, J. S. (1979) Relationship between the B-mitten EEG pattern and tardive dyskinesia. Arch. Gen. Psychiatry 36, 599 – 603.

Weiss, K. J., Ciraulo, D. A. and Shader, R. I. (1980) Physostigmine test in the Rabbit syndrome and tardive dyskinesia. Am. J. Psychiatry 137, 627 – 628.

Wilson, I.C., Garbutt, J. C., Lanier, C. F., Moylan, J., Nelson, W. and Prange, Jr., A. J. (1983) Is there a tardive dysmentia? Schiz. Bull. 9, 187 – 192.

Wolf, M. E., Jeste, D. V., Mosnaim, A. D. and Rawlings, R. (1983) The clinical association of tardive dyskinesia and Parkinsonism. Abstracts of the Annual Meeting of the Society of Biological Psychiatry, New York.

Burrows/Norman/Davies (eds) Antipsychotics

Chapter 16

Neuroleptics in children

MAGDA CAMPBELL

and

STEPHEN I. DEUTSCH

Department of Psychiatry, New York University Medical Center,
550 First Avenue, New York, NY 10016, U.S.A.

INTRODUCTION

In adult psychiatric patients the use of neuroleptics is restricted mainly to schizophrenic disorders and other psychoses. Neuroleptics have a less specific role in child psychiatry. They are used in a variety of diagnostic entities, including non-psychotic conditions; on the other hand, schizophrenic and bipolar disorders are very rare in prepubertal children. Whereas the advent of chlorpromazine and other neuroleptics changed the practice of psychiatry involving adult patients, the availability of the same class of drugs did not bring a dramatic or substantial change to the practice of child psychiatry. This can be attributed to several reasons: 1) the goal of treatment in children differs from that in adults; while in adults, treatment should yield decrease of symptoms, in children one also wishes to promote the delayed or stunted development with the various treatment approaches, and, in general, expectations from treatment are greater. 2) The efficacy of neuroleptics in adults was explored and demonstrated in large and well-controlled clinical trials, using carefully diagnosed and homogeneous patient samples; this was not the case in children, until the most recent years. 3) some of the untoward effects of neuroleptics, specifically excessive sedation, are expected to interfere with the child's functioning and learning; this undesirable effect of neuroleptics restricts their use in this population of patients. An overview of the literature will be given detailing the results of well-controlled clinical trials.

INDICATIONS

Throughout the text, DSM-III (1980) diagnostic categories will be used. They are often similar to, and, may overlap with ICD-9 categories (Thompson et al., 1983).

Schizophrenic disorders

These are rare conditions in prepubertal children and little research has been conducted in this area. It seems that the less sedative type of neuroleptics may be beneficial as part of a comprehensive treatment program, though clinical experience suggests that these drugs are less effective in schizophrenic children than in adults.

Bipolar disorder

To the best of our knowledge, no research has been done in assessing the efficacy of neuroleptics in this condition which is very rare before puberty.

Infantile autism

Recent systematic research has shown that neuroleptics will significantly decrease behavioral symptoms and enhance certain types of learning in normo- or hyperactive young autistic children, when administered in a structured educational/behavioral program setting.

Conduct disorder, undersocialized, aggressive

Recent review of the literature indicates that stimulant drugs are usually ineffective in reducing or controlling aggressiveness while certain types of neuroleptics, particularly haloperidol, may be a useful adjunct to other treatments.

Attention deficit disorder with hyperactivity

If such a child fails to respond to a stimulant drug, administration of a neuroleptic may be indicated.

Tourette's disorder

Of all drugs, perhaps haloperidol and pimozide seem to be most effective in this syndrome.

Mental retardation associated with behavioral symptoms

A subgroup of mentally retarded children exhibits behavioral symptoms, most commonly aggressiveness directed against others and/or self, hyperactivity and impulsivity. If behavioral approaches fail, a trial of neuroleptic treatment may be indicated. In residential institutions and community homes these drugs are used in the treatment of greater than 50% of the mentally retarded population (Breuning, 1982; Ferguson, 1982; Breuning et al., 1982, 1983). Some of these subjects are children or adolescents. In about 60% of these cases, thioridazine has been selected in an attempt to reduce aggressive, self-stimulatory, or psychotic behaviors (Breuning, 1982; Breuning et al., 1982, 1983). Despite their widespread use in this population, until recently, few studies have been conducted to evaluate their effects on intellectual performance, acquisition of habilitative behaviors and learning in mentally retarded subjects. Careful reviews of the literature indicate that many studies claiming the efficacy of these drugs are methodologically inadequate, while others indicate that the reduction of behavioral problems may be accompanied by decreases of cognitive functions, learning and performance (for review, see Sprague and Werry, 1971; Lipman et al., 1978).

METHODOLOGICAL CONSIDERATIONS AND MEASUREMENT OF DRUG EFFECTS

The decision for matching psychoactive agent to diagnostic classification depends upon solid empirical research. Studies investigating drug efficacy must have adequate samples and experimental controls and must have used appropriate assessment procedures, instruments and statistical analyses. Otherwise the interpretation and generalizability of results are in question.

Size and characteristics of the sample

A study will detect true differences in a population only if the following are suitably chosen: adequate sample size (Cohen, 1977), the critical value selected, and the magnitude of the expected difference. The choice of diagnostic criteria is a further confounding factor. Any sample selected will contain a range of developmental, intellectual, biological, physiological, medical (e.g. inpatient/outpatient) and social differences within the sample. In small groups there is greater probability that these characteristics will not be equally distributed across groups. For assessment, there are a number of instruments available designed to quantify relevant historical, medical, demographic and social data (Guy, 1976; Campbell, 1977; Campbell et al. 1985).

Finally, the choice of classification system and the means by which diagnosis and selection are determined influence between-studies comparability.

Assessment instruments and procedures

Appropriate assessment instruments should be selected on the basis of their known validity, reliability and sensitivity to drug effects. The effect of drug treatment on behavior may depend upon the ecological conditions under which the behavior is observed. Children may display many different behaviors across situations. Certain behaviors observed during free play may not be displayed in a classroom setting and vice versa, or in the doctor's office. It is important that behaviors of experimental interest be assessed in situations where they are most likely to occur.

Experimental design

The purpose of an experimental design is to construct an optimal environment and a means within that environment which will provide an adequate test of the research hypothesis. The design must also control for possible contaminating factors. For a review of methodological issues in children a chapter by Connors (1977), and a monograph by Campbell et al. (1985) are recommended.

THERAPEUTIC EFFICACY

Short-term behavioral effects

Review of the literature and clinical experience indicate that administration of neuroleptics can reduce certain symptoms including stereotypies, tics, withdrawal, hyperactivity and aggressiveness in disturbed children of normal and subnormal intelligence. There is only one double-blind and placebo-controlled study on the effect of neuroleptic drugs in schizophrenics: the patient sample consisted of adolescents.

Phenothiazines. The aliphatics and piperidines are the subclass of phenothiazines with more sedative-hypnotic actions, while the piperazine subclass has more activating and motor-stimulating qualities. Chlorpromazine and thioridazine are the most frequently used phenothiazines in children. However, they often produce sedation at doses that reduce symptoms, or, in certain diagnostic populations, such as the autistics, sedation may appear before any therapeutic change is observed. Chlorpromazine may lower the seizure threshold or may increase the frequency of seizures in epileptics (Tarjan et al., 1957). Though it is said that thioridazine lacks this effect (Freeman, 1970) there is no scientific evidence to substantiate this statement.

In reducing behavioral symptoms including hyperkinesis and aggressiveness, chlorpromazine was found effective (Werry et al., 1966), but equal to or less effective than dextroamphetamine (Rapoport et al., 1971). Similarly, Gittelman-Klein et al. (1976) found thioridazine effective, but inferior to the stimulant drug methylphenidate. These three clinical trials were in outpatient children of normal intelligence. In retarded children, however, Alexandris and Lundell (1968) in a well-controlled study found thioridazine more effective than placebo or amphetamine in reducing behavioral symptoms which included aggressiveness.

In a small sample of diagnostically heterogeneous children with a symptom profile of aggressiveness and explosiveness, chlorpromazine was as effective as haloperidol or lithium (Campbell et al., 1982a). In preschool autistic children, trifluoperazine (Fish et al., 1966), but not chlorpromazine (Campbell et al., 1972), resulted in improved behavior and increased verbal production. Therapeutic changes with trifluoperazine were seen only in the more impaired children, who also tolerated higher doses of the drug than those with speech. Two of the four speaking children became worse, even on low doses of drug. Fluphenazine was reported to improve the behaviors of autistic children (Engelhardt et al., 1973). The dosage used in these outpatients was high relative to doses used in a similar inpatient population (Faretra et al., 1970).

Some of the data and results from these trials are summarized in Table 1.

Butyrophenones. Trifluperidol is a butyrophenone derivative that produces more neurologic untoward effects than haloperidol, particularly acute dystonic reactions and extrapyramidal symptoms. In a small sample of autistic children, trifluperidol was more effective than chlorpromazine or trifluoperazine in decreasing symptoms of withdrawal, affective blunting, psychotic speech, irritability, impulsivity and anergy (Fish et al., 1969).

Behavioral symptoms were reduced in hyperactive and aggressive children at two daily dosages of haloperidol (Werry and Aman, 1975; Werry et al., 1975). Haloperidol was found to be similarly effective in several other studies, by Cunningham et al. (1968) and by Campbell et al. (1982a), who used chlorpromazine as a comparison drug, and by Campbell et al. (1982d, 1984), when it was compared with, and found equal to, lithium. In the Werry study, the active drugs were significantly superior to placebo; untoward effects were mild, but more common with the higher dose of haloperidol. Campbell et al. (1984) found more untoward effects with haloperidol than with lithium. Excessive sedation and acute dystonic reaction were the most common untoward effects with haloperidol, particularly during dosage regulation and at doses above optimal.

In schizophrenic adolescents haloperidol was effective in reducing certain symptoms when given under double-blind and placebo-controlled conditions, but extrapyramidal side effects were frequent, followed by sedation (Pool et al., 1976).

Haloperidol was systematically investigated in young autistic children after promising results from two pilot studies (Faretra et al., 1970; Engelhardt et al., 1973). In three double-blind studies involving preschool-age autistic children who participated in an inpatient structured educational program, haloperidol was significantly superior to placebo in reducing behavioral symptoms. In the first trial, we wished to assess critically the therapeutic potential of haloperidol and behavior

TABLE 1

Phenothiazines: features of representative literature.

Author(s)	Subjects		Intelligence and status	Symptoms and/or diagnosis	Drug and dose (mg/day)	Side effects	Effects on symptoms
	Age (yrs)	Total no.					
Rapoport et al., 1971	4.5 – 10.5	19	normal; outpatients	chronic restlessness, aggressiveness, distractibility	d-amphetamine 10 CPZ 75 placebo	drowsiness with CPZ	d-amphetamine >CPZ
Werry et al., 1966	$\bar{x} = 8$	39	normal; outpatients	hyperactivity, aggressiveness, excitability, distractibility	CPZ, $\bar{x} = 106$ placebo	sleepiness, photo-sensitization of skin	reduction
Gittelman-Klein et al., 1976	$\bar{x} = 102.59$ mths $\pm$ 24.25 (S.D.)	155	normal; outpatients	hyperkinetic reaction of childhood	TDZ 50 – 300, $\bar{x} = 160$ methylphenidate 10 – 60 $\bar{x} = 47$ placebo, combination	enuresis extreme drowsiness with TDZ GI complaints increased appetite	methylphenidate or combination > TDZ, all active drugs > placebo
Alexandris and Lundell, 1968	7 – 12	21	retarded; inpatients	hyperkinesis, aggressiveness, short attention span and other symptoms; hyperkinetic syndrome	TDZ 30 – 150 $\bar{x} = 95$ amphetamine 7.5 – 75 $\bar{x} = 52$ placebo		TDZ > amphetamine or placebo

Campbell et al., 1982a	6.58 – 10.33	15	normal and retarded; inpatients	aggressiveness, explosiveness	CPZ 100 – 200 HAL, Li_2CO_3	drowsiness with CPZ	CPZ = HAL = Li_2CO_3
Campbell et al., 1972	3 – 6	10	severely retarded to average; inpatients	infantile autism	CPZ 9 – 45 $\bar{x}$ = 17.3 Li_2CO_3	excessive sedation, motor excitation, irritability, catatonic-like states, insomnia	no significant improvement
Fish et al., 1966	2 – 6	22	retarded to low normal; inpatients	infantile autism	trifluoperazine 2 – 20; amphetamine	lethargy, diminished interest and speech in less language impaired	improved alertness, verbal production, and less withdrawal in more severely language impaired
Faretra et al., 1970	5 – 12	60	retarded (?); inpatients	psychotic	fluphenazine 0.75 – 3.75 HAL	akathisia, rash	HAL > fluphenazine for symptom reduction
Engelhardt et al., 1973	6 – 12	30	retarded; outpatients	infantile autism	fluphenazine $\bar{x}$ = 10.4 HAL	increased salivation, drowsiness	fluphenazine = haloperidol

Abbreviations: CPZ = chlorpromazine; TDZ = thioridazine; HAL = haloperidol; Li_2CO_3 = lithium carbonate.

therapy on behavioral symptoms and on language acquisition, and the interaction of the two treatments (Campbell et al., 1978). Haloperidol significantly reduced withdrawal and stereotypies in children above 4.5 years of age. The combination of the two treatments resulted in significant increase of language acquisition. Untoward effects were observed only above optimal doses. The same effects of haloperidol were replicated in 10 subjects by Cohen et al. (1980). A third study was undertaken to explore further the therapeutic efficacy of haloperidol in a larger patient sample (40 children), using additional rating scales under various ecological conditions. Haloperidol was significantly superior to placebo in reducing symptoms of withdrawal, stereotypies, abnormal object relations, fidgetiness, hyperactivity, negativism, irritability and lability of affect (Campbell et al., 1982c; Anderson et al., 1984). There was a significant relationship between reduction of symptoms and haloperidol levels in serum (Poland et al., 1982). At optimal doses, under careful clinical monitoring, no untoward effects were rated; above optimal doses or during dosage regulation, the most common untoward effects were excessive sedation and acute dystonic reaction, during the 14 week clinical trial. It is of interest, that in other diagnostic categories administration of haloperidol may result in untoward effects, mainly sedation, at therapeutic doses. The presence of adverse effects detracts from the efficacy of haloperidol in conduct disorder, Tourette's and schizophrenic disorder (Pool et al., 1976; Borison et al., 1982; Campbell et al., 1982d; Shapiro and Shapiro, 1982a). It is possible that the presence or absence of untoward effects at therapeutic doses is a function of diagnosis. As to the mechanism of effectiveness of haloperidol in autistic children, it seems that this potent antidopaminergic drug is particularly effective in reducing those symptoms associated with excess dopaminergic activity in intellectually subnormal autistics: namely severe hyperactivity and stereotypies (Cohen et al., 1974, 1977).

Table 2 presents a brief summary of these studies with butyrophenones in children.

Thioxanthenes. Thiothixene was explored in a few studies involving mainly schizophrenic and a small number of autistic children (Wolpert et al., 1967; Campbell et al., 1970; Waizer et al., 1972; Simeon et al., 1973) and schizophrenic adolescents (Realmuto et al., 1984). The sample sizes were modest or small; the studies were pilot, open, single, or double-blind; placebo was not employed. However, in these patients who were 3 – 18 years of age, thiothixene appeared to be a promising therapeutic agent in doses of 1 – 42.6 mg/day: decreases of withdrawal, stereotypies, psychotic speech, hallucinations, anxiety and excitability were some of the changes rated. At doses above optimal untoward effects were observed, which included excessive sedation and extrapyramidal symptoms.

Dihydroindolones. Molindone was administered to children with infantile autism and conduct disorder, aggressive type. Like the clinical trials of thiothixene, these studies too have some methodological flaws and therefore the results are inconclusive. In a sample of 10 children, ages 3 – 5 years, 8 of whom were autistic, at doses of 1 – 2.5 mg/day, reduction of withdrawal, negativism, and stereotypies, and increases in affective responsiveness and attention span were rated (Campbell et al., 1971). Stimulating effects were observed on lower doses, and sedative effects on higher doses, or, an admixture of both. Untoward effects included behavioral toxicity, sedation, acute dystonic reaction and parkinsonian signs. As in trifluoperazine and thiothixene, the therapeutic margin for molindone was wider than the relatively narrow margin in autistic children for chlorpromazine and trifluperidol (Campbell et al., 1971). Molindone is currently being studied in hospitalized school-age aggressive children, diagnosed as conduct disorder (Greenhill et al., 1981). The daily doses ranged from 18 up to 155 mg (mean, 40.5).

Dibenzoxazepines. To the best of our knowledge, there is only one double-blind and placebo-controlled study on the use of neuroleptics in youngsters diagnosed as schizophrenic disorder; the drugs investigated were loxapine succinate and haloperidol (Pool et al., 1976). The 75 subjects, ages 13 – 18 years, were hospitalized with acute schizophrenia, or chronic schizophrenia with acute exacerbation. They were randomly assigned to one of the three treatments. On all three, there were marked improvements on the Brief Psychiatric Rating Scale (BPRS) and on the Nurse's Observation Scale for Inpatient Evaluation (NOSIE). However, loxapine was significantly more effective than placebo at week 4 on a number of items of the BPRS. Extrapyramidal symptoms and sedation were common with both active agents; haloperidol was less sedative than loxapine.

Diphenylbutylpiperidines. Pimozide (1 – 2 mg/day) was reported to be therapeutic without evidence of toxicity in 10 children, ages 9 – 14 years, most of whom were diagnosed as having schizophrenia or 'schizophrenia-like symptomatology' (Pangalila-Ratulangi, 1973). More recently, the efficacy and safety of pimozide was investigated in a multi-center study involving in- and outpatients (Naruse et al., 1982). Of the 87 children who participated in the study, 34 were diagnosed as 'autistic disturbance', 27 as 'hyperkinetic syndrome', and 17 as 'mentally retarded'. They were randomly assigned to pimozide, haloperidol or placebo. Both pimozide (1 – 7 mg/day) and haloperidol (0.75 – 6.75 mg/day) were significantly more effective than placebo; there was no difference between the two drugs. Clinically, pimozide appeared to be superior to haloperidol.

In at least two large series exploring pimozide's effectiveness in suppressing tics in children, it was shown to be effective and with less sedation or extrapyramidal side effects than haloperidol (Debray et al., 1972; Messerschmitt, 1972). A short-term (12 days) double-blind, placebo-controlled crossover comparison of pimozide with haloperidol in nine patients showed both drugs to be equieffective in suppressing symptoms of Tourette's disorder (Ross and Moldofsky, 1978). However, patients reported blindly less lethargy and sedation while receiving pimozide. In an

TABLE 2

Butyrophenones: features of representative literature.

Author(s)	Subjects		Intelligence and status	Symptoms and/or diagnosis	Drug and dose (mg/day)	Side effects	Effects on symptoms
	Age (yrs)	Total no.					
Cunningham et al., 1968	7.66 – 12.83	12	normal; inpatients	aggressive hyperactive, or destructive; severe behavior disorder	HAL 3 placebo	apathy, sleepiness, transient muscular pains or spasms	reduction of target symptoms
Fish et al., 1969	2 – 5	10	retarded; inpatients	infantile autism	trifluperidol 0.17 – 0.67 $\bar{x}$ = 0.37 CPZ, trifluoperazine	irritability, excessive sedation, excitement	trifluperidol > CPZ or trifluoperazine
Werry and Aman, 1975; Werry et al., 1975	4.92 – 12.33	32	normal; outpatients	hyperactivity aggressiveness; conduct disorder and hyperkinesis	HAL 0.05 mg/kg or 0.025 mg/kg, methylphenidate, placebo	more with high HAL: drowsiness, acute dystonic reaction	methylphenidate or either HAL dosage > placebo
Pool et al., 1976	13 – 18	75	normal (?); inpatients	acute schizophrenia or chronic with acute exacerbation	HAL 2 – 16 $\bar{x}$ = 9.8 loxapine placebo	extrapyramidal side effects and sedation	reduction
Campbell et al., 1978	2.6 – 7.2 $\bar{x}$ = 4.5	40	retarded; inpatients	infantile autism	HAL 0.5 – 4.0, $\bar{x}$ = 1.65 + behavior therapy, placebo	above optimal doses excessive sedation and dystonic reaction	facilitation of language learning with combination; reduced withdrawal and stereotypy with HAL. No change in

Cohen et al., 1980	2.1 – 7.0	10	retarded; inpatients	infantile autism	HAL $\bar{x} = 1.78$, placebo	above optimal doses excessive sedation and dystonic reaction	reduced withdrawal and stereotypies
Anderson et al., 1984; Campbell et al., 1982c	2.33 – 6.92	40	retarded; inpatients	infantile autism	HAL 0.5 – 3, $\bar{x} = 1.11$, or 0.019 – 0.217 mg/kg, $\bar{x} = 0.050$, placebo	above optimal doses or during regulation excessive sedation, acute dystonic reaction	HAL > placebo in reducing stereotypies, withdrawal, hyperactivity, etc.
Campbell et al., 1982a	6 – 10.66	15	normal and retarded; inpatients	aggressiveness, explosiveness	HAL 4.0 – 16.0, $\bar{x} = 9.2$ CPZ Li_2CO_3	drowsiness, drooling, slurred speech, dystonic reaction	reduction of target symptoms
Campbell et al., 1982d, 1984	5.2 – 12.9	61	normal; inpatients	aggressiveness, explosiveness; conduct disorder	HAL 1.0 – 6.0, $\bar{x} = 2.95$ or 0.04 – 0.21 mg/kg, $\bar{x} = 0.096$ Li_2CO_3, placebo	sedation, acute dystonic reaction, parkinsonian side effects, during dose regulation or above optimal dose	HAL = Li_2CO_3 and > placebo reduction of symptoms

Abbreviations: CPZ = chlorpromazine; TDZ = thioridazine; HAL = haloperidol; Li_2CO_3 = lithium carbonate.

open-label study of 42 patients, Shapiro and Shapiro (1982a) reported reduction of symptoms with pimozide (2 – 30 mg/day), and fewer adverse effects than with haloperidol.

Penfluridol is a long-acting oral diphenylbutylpiperidine derivative which could be administered weekly due to its long half-life. In at least two studies (Holomboe, 1977; Shapiro and Shapiro, 1982a), examining penfluridol's effectiveness in a total of 15 patients with Tourette's disorder in a weekly dosage range of 15 to 120 mg, it appeared to be equieffective with haloperidol with less severe sedative or akinesic side effects. However, the drug has been withdrawn from investigation in the U.S.A. due to the induction of tumors in laboratory rats.

Long-term efficacy

In daily practice and in institutions neuroleptics are frequently administered over a prolonged period of time to children with psychiatric disorders and to the mentally retarded (Lipman et al., 1978). However, there is little knowledge about their long-term efficacy based on systematic research.

Weiss and associates (1979) report that of 75 hyperactive children, the 17 subjects who were receiving chlorpromazine for 18 – 48 months did not differ at 10-year follow-up from those who received medication for less than 6 months. In a clinical trial of hyperactive school children, thioridazine was less effective after 12 weeks than at week 4 according to the ratings of teachers and psychiatrists (Gittelman-Klein et al., 1976).

In a group of 28 hyperactive and aggressive outpatients, all of whom were under 12 years of age, haloperidol (0.05 mg/kg per day) was clinically effective over a period of 6 months in reducing the target symptoms, as compared to placebo (Wong and Cock, 1971). In those children who improved on haloperidol, the gains were maintained throughout the study period, whereas the children who improved on placebo exhibited a fluctuating course. However, differences between the two treatments did not reach statistical significance, and there was only a trend towards improvement with haloperidol.

The long-term efficacy of haloperidol was investigated in a prospective fashion in young autistic children, most of whom are of preschool-age. The daily doses of haloperidol range from 0.5 to 3.0 mg. The drug was discontinued every 6 months and replaced by placebo for 4 weeks. Ratings were carried out on the Children's Psychiatric Rating Scale (CPRS) and Clinical Global Impressions (CGI) on baseline and at fixed intervals; these ratings were videotaped. Behavioral ratings were analyzed for 22 children at month 6 (Campbell et al., 1982b). The reduction of symptoms was maintained at that time; however, one week after the discontinuation of haloperidol, significant increases of withdrawal, stereotypies, hyperactivity, fidgetiness and abnormal object relations were rated on the CPRS, as well as significant worsening on the CGI.

Shapiro and Shapiro (1981) performed a 7 month to 8.5 year follow-up study of their first 80 patients with Tourette's disorder, some of whom were children, in order to evaluate the efficacy of haloperidol. Almost 75% of the patients who continued to use the medication during the course of the follow-up period showed an 80% decrease of symptoms, but 13% of the original sample discontinued treatment because of adverse side effects. In treating over 600 patients with haloperidol, these authors report the same approximate degree of improvement (Shapiro and Shapiro, 1981). They recommend a low dosage regimen with a usual range between 2 and 10 mg. Their method of drug administration involves 0.25 mg increments every fifth day until a 70% decrease in symptomatology is observed. In 16 patients with Tourette's disorder, blood levels of haloperidol were significantly correlated with dosage administered, but not with clinical response or adverse side effects (Shapiro and Shapiro, 1981). Thus, the therapeutic effect of haloperidol may be more closely related to its interaction with striatal dopamine (D_2) receptors than to its absolute levels in sera. Apparently, haloperidol is more effective than pimozide in reducing vocal tics, while both are equally effective in controlling motor tics (Normura and Segawa, 1982).

EFFECTS ON COGNITION AND LEARNING

Short-term effects

The effects of neuroleptics on cognition have not been adequately assessed in children. This is unfortunate, because learning problems are common in children who have serious behavioral problems requiring administration of neuroleptics. In general, it is believed that the neuroleptics, because of their tranquilizing-sedative effects, have an adverse effect on cognitive functions and learning. However, there is no strong evidence based on carefully diagnosed patients employing sound and sophisticated methodology to support this belief. Many studies were conducted in institutionalized and intellectually subnormal individuals; the drugs most frequently investigated were the sedative types of neuroleptics, chlorpromazine and thioridazine. There is some suggestion that the effects of this class of drugs in children may be dose-related (Werry and Aman, 1975; Campbell et al., 1978; Greenhill et al., 1981) or that their effects may depend on the diagnostic category under study (Werry et al., 1966; Platt et al., 1981, 1984; Campbell et al., 1982c; Anderson et al., 1984).

In hyperactive and aggressive children of normal intelligence, low dose haloperidol (0.025 mg/kg per day) facilitated performance on a number of laboratory measures; high dose (0.05 mg/kg per day) yielded deterioration of a short-term memory task and had no effect on other measures (Werry and Aman, 1975). In 48 outpatients with a similar behavioral profile, 8 weeks of chlorpromazine administration (mean daily dose of 106 mg) resulted in a trend toward improvement on the Continuous Performance Test, and possible deterioration on the WISC comprehension subtest and on the Bender Gestalt orientation quotient (Werry et al., 1966). Outside of the laboratory, there was a decrease of hyperactivity and improved attention. In four severely aggressive and explosive conduct disorder children there was no effect of chlorpromazine on a cognitive battery on daily doses of 100 – 200 mg (2.80 – 5.79 mg/kg); the same was true for haloperidol (4 – 16 mg, 0.12 – 0.75 mg/kg) (Campbell et al., 1982a). However, the samples were too small and therefore no conclusions can be made based on this pilot study. In a subsequent, placebo-controlled clinical trial of haloperidol involving a large sample of children with the same behavioral profile and diagnosis and of normal intelligence, haloperidol had mild effects on cognitive functions (Platt et al., 1984). In the 20 inpatients who received haloperidol (1.0 – 6.0 mg/day, mean, 2.95, or 0.04 – 0.21 mg/kg per day, mean, 0.096) there were significant decreases in Porteus Maze test quotient scores and a slowing of reaction time (RT) on a simple RT task. No significant effects were found for the Matching Familiar Figures Test, short-term recognition memory, concept attainment task, or the Stroop Test. The dosage used in this study is higher than that used by Werry and Aman (1975); however, these levels were the minimum required for clinical efficacy in this severely disturbed inpatient population, who failed to respond to previous outpatient treatments including psychoactive drugs.

In young autistic children haloperidol had no effect or had a positive effect on cognition and learning in the laboratory. It was demonstrated that the combination of haloperidol and language training was significantly more effective than language training or haloperidol alone in increasing language acquisition (Campbell et al., 1978; see Table 2). Subsequently, a study was designed to assess objectively the effects of haloperidol on discrimination learning and to determine whether haloperidol facilitates learning by reduction of symptoms which interfere with learning, or by more directly affecting attentional mechanisms. In this clinical trial, haloperidol was administered to 40 autistic children (Campbell et al., 1982c; Anderson et al., 1984). Following a 2-week placebo period, the children were randomly assigned to one of the two treatment sequences: haloperidol-placebo-haloperidol or placebo-haloperidol-placebo. Daily doses of haloperidol ranged from 0.5 to 2.0 mg/day (mean, 0.97) or 0.020 – 0.122 mg/kg (mean, 0.05). Each treatment period was of 4 weeks duration; the entire study lasted 14 weeks. Thirty-two children, mildly to profoundly retarded, ages 2.33 – 6.92 years (mean, 4.6), completed the discrimination training and their data were analyzed. At the doses administered, haloperidol facilitated discrimination learning and its retention. Children receiving haloperidol performed as well as those children whose DQ scores were 20 points higher and who were on placebo.

Long-term effects

There is still less known about the long-term effects of this class of drug on cognitive functions in children. In a retrospective study involving 125 hospitalized children, ages 4 – 16 years, who were diagnostically heterogeneous, the long-term effects of drugs were assessed on a variety of measures (McAndrew et al., 1972). In three aggressive, nonpsychotic children of normal intelligence, ages 12 and 13, who were receiving thioridazine for 1 – 4 years (doses varied from 50 to 400 mg/day) there was a significant increase in scores on the Stanford Achievement battery after the drug was discontinued. Similar effects of neuroleptic discontinuation were reported in mentally retarded adults (Breuning and Davidson, 1981) and 40 mentally retarded adolescents (Breuning et al., 1983). In a prospective study of 28 children under 12 years of age, with severe symptoms of aggressiveness and hyperkinesis, the behavioral efficacy of haloperidol was compared to placebo. The children were diagnostically heterogeneous, of normal intelligence and nonpsychotic. There was no adverse effect of haloperidol (0.05 mg/kg per day) on intellectual functioning or visuomotor tasks; actually there were significant increases in IQs in both treatment groups (Wong and Cock, 1971).

The long-term effects of haloperidol were assessed in eight autistic children, ages 4.2 – 9 years, who functioned on a borderline to profoundly retarded level (Die et al., 1984). The daily doses of haloperidol ranged frcm 0.5 to 3.0 mg (mean, 1.4); the drug was administered over a period of 10 months to 2 years 10 months (mean, 1.7 years). Three children showed marked increases in IQ or DQ scores; in two of these there was a significant improvement in language. Two children showed no change, while three moved to a lower overall category. In general, the improvements were in the language area, while decrements occurred in adaptive behavior. Stability of IQ scores throughout life has been reported in many autistic children; any change is of great importance. Whether the changes were a result of drug effects, individual differences or differences in psychosocial environment may be only determined by using a control group.

Although some short-term studies examining the effects of haloperidol on cognitive functioning show impairment, a recent study designed to test subtle effects of low dosages, which were gradually titrated and used to treat motor and vocal tics of patients with Tourette's disorder for long periods, failed to show significant adverse effects on higher cognitive processes (Bogomolny et al., 1982). In this study the total dosage ranged from 0.5 to 3.0 mg/day. Thus, when the usually effective dosage range of haloperidol for Tourette's disorder is adhered to and cognitive testing conducted after a period of accommdation to a stable dosage, litte, if any, impairment of these functions may be manifest.

The effect of neuroleptics on IQs of mentally retarded persons was also investigated. In a sample of 162, some of whom were adolescents (age range from 11 to 71), a comparison of a behavioral procedure (i.e. the loss of a token for engaging in aggressive and psychotic behaviors) with a variety of different neuroleptics (dosage range of 200 to 1500 mg/day CPZ equivalents) showed that the behavioral procedure alone was more effective than the drug alone in controlling targeted aggressive and psychotic behaviors (Ferguson, 1982). Moreover, an absence of a beneficial synergistic effect between drug and behavioral procedure was also suggested by the results. Mean IQ scores were shown to increase about 30 IQ points when mentally retarded subjects weaned completely from all neuroleptics for 39 days were tested under a condition of positive reinforcement (Ferguson, 1982). These persons received an edible reinforcement for each correct response. This increase contrasted with an almost 7-point increase in IQ in a comparison group of subjects only weaned from neuroleptics but not receiving any reinforcement.

In a study of a sample of 40 mentally retarded subjects (age range 11 to 25 years), Breuning et al. (1983) corroborated their finding that IQ scores obtained under a reinforcement condition increased significantly following thioridazine discontinuation. Moreover, the frequency of a variety of inappropriate behaviors, which included aggressive, destructive and yelling behaviors, decreased significantly upon drug discontinuation in a group of subjects for whom these target behaviors were felt to be nonresponsive to thioridazine. Thus, in addition to having no beneficial effect upon their intellectual performance, thioridazine may contribute to the emergence of inappropriate behaviors in subjects designated as nonresponders. Of note is the fact that the thioridazine responders and nonresponders in this study were selected from an earlier study of thioridazine discontinuation in 142 chronically medicated mentally retarded persons. In the earlier study, 86% of this original sample of 142 individuals were identified as nonresponders, i.e. they either showed no change or a decrease in the frequency of inappropriate behaviors upon drug discontinuation.

In addition to the poorer workshop performance of medicated, as compared to unmedicated, mentally retarded persons and the emergence of inappropriate behaviors in medicated thioridazine nonresponders, withdrawal dyskinesias have also been noted upon drug discontinuation in this population (Breuning et al., 1982). These dyskinesias were shown to adversely affect workshop performance.

UNTOWARD EFFECTS

The assessment of untoward effects has been reviewed by Campbell et al. (1985).

Immediate untoward effects

Behavioral toxicity is the most frequently observed immediate untoward effect in children, particularly in the younger age group. This is usually manifested as worsening of pre-existing symptoms (e.g. irritability, hyperactivity, apathy, insomnia) or newly emerging symptoms (e.g. like in a daze, hypoactivity, decrease of verbal production). The potential ability of haloperidol to precipitate dysphoric states, lethargy, cognitive impairment and school avoidance or school phobias in patients with Tourette's disorder has received special consideration (Ross and Moldofsky, 1978; Mikkelsen et al., 1981; Bogomolny et al., 1982; Brunn, 1982; Shapiro and Shapiro, 1982a). A careful and stable baseline assessment of the child is required in order to assess behavioral toxicity.

Adverse effects on cognitive functions and learning were reported, particularly in the mentally retarded, and most frequently with chlorpromazine and thioridazine (see above; for review, see Werry and Aman, 1975; Winsberg and Yepes, 1978; Werry 1981). Administration of haloperidol to children diagnosed as Tourette's disorder may produce sedation which in turn leads to deterioration in school performance (Shapiro et al., 1978).

CNS untoward effects include acute dystonic reactions, parkinsonian signs and akathisia. Acute dystonic reactions may be avoided by a low starting dose and gradual dose increments; they can be readily relieved by administration of Benadryl, orally or intramuscularly (25 mg). Parkinsonian untoward effects can be diminished or controlled by lowering the dosage; they are less frequently observed in preschool-age children, than in those of school-age and adolescents. Administration of chlorpromazine was reported to be associated with onset of grand mal seizures or increase in frequency of seizures in patients with pre-existing seizure disorders (Tarjan et al., 1957).

Liver damage and blood dyscrasias related to neuroleptics appear to be rare in children (for review, see DiMascio et al., 1970; Engelhardt and Polizos, 1978).

Long-term untoward effects

The rabbit syndrome is a late onset extrapyramidal untoward effect; it consists of rapid perioral muscular movements (Villeneuve, 1972). Tardive and neuroleptic withdrawal dyskinesias, both reversible and permanent were reported in children. The assessment of these drug-related movement disorders represents an even greater challenge in this age population than in adult psychiatric patients (for review, see Campbell et al., 1983c). Only a few reports exist in the literature on studies of neuroleptic-related dyskinesias in children (for review, see Gualtieri et al., 1980; Campbell et al., 1983c). According to various investigators, the prevalence of tardive or withdrawal dyskinesias in children ranges from 8 to 51% (McAndrew et al., 1972; Engelhardt and Polizos, 1978; Polizos and Engelhardt, 1980; Campbell et al., 1982b, 1983a, c; Gualtieri et al., 1982). All but one of these studies are retrospective; in most, baseline or prior-to-neuroleptic evaluations were not carried out; or the assessment methods were not specified. The majority of the subjects were autistic or mentally retarded and therefore they may have exhibited abnormal movements in the form of stereotypies, mannerisms or rocking as part of their clinical picture, when unmedicated. With an antidopaminergic agent, such as the neuroleptics, these movements may be suppressed, only to re-emerge when the drug is discontinued; this has been demonstrated in placebo-controlled studies using an ABAB or ABA design (Cohen et al., 1980; Campbell et al., 1982c). Often these movements are difficult or impossible to differentiate accurately from the neuroleptic-induced dyskinesias. This in turn renders it difficult to determine the true prevalence of tardive or withdrawal dyskinesias in patients treated with neuroleptics (Gualtieri et al., 1980; Breuning et al., 1982). In addition, normal young children too may exhibit stereotypic-like movements (Campbell et al., 1983c; Werry et al., 1983).

In a prospective study designed to assess the long-term therapeutic effects of haloperidol and its safety, 9 of 44 patients developed neuroleptic-related movements (Campbell et al., 1982b, 1983a; unpublished data). The children participating in this study were diagnosed as infantile autism; their ages ranged from 2.6 to 7.10 years. They all responded markedly to haloperidol. Dosage ranged from 0.5 to 3.0 mg/day in all but one child (a 7.9-year-old boy, who received 7.5 mg of haloperidol per day). No antiparkinsonian or other psychoactive drugs were administered concomitantly. Every 6 months haloperidol was discontinued and for 4 weeks replaced by placebo, to determine whether the child required continuation of haloperidol for the reduction of behavioral symptoms and to assess withdrawal phenomena. Assessment of behavioral symptoms and abnormal movements was carried out at fixed intervals. The Abnormal Involuntary Movement Scale (AIMS) developed by the NIMH (Fann et al., 1980) and the Rockland Research Institute Abbreviated Dyskinesia Rating Scale (Simpson et al., 1979) were the instruments employed. Of the 44 children who participated in the study (36 male, 8 female), 9 developed movements (5 male, 4 female) (unpublished data). In 7 of the 9 children the movements were de novo and in 2 there was a change in the topography and/or severity and frequency of the pre-existing abnormal movements (stereotypies). Haloperidol was administered for 3 – 18 months prior to the onset or change of movements. In 4 children the movements developed while on haloperidol, and in 5 during the placebo period. The movements ceased in less than one month up to 9 months; the exception is one child who recently developed tongue movements within the oral cavity. The movements ceased on haloperidol in 2 children, on placebo in 4, and in 2 while no medication was received. In this prospective study, 20.4% of children who had a high baseline rate of stereotypies developed medication-related movements, mainly in the area of the mouth. Thus, haloperidol is a relatively safe drug for this population of children when prescribed judiciously and administered under careful clinical monitoring.

There is little if any systematic investigation of the effects of neuroleptics on linear growth; on the basis of small and retrospective studies it appears that growth is not affected adversely (for review, see Campbell et al., 1983b).

DOSAGE REGULATION

In children, the administration of antipsychotic medications must be viewed as only an adjunctive mode of treatment which should not interfere with normal maturational development. The dosages must be carefully titrated so as not to impede the acquisition of new information and social skills. In agitated psychotic adults, sedation caused by many neuroleptics may by viewed as a positive therapeutic effect; however, in children sedation may impair learning and school participation. Therefore, all drugs should be instituted with low, therapeutically ineffective doses with a stepwise progression of gradual increments occurring at regular intervals. The usual error in the management of children is the administration of excessively high dosages which interfere with functioning. Moreover, due to the common expression of behavioral side effects of an affectomotor nature in children, there is a need for daily observation to ascertain positive and negative effects. These behavioral side effects include irritability, alteration in level of motor activity and loss of appetite. In addition, the more widely appreciated dystonic, akinesic, akathisic and extrapyramidal side effects occur as well. Such side effects of drug usage may or may not be detrimental to the overall psychological and physical well-being of the patient. Careful clinical observation and quantitative assessment of these effects must be made. Depending upon what properties and possible side effects are already known about the drug, certain assessments of behavior and physiology should be made prior to and throughout treatment. For example, baseline and experimental evaluations of blood pressure, pulse rate, body weight, irritability, and sleepiness may be important in determining the extent of drug side effects. Daily observations during the phase of dosage regulation are more easily performed in inpatient settings; whereas, dosage regulation in outpatients often requires the close cooperation of parents and teachers. The possible long-term effects of drug on physical growth and behavior should also be taken into consideration.

There are two major principles which should guide the clinician in his dosage regulation of childhood disorders. The first is the recognition of individual variation in both the maximum tolerated and 'optimal' dosage between children of the same approximate size and weight with the same illness and severity. The second is that the effective dosage range for a given agent may vary according to the specific disorder. For example, the treatment of Tourette's disorder requires lower doses of haloperidol than the treatment of many acute psychotic disorders in adolescents. Moreover, specific self-stimulatory or aggressive symptoms in mentally retarded individuals are responsive to different 'optimal' dosages which must be carefully titrated so as not to interfere with workshop or intellectual performance.

The efficacy of a drug, the comparability of findings across studies and the magnitude and manifestation of a particular type of side effect may be related to dosage level. Werry and Aman (1975) found that while high (0.05 mg/kg per day) and low (0.025 mg/kg per day) doses of haloperidol effectively reduced behavioral symptoms, cognitive performance deteriorated only under high doses. Dosage level determination may depend upon the type of patient population. Children in institutions often receive various psychoactive drugs over time and have a more prolonged history of drug administration than outpatients. In conjunction with dietary factors, this may alter drug absorption, excretion, and metabolism and decrease the efficacy of drug (Werry and Sprague, 1970; Christensen, 1979). In general, there is a linear or curvilinear association between the logarithm of the dose and its effect (Haas et al., 1963). Studies which permit only a single fixed dosage level must assume an extremely homogeneous sample and relatively identical rates of responding. Assuming that all individuals in the study will not respond at an optimal level, the expectation is that the overall average effect of test drug will be significantly greater than placebo or a comparison drug.

The problem with using a single fixed dosage is that if enough subjects do not respond at a level greater than placebo, 'the resulting data can easily give the impression that the medication tested lacks efficacy' (Chassan, 1979; p. 189). In clinical practice, no physician administers a single fixed dose to all patients in the same diagnostic category. Individualized dosage regulation (i.e. gradual incremental steps) with the proper controls can be implemented without losing the double blind. This is particularly important in studies testing the efficacy of pharmacological agents in children where maturational and developmental factors may interact with drug treatment and/or dosage level.

Finally, the relationship of serum levels to therapeutic efficacy of neuroleptics is unclear at this time. Blood levels may signify adequate drug absorption, but actual drug effect is due to the interaction of the antipsychotic agent with specific receptors within the CNS.

TABLE 3

Representative neuroleptics and dosages in children under 12 years of age.

		Oral dose range (mg/day)
I.	*Phenothiazines*	
	1. Aliphatics	
	chlorpromazine	10 – 200
	2. Piperidines	
	thioridazine	10 – 200
	3. Piperazines	
	fluphenazine	0.25 – 16
	trifluoperazine	1 – 20
II.	*Butyrophenones*	
	trifluoperidol	0.17 – 0.67
	haloperidol	0.5 – 16
III.	*Thioxanthenes*	
	thiothixene	1 – 40
IV.	*Dihydroindolones*	
	molindone	1 – 40*
V.	*Diphenylbutylpiperidines*	
	pimozide	1 – 7

* Greenhill et al. (1981) administered up to 155 mg/day.

CONCLUSIONS

In child psychiatry the neuroleptics have not had the same revolutionary effect that they have had in adult psychiatry. In childhood, psychoses are rare and neuroleptics are usually prescribed for a variety of behavioral symptoms (overactivity, aggressivity, withdrawal, attentional deficits, tics and stereotypies). Although often critical to a successful treatment plan, neuroleptics are viewed as an adjunctive mode of therapy designed to supplement other psychotherapeutic, social and special educational interventions. They are to be used in highly individualized dosages which do not interfere with maturational processes, learning and acquisition of social skills. The appropriate therapeutic dose will often differ between individuals with the same diagnosis of the same approximate size and weight. Also, dosage selection will depend upon the specific disorder and targeted symptoms under consideration. The most frequent problem with the use of neuroleptics in the clinical practice of child psychiatry is overmedication.

The clinician still does not have a large array of empirical studies from which he or she can choose the 'best' drug (and dosage level) to be used for a particular diagnostic population. While there is a growing number of drug studies in children, many of these clinical trials are afflicted with serious methodological problems. Studies which seem methodologically adequate need to be replicated before full support can be given to their conclusions. Furthermore, we know very little about the relationship among contributing factors, such as biological, psychosocial, environmental, genetic and other treatment modalities to drug action and behavioral change in children. More comprehensive studies using large patient samples are needed in this area.

Neuroleptics may have long-term effects on growth and cognitive functions; they are known to induce dyskinesias in some patients. Therefore, a careful analysis of the risk-to-benefit ratio should be made for every individual prior to the implementation of drug treatment.

ACKNOWLEDGEMENT

This work was supported in part by Public Health Service Grant MH-32212 from the National Institute of Mental Health.

REFERENCES

Alexandris, H. and Lundell, F. (1968) Effect of thioridazine, amphetamine and placebo on the hyperkinetic syndrome and cognitive area in mentally deficient children. Can. Med. Assoc. J. 98, 92 – 96.

Anderson, L. T., Campbell, M., Grega, D. M., Perry, R., Small, A. M. and Green, W. H. (1984) Haloperidol in the treatment of infantile autism: effects on learning and behavioral symptoms. Am. J. Psychiatry, 141, 1195 – 1202.

Bogomolny, A., Erenberg, G. and Rothner, A. D. (1982) Behavioral effects of haloperidol in young Tourette syndrome patients. In: A. J. Friedhoff and T. N. Chase (Eds), Advances in Neurology, Vol. 35: Gilles de la Tourette Syndrome. Raven Press, New York, pp. 427 – 432.

Borison, R. L., Ang. L., Chang, S., Dysken, M., Comaty, J. E. and Davis, J. M. (1982) New pharmacological approaches in the treatment of Tourette syndrome. In: A. J. Friedhoff and T. N. Chase (Eds), Advances in Neurology, Vol. 35: Gilles de la Tourette Syndrome. Raven Press, New York, pp. 377 – 382.

Breuning, S. E. (1982) An applied dose-response curve of thioridazine with the mentally retarded: aggressive, self-stimulatory, intellectual, and workshop behaviors – a preliminary report. Psychopharmacol. Bull. 18, 57 – 59.

Breuning, S. E. and Davidson, N. A. (1981) Effects of psychotropic drugs on the intelligence test performance of institutionalized retarded adults. Am. J. Ment. Defic. 85, 575 – 579.

Breuning, S. E., Davis, V. J., Matson, J. L. and Ferguson, D. G. (1982) Effects of thioridazine and withdrawal dyskinesias on workshop performance of mentally retarded young adults. Am. J. Psychiatry 139, 1447 – 1454.

Breuning, S. E., Ferguson, D. G., Davidson, N. A. and Poling, A. D. (1983) Effects of thioridazine on the intellectual performance of mentally retarded drug responders and nonresponders. Arch. Gen. Psychiatry 40, 309 – 313.

Bruun, R. D. (1982) Dysphoric phenomena associated with haloperidol treatment of Tourette syndrome. In: A. J. Friedhoff and T. N. Chase (Eds), Advances in Neurology, Vol. 35: Gilles de la Tourette Syndrome. Raven Press, New York, pp. 433 – 436.

Campbell, M. (1977) Demographic parameters of disturbed children: a template to the CPDI and CSH, its rationale and significance. Psychopharmacol. Bull. 13, 30 – 33.

Campbell, M., Fish, B., Shapiro, T. and Floyd, Jr., A. (1970) Thiothixene in young disturbed children: a pilot study. Arch. Gen. Psychiatry 23, 70 – 72.

Campbell, M., Fish, B., Shapiro, T. and Floyd, Jr., A. (1971) Study of molindone in disturbed preschool children. Curr. Ther. Res. 13, 28 – 33.

Campbell, M., Fish, B., Korein, J., Shapiro, T., Collins, P. and Koh, C. (1972) Lithium and chlorpromazine: a controlled crossover study of hyperactive severely disturbed young children. J. Autism Child. Schizophr. 2, 234 – 263.

Campbell, M., Anderson, L. T., Meier, M., Cohen, I. L., Small, A. M., Samit, C. and Sachar, E. J. (1978) A comparison of haloperidol and behavior therapy and their interaction in autistic children. J. Am. Acad. Child Psychiatry 17, 640 – 655.

Campbell, M., Cohen, I. L. and Small, A. M. (1982a) Drugs in aggressive behavior. J. Am. Acad. Child Psychiatry 21, 107 – 117.

Campbell, M., Anderson, L. T., Cohen, I. L., Perry, R., Small, A. M., Green, W. H., Anderson, L. and McCandless, Jr., W. H. (1982b) Haloperidol in autistic children: effects on learning, behavior, and abnormal involuntary movements. Psychopharmacol. Bull. 18, 110 – 112.

Campbell, M., Anderson, L. T., Small, A. M., Perry, R., Green, W. H. and Caplan, R. (1982c) The effects of haloperidol on learning and behavior in autistic children. J. Autism Dev. Dis. 12, 167 – 175.

Campbell, M., Small, A. M., Green, W. H., Jennings, S. J., Perry, R., Padron, M. and Bennett, W. G. (1982d) Lithium and haloperidol in hospitalized aggressive children. Psychopharmacol. Bull. 18, 126 – 129.

Campbell, M., Perry, R., Bennett, W. G., Small, A. M., Green, W. H., Grega, D., Schwartz, V. and Anderson, L. (1983a) Long-term therapeutic efficacy and drug-related abnormal movements: a prospective study of haloperidol in autistic children. Psychopharmacol. Bull. 19, 80 – 83.

Campbell, M., Green, W. H., Perry, R. and Anderson, L. T. (1983b) Pharmacotherapy. In: C. E. Walker and M. C. Roberts (Eds), Handbook of Clinical Child Psychology. John Wiley & Sons, New York, pp. 1109 – 1130.

Campbell, M., Grega, D. M., Green, W. H. and Bennett, W. G. (1983c) Neuroleptic-induced dyskinesias in children. Clin. Neuropharmacol. 6, 1425 – 1438.

Campbell, M., Small, A. M., Green, W. H., Jennings, S. J., Perry, R., Bennett, W. G. and Anderson, L. (1984) Behavioral efficacy of haloperidol and lithium carbonate. A comparison in hospitalized aggressive children with conduct disorder. Arch. Gen. Psychiatry 41, 650 – 656.

Campbell, M., Green, W. H., Deutsch, S. I. and Anderson, L. T. (1985) Childhood Pharmacotherapy. Sage Publications, Beverly Hills, California.

Chassan, J. B. (1979) Research Design in Clinical Psychology and Psychiatry, 2nd Edn. Irvington Publishers, New York.

Christensen, D. E. (1973) Combined Effects of Methylphenidate (Ritalin) and a Classroom Behavior Modification Program in Reducing the Hyperkinetic Behaviors of Institutionalized Mental Retardates. Thesis Submitted for the Degree of Doctor of Philosophy in Psychology, University of Illinois at Urbana-Champaign.

Cohen, D. J., Shaywitz, B. A., Johnson, W. T. and Bowers, M. (1974) Biogenic amines in autistic and atypical children: cerebrospinal fluid measures of homovanillic acid and 5-hydroxyindoleacetic acid. Arch. Gen. Psychiatry 31, 845 – 853.

Cohen, D. J., Caparulo, B. K., Shaywitz, B. A. and Bowers, M. (1977) Dopamine and serotonin metabolism in neuropsychiatrically disturbed children: CSF homovanillic acid and 5-hydroxyindoleacetic acid. Arch. Gen. Psychiatry 34, 545 – 550.

Cohen, I. L., Campbell, M., Posner, D., Small, A. M., Triebel, D. and Anderson, L. T. (1980) Behavioral effects of haloperidol in young autistic children. An objective analysis using a within-subjects reveral design. J. Am. Acad. Child Psychiatry 19, 665 – 677.

Cohen, J. (1977) Statistical Power Analysis in the Behavioral Sciences, Revised edition. Academic Press, New York.

Conners, C. K. (1977) Drug research with children. In: J. M. Wiener (Ed.), Psychopharmacology in Childhood and Adolescence. Basic Books, Inc., New York, pp. 58 – 83.

Cunningham, M. A., Pillai, V. and Rogers, W. J. B. (1968) Haloperidol in the treatment of children with severe behavior disorders. Br. J. Psychiatry 114, 845 – 854.

Debray, P., Messerschmitt, P., Lonchap, D. and Herbault, M. (1972) L'utilization du pimozide en pédo-psychiatrie. Nouv. Presse Med. 1, 2917.

Diagnostic and Statistical Manual of Mental Disorders (DSM-III) (1980) 3 rd Edition. American Psychiatric Association, Washington, D. C., U.S.A.

Die Trill, M., Wolsky, B. B., Shell, J., Green, W. H., Perry, R. and Campbell, M. (1984) Effects of long-term haloperidol treatment on intellectual functioning in autistic children: a pilot study. Paper presented at the 31st Annual Meeting of the American Academy of Child Psychiatry, Toronto, Canada, October 10 – 14, 1984.

DiMascio, A., Soltys, J. J. and Shader, R. I. (1970) Psychotropic drug side effects in children. In: R. I. Shader and A. DiMascio (Eds), Psychotropic Drug Side Effects. Williams and Wilkins Company, Baltimore, pp. 235 – 260.

Engelhardt, D. M. and Polizos, P. (1978) Adverse effects of pharmacotherapy in childhood psychosis. In: M. A. Lipton, A. DiMascio, and K. F. Killam (Eds), Psychopharmacology: A Generation of Progress. Raven Press, New York, 1463 – 1469.

Engelhardt, D. M., Polizos, P., Waizer, J. and Hoffman, S. P. (1973) A double-blind comparison of fluphenazine and haloperidol in outpatient schizophrenic children. J. Autism Child Schizophr. 3, 128 – 137.

Fann, W. E., Smith, R. C., Davis, J. M. and Domino, E. F. (Eds.) (1980) Tardive Dyskinesia: Research and Treatment. Spectrum Publications, Jamaica, New York.

Faretra, G., Dooher, L. and Dowling, J. (1970) Comparison of haloperidol and fluphenazine in disturbed children. Am. J. Psychiatry 126, 1670 – 1673.

Ferguson, D. G. (1982) Effects of neuroleptic drugs on the intellectual and habilitative behaviors of mentally retarded persons. Psychopharmacol. Bull. 18, 54 – 56.

Fish, B., Shapiro, T. and Campbell, M. (1966) Long term prognosis and the response of schizophrenic children to drug therapy: a controlled study of trifluoperazine. Am. J. Psychiatry 123, 32 – 39.

Fish, B., Campbell, M., Shapiro, T. and Floyd, Jr., A. (1969) Comparison of trifluperidol, trifluoperazine and chlorpromazine in preschool schizophrenic children: the value of less sedative antipsychotic agents. Curr. Ther. Res. 11, 589 – 595.

Freeman, R. D. (1970) Psychopharmacology and the retarded child. In: F. Menolascino (Ed.), Psychiatric Approaches to Mental Retardation. Basic Books, New York, pp. 294 – 368.

Gittelman-Klein, R., Klein, D. F., Katz, S., Saraf, K. R. and Pollack, E. (1976) Comparative effects of methylphenidate and thioridazine in hyperkinetic children. I. Clinical results. Arch. Gen. Psychiatry 33, 1217 – 1231.

Greenhill, L. L., Barmack, J. E., Spalten, D., Anderson, M. and Halpern, F. (1981) Molindone hydrochloride in the treatment of aggressive, hospitalized children. Psychopharmacol. Bull. 17, 125 – 126.

Gualtieri, C. T., Barnhill, J., McGimsey, J. and Schell, D. (1980) Tardive dyskinesia and other movement disorders in children treated with psychotropic drugs. J. Am. Acad. Child Psychiatry 19, 491 – 510.

Gualtieri, C. T., Breuning, S. E., Schroeder, S. R. and Quade, D. (1982) Tardive dyskinesia in mentally retarded children, adolescents, and young adults: North Carolina and Michigan Studies. Psychopharmacol. Bull. 18, 62 – 65.

Guy, W. (1976) ECDEU Assessment Manual for Psychopharmacology, revised. DHEW Publication No. (ADM) 76-338, Rockville, Md.

Haas, H., Fink, H. and Hartfelder, G. (1963) The placebo problem. Psychopharmacol. Serv. Cent. Bull, 2, (8), 1 – 65.

Hersen, M. and Barlow, D. H. (1976) Single Case Experimental Designs: Strategies for Studying Behavior Change. Pergamon Press, New York.

Holmboe, R. (1977) Paper presented at VI World Congress of Psychiatry, Honolulu, Hawaii.

Kazdin, A. E. (1976) Statistical analyses for single-case experimental designs. In: M. Hersen and D. H. Barlow (Eds), Single Case Experimental Designs: Strategies for Studying Behavior Change. Pergamon Press, New York.

Lipman, R. S., DiMascio, A., Reatig, N. and Kirson, T. (1978) Psychotropic drugs and mentally retarded children. In: M. A. Lipton, A. DiMascio and K. F. Killam (Eds), Psychopharmacology: A Generation of Progress. Raven Press, New York pp. 1437 – 1449.

McAndrew, J. B., Case, Q. and Treffert, D. A. (1972) Effects of prolonged phenothiazine intake on psychotic and other hospitalized children. J. Autism Child Schizophr. 2, 75 – 91.

Messerschmitt, P. L. (1972) L'utilization du pimozide en pédo-psychiatrie (á propos de 186 malades). Theses, Faculté de Médicine de Paris.

Mikkelsen, E. J., Detlor, J. and Cohen, D. J. (1981) School avoidance and social phobia triggered by haloperidol in patients with Tourette's disorder. Am. J. Psychiatry 138, 1572 – 1576.

Naruse, H., Nagahata, M., Nakane, Y., Shirahashi, K., Takesada, M. and Yamazaki, K. (1982) A multi-center double-blind trial of pimozide (Orap), haloperidol and placebo in children with behavioral disorders, using crossover design. Acta Paedopsychiatr. (Stockholm) 48, 173 – 184.

Normura, Y. and Segawa, M. (1982) Tourette syndrome in Oriental children: clinical and pathophysiological considerations. In: A. J. Friedhoff and T. N. Chase (Eds.), Advances in Neurology, Vol. 35: Gilles de la Tourette Syndrome. Raven Press, New York, pp. 277 – 280.

Pangalila-Ratulangi, E. A. (1973) Pilot evaluation of Orap (pimozide, R6238) in child psychiatry. Psychiatr. Neurol. Neurochir. 76, 17 – 27.

Platt, J. E., Campbell, M., Green, W. H., Perry, R. and Cohen, I. L. (1981) Effects of lithium carbonate and haloperidol on cognition in aggressive hospitalized school-age children. J. Clin. Psychopharmacol. 20 (1), 8 – 13.

Platt, J. E., Campbell, M., Green, W. H. and Grega, D. M. (1984) Cognitive effects of lithium carbonate and haloperidol in treatment resistant aggressive children. Arch. Gen. Psychiatry 41, 657 – 662.

Poland, R. E., Campbell, M., Rubin, R. T., Perry, R. and Anderson, L. (1982) Relationship of serum haloperidol levels and clinical response in autistic children. Abstracts. Vol. II. 13th C.I.N.P. Congress, p. 591.

Polizos, P. and Engelhardt, D. M (1980) Dyskinetic and neurological complications in children treated with psychotropic medication. In: W. E. Fann, R. C. Smith, J. M. Davis and E. F. Domino (Eds), Tardive Dyskinesia. Research and Treatment. Spectrum Publications, Jamaica, New York, pp. 193 – 199.

Pool, D., Bloom, W., Mielke, D. H., Roniger, J. J. and Gallant, D. M. (1976) A controlled evaluation of loxitane in seventy-five adolescent schizophrenic patients. Curr. Ther. Res. 19, 99 – 104.

Rapoport, J., Abramson, A., Alexander, D. and Lott, I. (1971) Playroom observations of hyperactive children on medication. J. Am. Acad. Child Psychiatry 10, 524 – 534.

Realmuto, G. M., Erickson, W. D., Yellin, A. M., Hopwood, J. H. and Greenberg, L. M. (1984) Clinical comparison of thiothixene and thioridazine in schizophrenic adolescents. Am. J. Psychiatry 141, 440 – 442.

Ross, M. S. and Moldofsky, H. (1978) A comparison of pimozide and haloperidol in the treatment of Gilles de la Tourette's syndrome. Am. J. Psychiatry 135, 585 – 587.

Shapiro, A. K. and Shapiro, E. S. (1981) The treatment and etiology of tics and Tourette syndrome. Compr. Psychiatry 22, 193 – 205.

Shapiro, A. K. and Shapiro, E. (1982a) Clinical efficacy of haloperidol, pimozide, penfluridol, and clonidine in the treatment of Tourette syndrome. In: A. J. Friedhoff and T. N. Chase (Eds), Advances in Neurology, Vol. 35: Gilles de la Tourette Syndrome. Raven Press, New York, pp. 383 – 386.

Shapiro, A. K. and Shapiro, E. (1982b) Tourette syndrome: history and present status. In: A. J. Friedhoff and T. N. Chase (Eds), Advances in Neurology, Vol. 35: Gilles de la Tourette Syndrome. Raven Press, New York, pp. 17 – 23.

Shapiro, A. K., Shapiro, E. S., Brunn, R. D. and Sweet, R. C. (1978) Gilles de la Tourette Syndrome. Raven Press, New York.

Shapiro, E. S. and Shapiro, A. K. (1982) Tardive dyskinesia and chronic neuroleptic treatment of Tourette patients. In: A. J. Friedhoff and T. N. Chase (Eds), Advances in Neurology, Vol. 35: Gilles de la Tourette Syndrome. Raven Press, New York, p. 413.

Sidman, M. (1960) Tactics of Scientific Research. Basic Books, New York.

Simeon, J., Saletu, B., Saletu, M., Itil, T. M. and Da Silva, J. (1973) Thiothixene in childhood psychoses. Paper presented at the Third International Symposium on Phenothiazines, Rockville, Maryland, U.S.A.

Simpson, G. M., Lee, J. H., Zoubok, B. and Gardos, G. (1979) A rating scale for tardive dyskinesia. Psychopharmacology 64, 171 – 179.

Sprague, R. L. and Werry, J. S. (1971) Methodology of psychopharmacological studies with the retarded. In: N. R. Ellis (Ed.), International Review of Research in Mental Retardation. Academic Press, New York, pp. 147 – 219.

Tarjan, G., Lowerey, V. E. and Wright, S. W. (1957) Use of chlorpromazine in two hundred seventy-eight mentally deficient patients. J. Dis. Child. 94, 294 – 300.

Thompson, J. W., Green, D. and Savitt, H. L. (1983) Preliminary report on a crosswalk from DSM-III to ICD-9-CM. Am. J. Psychiatry 140, 176 – 180.

Turner, D. A., Purchatzke, G., Gift, T., Farmer, C. and Uhlenhuth, E. H. (1974) Intensive design in evaluating anxiolytic agents. In: F. G. McMahon (Ed.), Principles and Techniques of Human Research and Therapeutics. J. Levine, B. C. Schiele, W. J. R. Taylor (Eds), Vol. VIII: Psychopharmacological Agents. Futura Publishing Company, Mt. Kisco, N. Y., pp. 105 – 118.

Villeneuve, A. (1972) The rabbit syndrome: a peculiar extrapyramidal reaction. Can. Psychiatr. Assoc. J. 17, 69 – 72.

Waizer, J., Polizos, P., Hoffman, S. P., Engelhardt, D. M. and Margolis, R. A. (1972) A single-blind evaluation of thiothixene with outpatient schizophrenic children. J. Autism Child. Schizophr. 2, 378 – 386.

Weiss, G., Hechtman, L., Perlman, T., Hopkins, J. and Wener, A. (1979) Hyperactives as young adults. A controlled prospective ten-year study follow-up of 75 children. Arch. Gen. Psychiatry 36, 675 – 681.

Werry, J. S. (1981) Drugs and learning. J. Child. Psychol. 22, 283 – 290.

Werry, J. S. and Aman, M. G. (1975) Methylphenidate and haloperidol in children. Arch. Gen. Psychiatry 32, 790 – 795.

Werry, J. S., Aman, M.G. and Lampen, E. (1975) Haloperidol and methylphenidate in hyperactive children. Acta Paedopsychiatr. (Stockholm) 42, 26 – 40.

Werry, J. S., Weiss, G., Douglas, V. and Martin, J. (1966) Studies on the hyperactive child. III. The effect of chlorpromazine upon behavior and learning ability. J. Am. Acad. Child. Psychiatry 5, 292 – 312.

Werry, J. S., Carlielle, J. and Fitzpatrick, J. (1983) Rhythmic motor activities (stereotypies) in children under five: etiology and prevalence. J. Am. Acad. Child. Psychiatry 22, 329 – 336.

Winsberg, B. G. and Yepes, L. E. (1978) Antipsychotics. In: J. S. Werry (Ed.), Pediatric Psychopharmacology. Brunner Mazel, New York, pp. 234 – 273.

Wolpert, A., Hagamen, M. B. and Merlis, S. (1967) A comparative study of thiothixene and trifluoperazine in childhood schizophrenia. Curr. Ther. Res. 9, 482 – 485.

Wong, G. H. and Cock, R. J. (1971) Long-term effects of haloperidol on severely emotionally disturbed children. Aust. N.Z. J. Psychiatry 5, 296 – 300.

Burrows/Norman/Davies (eds) Antipsychotics

Chapter 17

The use of antipsychotic agents in the elderly

WILLIAM M. PETRIE

and

THOMAS A. BAN

Tennessee Neuropsychiatric Institute, 1501 Murfreesboro Road, Tennessee, TN 37217, U.S.A.

INTRODUCTION

Antipsychotics are widely used in aged populations. They are primarily employed for schizophrenic illnesses extending into later life, paranoid disorders in the elderly, manic symptoms, and agitated restless, or hostile behavior in degenerative dementias. Despite the patterns of extensive use, research on antipsychotics in non-schizophrenic, elderly patients has been limited.

In hospitalized patients, survey data have indicated that antipsychotics were prescribed four times more frequently than any other psychotropic agent. In the survey of Prien and Cole (1978), thioridazine was the most widely prescribed agent. In the ambulatory elderly, however, neuroleptic use is considerably lower, estimated at less than 1% in one survey (Stewart et al., 1982).

Among nursing homes, there were wide variations in prescribing patterns, with the percentage of patients receiving daily antipsychotics varying from 0 to 46% of nursing home populations. In a survey of Tennessee nursing homes including patients residing for more than one year, 43% received antipsychotics – 9% received daily doses of antipsychotics throughout the year (Ray et al., 1980). Another survey of chronically ill elderly patients revealed that withdrawn patients frequently received antipsychotics (Achong et al., 1978).

Patients treated with antipsychotics frequently receive other drugs. In his survey of hospitalized patients, Prien (1975) found that one of six patients was treated with two psychotropic agents simultaneously, with the most frequent combination an antipsychotic and a sedative-hypnotic drug (Prien, 1975). There is a high incidence of concomitant physical illnesses in aged psychiatric patients (Shanas, 1974), and the extent of polypharmacy is greater in the elderly than in adult populations (Fracchia et al., 1971; Lamy and Vestal, 1976).

PHARMACOKINETICS

The elderly may respond quite differently to antipsychotic therapy than younger patients. Debilitating, degenerative illnesses may accentuate this difference.

The possibility that pharmacokinetic changes are responsible for the different responses to antipsychotics was raised because there is reduction in gastric pH, delayed gastric emptying, decreased intestinal motility, and a reduction in the vascular supply of the intestine in the elderly (Bender, 1968). However, these factors do not sufficiently explain the altered pharmacologic effects of antipsychotics in the aged (Cooper and Robinson, 1981). Because enzymatic degradation of neuroleptics occurs within the intestinal lumen, delayed gastric emptying may result in a decrease in the bioavailability of chlorpromazine (Rivera-Calimlim et al., 1978). On the other hand, metabolism may be speeded by changes in the intestinal wall and by altered microflora of the small intestine (Scheline, 1973); therefore metabolites may be more readily absorbed, possibly accounting for the more frequent adverse effects in older patients (Hollister et al., 1970).

Drug distribution is affected by changes in weight and body composition in the elderly. Total body water is decreased while body fat is increased (Edelman and Liebman, 1959; Novak, 1972). Blood flow to the kidney and liver is decreased, and cardiac output reduced while blood flow to the brain, heart and muscle is increased (Cooper and Robinson, 1981). The blood-brain barrier may also become more permeable to drugs, resulting in greater CNS effects. A reduction of red cell binding in the elderly has been noted with other drugs (Chan et al., 1975), and may also be significant with neuroleptics.

Neuroleptics are metabolized in hepatic tissue, and with reduction in the function of the cytochrome P450 system, elimination half-lives of antipsychotics are increased. This corresponds to findings of Klein and Davis (1969) who observed a positive correlation between age and plasma levels of thioridazine in 18 schizophrenic patients. However, Muusze and Vanderheeren (1977) found no correlation between plasma levels of thioridazine or its metabolites with age; Martensson and Roos (1973) noted a positive relationship, but only at doses below 5 mg/kg; and Axelsson and Aspenstrom (1982) found only a weak correlation between age and plasma levels. A study of haloperidol plasma concentrations and age failed to reveal any significant relationship to age (Forsman and Ohman, 1976).

THERAPEUTIC EFFECTS

While nearly all the antipsychotics have been employed in elderly patients, most of the clinical trials have lumped patients into the general category of 'organic brain syndrome', or 'psychogeriatric patients'. Recent studies have paid more careful attention to the importance of diagnosis in the geriatric population.

Phenothiazines

Chlorpromazine has been used widely in geriatrics. It has been observed to improve personal hygiene, eating habits and insomnia in geriatric patients (Kurland, 1955; Pollack, 1956). In a placebo-controlled study of elderly patients with the diagnoses of chronic schizophrenia and agitated organic brain syndrome, Seager (1955) found chlorpromazine in doses of 150 – 225 mg superior to an inactive substance. In another study of hospitalized organic and schizophrenic patients, Barton and Hurst (1966) also found chlorpromazine more effective than placebo in controlling psychotic, agitated behavior. However, in other studies with mixed populations, no significant difference between chlorpromazine (50 – 200 mg) and placebo could be revealed (Abse and Dahlstrom, 1960; Robinson, 1969; Birkett and Boltuch, 1972). Even more, one study reported deterioration with active drug treatment compared to placebo (Robinson, 1969).

Acetophenazine, a piperazine phenothiazine, shares common properties with other phenothiazines (Marler, 1967). Because of the low incidence of extrapyramidal and hypotensive effects with acetophenazine, it was thought to be useful in geriatrics. While in one clinical study with chronically hospitalized geriatric patients, acetophenazine (40 – 60 mg/day) was superior to placebo (Hamilton and Bennet, 1962b), in another clinical study with schizophrenic patients, acetophenazine (mean dose: 79 mg/day) was superior to chlorpromazine (mean dose: 98 mg/day) in controlling delusions (Sheppard et al., 1964), although it is clear that the acetophenazine dose was relatively higher than the chlorpromazine dose.

Trifluoperazine has not been extensively studied in the aged, and available studies have provided equivocal results when compared with placebo (Hamilton and Bennett, 1962a). In a collaborative study of the United States Veterans Administration hospitals, acetophenazine (20 – 125 mg/day) was as effective as trifluoperazine (7 – 12 mg/day) in the control of agitation and psychosis, and more effective in decreasing excitement and improving social competence (Honigfeld et al., 1965).

Thioridazine has been the phenothiazine most widely utilized in geriatric populations. In dosages of 20 – 200 mg per day (well below accepted antipsychotic doses in adults), thioridazine has produced improvement in combative, agitated behavior in hospitalized and institutionalized patients (Reedy, 1967; Fraiberg, 1972; Barksdale, 1971). In placebo-controlled studies, thioridazine has generally proved superior to placebo (Judah et al., 1959). In two studies, thioridazine yielded more positive results than diazepam on social activity and retardation (Kirven and Montero, 1973; Cervera, 1974). Studies comparing thioridazine to other antipsychotics (chlorpromazine, thiothixene, and haloperidol) have failed to provide significant overall differences, although depression usually responded more favorably to thioridazine than to the other drugs (Tsuang et al., 1971; Altman et al., 1973; Katz and Itil, 1974).

Loxapine has received recent research attention with two controlled studies. In the nursing home study of Barnes et al. (1982), loxapine and thioridazine were equal in therapeutic effectiveness and superior to placebo in demented patients. Another study of hospitalized geriatrics (Petrie et al., 1982) compared loxapine to haloperidol and placebo in dementia patients with agitation and hostility. Both active drugs were superior to placebo; loxapine showed some superiority to haloperidol in nursing assessments. Both studies demonstrated significant but limited improvement in the behavior of carefully screened demented patients in nursing home and hospital settings compared to deterioration on placebo.

Reports of uncontrolled studies have described favorable changes in geriatric patients with fluphenazine hydrochloride (Chesrow et al., 1962), fluphenazine decanoate (Raskind et al., 1979), perphenazine (Silverman et al., 1959), and mesoridazine (Goldstein, 1974).

Thioxanthenes

Thiothixene shares many properties with the piperazine phenothiazines. Uncontrolled, but systematic, trials have demonstrated the effectiveness of thiothixene in hospitalized geriatric patients in doses of 2 – 15 mg/day; patients (Lehmann and Ban, 1970; Birkett et al., 1972) had diagnoses of both schizophrenia and dementia. Thiothixene has been more effective than placebo in one double-blind trial of organic brain syndrome patients (Rada and Kellner, 1976). A double-blind, comparative study of thiothixene and thioridazine in 40 organic brain syndrome patients, reported significant improvement in Brief Psychiatric Rating Scale (BPRS) scores with both drugs, without clinically significant differences (Katz and Itil, 1974). Thiothixene has also been used for the 'sundowner syndrome' and for acute confusional states associated with dementia (Charatan, 1978; Sloane, 1978).

Butyrophenones

In addition to thioridazine, haloperidol has received perhaps the greatest attention in the geropsychiatric literature. The first reports of the use of haloperidol in the aged appeared in 1961, when Gerle et al. (1961) reported moderate to marked improvement in therapy-refractory psychogeriatric patients with relatively low doses (0.4 – 0.6 mg) of the drug. Many other uncontrolled studies have consistently described significant therapeutic effects (Ban and Pecknold, 1975), although one study noted only modest improvement with haloperidol, which was less impressive than that observed with *cis*(Z)clopenthixol (Gotestam et al., 1981). Comparisons to thioridazine in organic brain syndrome patients have been most common in double-blind trials. Improvement has generally been comparable in both haloperidol and thioridazine-treated patients (Stotsky, 1972). While Smith et al. (1974) reported slightly greater improvement with haloperidol than with thioridazine, Cowley and Glen (1979) found thioridazine superior to haloperidol. Rosen (1979) reported greater improvement on the Wechsler Memory Scale in haloperidol than in thioridazine patients, although this probably reflects a difference in adverse effects.

OTHER NEUROLEPTICS

Reserpine has been utilized in the elderly, with improvement reported in a variety of dementia patients, especially those with irritability and hostility (Ban, 1969). One report suggested that tranquilization with reserpine was less rapid and less effective than with the phenothiazines (Dale, 1961). Reserpine has been utilized in combination with nicotinic acid (Proctor et al., 1958), methylphenidate (Ferguson and Funderburk, 1956) and thyroglobulin (Puls, 1967).

β-Adrenergic blocking drugs have been employed in isolated reports with psychotic, agitated patients when conventional antipsychotics have been ineffective (Petrie and Ban, 1981; Yudovsky et al., 1981). These agents produce less sedation, less impairment in psychomotor function, and are free of extrapyramidal effects.

TREATMENT ISSUES

Hallucinations, paranoid ideation, hostility, and uncooperativeness are generally more responsive to antipsychotic therapy than grandiosity, anxiety, tension and agitation. While there are important interactive effects of drugs and social therapies in the young (Schooler, 1978), we suggest that these interactions may be even more important in aged patients, where social isolation and withdrawal is common. Noncompliance is almost certainly a major limiting factor with elderly patients, except when family members supervise drug administration. The use of depot form antipsychotics is of clinical value in these cases (Raskind et al., 1979).

Because many elderly patients are involved with chronic treatment, the question of drug withdrawal or discontinuation will be continually raised. Most studies suggest that, in cases of psychotic relapse during drug discontinuation, resuming medication will result in rapid alleviation of symptoms (Gardos and Cole, 1978). This is particularly the case in the organic psychoses where symptoms are generally less systematized and persistent. However, the elderly may present legitimate risks of harm to others, and antipsychotics may reduce aggressive and violent behavior (Petrie et al., 1982).

ADVERSE EFFECTS

In summarizing, clearly, no drug emerges as statistically superior to others. The choice of drug will at times depend on the profile of adverse effects. Hurwitz found a general incidence rate of drug side effects of 21.3% in patients aged 70 – 79 and a rate of 25% in people over 80 compared to figures of 7% in ages 40 – 49, and 11% in ages 41 – 50 (Hurwitz, 1969).

Almost all the adverse effects of antipsychotics are more frequently reported in the elderly. When adverse effects do occur, they may be of such significance that therapy must be altered or changed altogether. Even more than in younger patients, the choice of antipsychotics is based on the profile of these adverse effects. Adverse effects with particular relevance to the elderly will be considered here.

Neurologic side effects

Motor side effects are especially problematic in the elderly. While acute dystonia and akathisia are more common in younger patients, Parkinsonian symptoms and tardive dyskinesia are more frequent in the aged. It has been estimated that 50% of patients between 60 and 80 develop drug-induced Parkinsonism (Ayd, 1961). When it occurs in the elderly it may be mistaken for sedation, depression or loss of social interest, and has serious consequences for patients whose ability to move and express themselves easily may be already compromised by their illness. In addition, the loss of coordination may predispose the elderly to more falls, and limit their ability to write, feed themselves, etc. For those elderly patients with ideopathic Parkinson's disease or with Parkinsonian symptoms associated with dementia, antipsychotics may produce unacceptable akinesia, rigidity and tremor. The predisposition of all elderly to develop extrapyramidal symptoms explains in part the popularity in the elderly of drugs with a lower incidence of extrapyramidal symptoms like thioridazine (Prien, 1975; Branchey et al., 1978).

Antiparkinson drugs, such as benztropine, procyclidine, or trihexyphenidyl are standard treatments for EPS, but produce serious anticholinergic effects, especially in combination with other psychotropic agents. The fact that they can exacerbate memory and cognition disturbances in the aged is particularly troubling. While withdrawal of anticholinergics is advisable when possible, extrapyramidal symptoms as well as psychopathological symptoms have been observed following discontinuation of antiparkinson agents (Manos et al., 1981).

Tardive dyskinesia results with high exposure rates to antipsychotic drugs, and because of its resistance to treatment or remission, represents one of the most serious drawbacks to antipsychotic therapy. Although it may occur with brief exposure, characteristically patients with tardive dyskinesia (TD) have been on antipsychotics for years. The prevalence of spontaneous lingual-facial-buccal movements in elderly without neuroleptic exposure or known CNS disease is 0.8% between 50 and 59, 6% between 60 and 69, and 7.8% between age 70 and 79 (Klawans and Barr, 1982). On the basis of prevalence surveys of tardive dyskinesia, Kane and Smith (1982) found that it is present in 20% of neuroleptic-treated patients in therapy compared to a 5% rate of 'spontaneous' dyskinesia in drug-free controls. Although increasing neuroleptic exposure and exposure to antiparkinson drugs have been suggested as contributing factors, the strongest associations are female sex and advancing age (Kane and Smith, 1982). In a study of two French retirement homes, female residents had twice the incidence (27%) of dyskinesia as did males (12%). While 18% of subjects without neuroleptic exposure had TD, 42% of those with neuroleptic exposure had TD (Bourgeois et al., 1980). Smith and Baldessarini (1980) found strong correlations between age and the severity and prevalence of TD, although neither increased after age 70. Their data suggested an increasing sensitivity of the aging brain to neuroleptics with a much reduced rate of improvement in the elderly (Smith and Baldessarini, 1980).

Careful examination of patients and cautious use of antipsychotics may be useful in reducing the risk of TD; the development of novel antipsychotics (e.g. clozapine) without the liability to produce frequent TD would be of use in the elderly.

All the antipsychotics lower the seizure threshold, although this occurs infrequently. With elderly or organic patients, this will be observed more frequently. Seizures have been associated with parenteral administration and rapid increase in drug dosage (Sovner and DiMascio, 1978). While seizures induced by antipsychotics may be controlled by increases or initiation of anticonvulsants, it should be remembered that phenothiazines have been reported to elevate phenytoin levels to toxic amounts (Vincent, 1980).

Hematologic

Agranulocytosis is more common in individuals over 40, but still occurs in less than 1 in 1000. Women are more frequently involved, and the aliphatic phenothiazines are the most common offenders (Cole et al., 1976). While usually observed in the first months of therapy, agranulocytosis becomes a risk whenever patients are switched to a different antipsychotic.

Retinitis pigmentosa has been observed with high (1200 mg/day) doses of thioridazine and lenticular and corneal opacities have been observed with the slit-lamp in patients on long-term antipsychotic therapy. These latter changes occur most frequently with chlorpromazine in high dosage (Klein and Davis, 1969), and generally recede when treatment is terminated.

Cardiovascular side effects

Hypotension may occur following treatment with the aliphatic and piperidine phenothiazines. With chlorpromazine, hypotension occurs in about 4% of patients, and with thioridazine in 2.4% (Klein and Davis, 1969). Parenteral use of the antipsychotics increases this effect; 25 – 50 mg of chlorpromazine i.m. produced a 15% fall in systolic pressure in supine patients (Foster et al., 1954). This is hazardous to the elderly as they may suffer confusional episodes or transient ischemic attacks following drug-induced hypotensive episodes (Verwoerdt, 1976).

Orthostatic hypotension, resulting from peripheral vasodilation secondary to α-adrenergic blockade is seen more frequently with aliphatic and piperidine phenothiazines than with piperazine phenothiazines. Haloperidol, thiothixene and other 'high potency' neuroleptics minimize this risk to patients.

Antipsychotics may also produce cardiomegaly, congestive heart failure and arrhythmias in the elderly. Of these cardiac effects, sinus tachycardia and EKG changes are the most common. Flattening or notching of T-waves, prolongation of the QT interval, PR changes and occasional U wave may be noted most commonly with piperidine and aliphatic phenothiazines (Goldstein et al., 1968). Thioridazine may also produce quinidine-like myocardial depressant effects (Kelly et al., 1963) which have been linked to episodes of sudden death. More benign thioridazine-induced changes in the EKG (leveling or notching of T-waves) have been correlated to plasma levels of the drug (Axelsson and Aspenstrom, 1982). In aged patients with pre-existing QT lengthening, antipsychotic-induced changes in PVCs or QT intervals could initiate lethal events. Even young healthy individuals have suffered fatalities due to arrhythmias while on chlorpromazine or thioridazine (Risch et al., 1982). Malignant ventricular arrhythmias following the use of thioridazine have responded to correction of hypokalemia, hypocalcemia and withdrawal of drug (Khan et al., 1981).

While the adverse effects of antipsychotics are often emphasized, it should not be overlooked that drugs such as chlorpromazine may have therapeutic benefits in post-myocardial infarction patients. When administered intravenously, a decrease in myocardial oxygen demand, a reduction of systemic vascular resistance and a reduction in pulmonary capillary wedge pressure have been reported, all of benefit to patients with congestive heart failure and cardiogenic shock (Lal and Bahl, 1967; Elkayam et al., 1977).

With the quinidine-like effects of certain antipsychotics, it is not surprising that certain arrhythmias might be suppressed. In experimental animals, both atrial (Singh and Sharma, 1969) and ventricular (Singh and Sharma, 1970) arrhythmias have responded to antipsychotic 'therapy', and in several patients, dehydrobenzperidol has been of clinical utility with ventricular arrhythmias refractory to pronestyl and lidocaine (Riss et al., 1969). These therapeutic uses of antipsychotics are not established and while of interest, require more substantial elucidation.

AUTONOMIC EFFECTS

Anticholinergic and α-adrenergic effects are present with all the antipsychotics. In the aging, gastrointestinal tract, antipsychotics will reduce motility and secretions causing constipation, and with maintenance therapy, produce ileus or even profound dilation of the intestines (Ritama et al., 1969). Paralytic ileus in the absence of fecal impaction is rare with single-antipsychotic agents. In the esophagus, dysphagia and achalasia have been reported. Urinary and sexual function is also governed by both central and peripheral autonomic mechanisms affected by antipsychotics. Because urinary and sexual function of many older patients is already compromised, there is a higher likelihood for the occurrence of urinary retention, or problems in erection or orgasm (Ghadirian et al., 1982).

Anticholinergics have long been recognized to produce confusional, delirious states. The vulnerability of the elderly to this has been one of the cornerstones of the cholinergic hypothesis of aging and dementia (Bartus et al., 1982). Because antipsychotics possess variable degrees of anticholinergic properties and are used frequently in elderly patients with dementia or memory disturbances, deleterious effects on memory may at times be suspected. The use of antipsychotics in combination with antiparkinson drugs will more frequently impair memory in the aged (Gershon et al., 1965). Piperidine and aliphatic phenothiazines carry the most potent anticholinergic effects, yet these are mild compared to anticholinergic effects of antiparkinson agents. While these antipsychotics may produce a full-blown delirium in some cases, a more insidious memory impairment occurs more frequently. Rosen (1979) noted more impairment on the Wechsler Memory Scale with thioridazine than with haloperidol in geriatric outpatients. It is possible that the differing anticholinergic effects of the two drugs account for this difference.

Sedation

Sedation is common with antipsychotic agents, and is marked in the early days of treatment. The most heavily sedating agents are the aliphatic phenothiazines (e.g. chlorpromazine), and piperidine derivatives (thioridazine), and certain thioxanthenes (e.g. chlorprothixene). Especially in the institutionalized elderly, sedation may reduce participation in social and behavioral therapies.

Ophthalmologic effects

The anticholinergic effects of antipsychotics impair visual accommodation, a function already taxed in the elderly due to reduced elasticity of the lens. Not only is vision blurred, but are cases, narrow-angle glaucoma may be precipitated. Open-angle glaucoma is present in over 1% of the elderly, but does not provide a contraindication to anticholinergic drugs.

SUMMARY

Antipsychotics have been widely utilized in aged patients for psychiatric illnesses with and without organic symptoms. Although overused in some settings, their value in carefully selected patients has been clearly shown, with improvement generally more marked in those without organic deterioration. Pharmacokinetic changes in the elderly alter dose requirements, but not as predictably as with other psychotropics. The phenothiazines – chlorpromazine, thioridazine, acetophenazine, and loxapine – have been most thoroughly studied in geriatrics as well as the thioxanthene, thiothixene and the butyrophenone, haloperidol. Of these agents, their profiles of adverse effects are important in the elderly, with drugs like thioridazine, chlorpromazine and acetophenazine utilized to minimize extrapyramidal effects, and drugs like thiothixene and haloperidol used to minimize autonomic and anticholinergic side effects. Tardive dyskinesia, and some shorter term extrapyramidal effects are more likely to occur with advancing age, and are treated with difficulty. The possibility of orthostatic hypotension, agranulocytosis and the induction of rhythm disturbances require special caution on the part of the geriatric practitioner.

REFERENCES

Abse, W. and Dahlstrom, W. G. (1960) The value of chemotherapy in senile mental disturbances. J. Am. Med. Assoc. 174, 2036 – 2042.

Achong, M. K., Bayne, J. R. Gershon, L. W. and Golshani, S. (1978) Prescribing of psychoactive drugs for chronically ill elderly patients. Can. Med. Assoc. J. 118, 1503 – 1508.

Altman, H., Mehta, D., Evenson, R. C. et al. (1973) Behavioral effects of drug therapy in psychogeriatric inpatients. I. Chlorpromazine and thioridazine. J. Am. Geriatr. Soc. 21, 241 – 248.

Axelsson, R. and Aspenstrom, G. (1982) Electrocardiographic changes and serum concentrations in thioridazine-treated patients. J. Clin. Psychiatry 43, 332 – 335.

Ayd, Jr., F. J. (1961) Tranquilizers and the ambulatory geriatric patient. J. Am. Geriatr. Soc. 8, 909 – 914.

Ban, T. A. (1969) Psychopharmacology. Williams and Wilkins, Baltimore.

Ban, T. A. and Pecknold, J. C. (1976) Other antipsychotic agents. In: E. Usdin and I. S. Forrest (Eds), Psychopharmacology Series, Vol. 2. Psychotherapeutic Drugs: Part II, Applications. Marcel Dekker, New York, pp. 971 – 995.

Barksdale, B. (1971) Behavior problems in nursing home patients. Treatment with thioridazine. Curr. Ther. Res. 13, 359 – 363.

Barnes, R., Veith, R., Okimoto, J., Raskind, M. and Gumbrecht, G. (1982) Efficacy of antipsychotic medications in behaviorally disturbed dementia patients. Am. J. Psychiatry 139, 1170 – 1174.

Barton, R. and Hurst, L. (1966) Unnecessary use of tranquilizers in elderly patients. Br. J. Psychiatry 112, 989 – 990.

Bartus, R. T., Dean, R. L., Beer, B. and Lippa, A. (1982) The cholinergic hypothesis of geriatric memory dysfunction. Science 217, 408 – 417.

Bender, A. D. (1968) Effect of age on intestinal absorption: implications for drug absorption in the elderly. J. Am. Geriatr. Soc. 16, 1331 – 1339.

Birkett, D. P. and Boltuch, B. (1972) Chlorpromazine in geriatric psychiatry. J. Am. Geriatr. Soc. 20, 403 – 406.

Birkett, D. P., Hirschfield, W. and Simpson, G. M. (1972) Thiothixene in the treatment of diseases of the senium. Curr. Ther. Res. 14, 775 – 779.

Bourgeois, M., Bouilh, P., Tignol, J. and Yesavage, J. (1980) Spontaneous dyskinesias vs neuroleptic-induced dyskinesias in 270 elderly subjects. J. Nerv. Ment. Dis. 168, 177 – 178.

Branchey, M. H., Lee, J. H., Amin, R. and Simpson, G. M. (1978) High- and low-potency neuroleptics in elderly psychiatric patients. J. Am. Med. Assoc. 239, 1860 – 1862.

Cervera, A. A. (1974) Psychoactive drug therapy in the senile patient. Controlled comparison of thioridazine and diazepam. Psychiatr. Digest 36, 15 – 21.

Chan, K., Kendall, M. J., Mitchard, M., Wells, W. D. E. and Vickers, M. D. (1975) The effect of aging on plasma pethidine concentration. Br. J. Clin. Pharmacol. 2, 297 – 302.

Charatan, F. B. (1978) Thiothixene in the treatment of elderly patients. In: L. Hollister (Ed.), A Decade of Thiothixene, Vol. 4: Proceedings from a Symposium. Biomedical Information Corporation, New York.

Chesrow, E. J., Kaplitz, S. E., Breme, J. T. et al. (1962) Use of a new benzodiazepine derivative (Valium) in chronically ill and disturbed elderly patients. J. Am. Geriatr. Soc. 10, 667 – 670.

Cole, J. O., Swett, Jr., C. and Pope, Jr., H. J. (1976) Agranulocytosis revisited. McLean Hosp. J. 1, 34 – 39.

Cooper, T. B. and Robinson, D. S. (1981) Pharmacokinetics of neuroleptic drugs in the aged. In: A. Raskin, D. S. Robinson and J. Levine (Eds), Age and the Pharmacology of Psychoactive Drugs. Elsevier/North-Holland, Inc., Amsterdam, pp. 181 – 192.

Cowley, L. M. and Glen, R. S. (1979) Double-blind study of thioridazine and haloperidol in geriatric patients with a psychosis associated with organic brain syndrome. J. Clin. Psychiatry 40, 411 – 419.

Dale, P. W. (1961) Current concepts in therapy. Medical management of mental problems in the aged. N. Engl. J. Med. 265, 84 – 85.

Edelman, I. S. and Liebman, J. (1959) Anatomy of body water and electrolytes. Am. J. Med. 27, 256 – 277.

Elkayam, U., Rotmensch, H. H., Terdiman, R. et al. (1977) Hemodynamic effects of chlorpromazine in patients with acute myocardial infarction and pump failure. Chest 72, 623 – 627.

Ferguson, J. T. and Funderburk, W. H. (1956) Improving senile behavior with reserpine and ritalin. J. Am. Med. Assoc. 160, 279 – 283.

Forsman, A. and Ohman, R. (1976) Pharmacokinetic studies on haloperidol in man. Curr. Ther. Res. 20, 319 – 336.

Foster, C. A., O'Mullane, E. J., Gaskell, P. and Churchill-Davidson, H. C. (1954) Chlorpromazine: a study of its action in man. Lancet 2, 614 – 617.

Fracchia, J., Sheppard, C. and Merlis, S. (1971) Combination medications in psychiatric treatment: patterns in a group of elderly hospital patients. J. Am. Geriatr. Soc. 19, 301 – 307.

Fraiberg, P. L. (1972) Control of behavioral symptoms in patients with long-term illness. Dis. Nerv. Syst. 33, 178 – 182.

Gardos, G. and Cole, J. O. (1978) Maintenance antipsychotic therapy: for whom and how long? In: M. A. Lipton, A. DiMascio and K. F. Killam (Eds), Psychopharmacology: A Generation of Progress. Raven Press, New York. pp. 1169 – 1178.

Gerle, B., Peterson, B. and Widmark, M. (1961) Clinical experiences with Haloperidol. Sven. Laekartidn. 58, 415 – 418.

Gershon, S., Neubauer, H. and Sundland, D. (1965) Interaction between some anticholinergic agents and phenothiazines. Potentiation of phenothiazine sedation and its antagonism. Clin. Pharmacol. Ther. 6, 749 – 756.

Ghadirian, A. M., Chouinard, G. and Annable, L. (1982) Sexual dysfunction and plasma prolactin levels in neuroleptic-treated schizophrenic outpatients. J. Nerv. Ment. Dis. 170, 463 – 467.

Goldstein, B. J., Clyde, D. J. and Caldwell, I. M. (1968) Clinical efficacy of the butyrophenones as antipsychotic agents. In: D. H. Efron (Ed.), Psychopharmacology, A Review of Progress

1957 – 1967. Public Health Service Publication 1836, Washington, D. C., Government Printing Office.

Goldstein, S. E. (1974) The use of mesoridazine in geriatrics. Curr. Ther. Res. 16, 316 – 323.

Gotestam, K. G., Ljunghal, S. and Olsson, B. (1981) A double-blind comparison of the effects of haloperidol and cis (Z)-clopenthixol in senile dementia. Acta Psychiatr. Scand. (Suppl.) 294, 46 – 53.

Hamilton, L. D. and Bennett, J. L. (1962a) The use of trifluoperazine in geriatric patients with chronic brain syndrome. J. Am. Geriatr. Soc. 10, 140 – 147.

Hamilton, L. D. and Bennett, J. L. (1962b) Acetophenazine for hyperactive geriatric patients. Geriatrics 17, 596 – 601.

Hollister, L. E., Curry, S. H., Derr, J. E. and Kanter, S. L. (1970) Studies of delayed-action medication. V. Plasma levels and urinary excretion of four different dosage forms of chlorpromazine. Clin. Pharmacol. Ther. 11, 49 – 59.

Honigfeld, G., Rosenblum, M. R., Blumenthal, I. J., Lambert, H. L. and Roberts, A. J. (1965) Behavioral improvement in the older schizophrenic patient. Drug and social therapies. J. Am. Geriatr. Soc. 13, 57 – 72.

Hurwitz, N. (1969) Predisposing factors in adverse reaction to drugs. Br. Med. J. 1, 536 – 539.

Judah, L., Murphree, D. and Seager, L. (1959) Psychiatric response of geriatric-psychiatric patients to Mellaril (TP-21 Sandoz). Am. J. Psychiatry 115, 1118 – 1119.

Kane, J. M. and Smith, J. M. (1982) Tardive dyskinesia: prevalence and risk factors, 1959 to 1979. Arch. Gen. Psychiatry 39, 473 – 481.

Katz, M. M. and Itil, T. M. (1974) Video methodology for research in psychopathology and psychopharmacology. Arch. Gen. Psychiatry 31, 204 – 210.

Kelly, G. H., Fay, J. E. and Laverty, S. G. (1963) Thioridazine hydrochloride (Mellaril): its effects on the electro-cardiographic abnormalities. Can. Med. Assoc. J. 89, 546 – 554.

Khan, M. M., Logan, K. R., McComb, J. M. and Adgey, A. A. (1981) Management of recurrent ventricular tachyarrhythmias associated with QT prolongation. Am. J. Cardiol. 47, 1301 – 1308.

Kirven, L. E. and Montero, E. F. (1973) Comparison of thioridazine and diazepam in the control of nonpsychotic symptoms associated with senility. Double-blind study. J. Am. Geriatr. Soc. 21, 546 – 551.

Klawans, H. L. and Barr, A. (1982) Prevalence of spontaneous lingual-facial-buccal dyskinesias in the elderly. Neurology (NY) 32, 558 – 559.

Klein, D. F. and Davis, J. M. (1969) Diagnosis and Drug Treatment of Psychiatric Disorders. Williams and Wilkins, Baltimore.

Kurland, A. A. (1955) Chlorpromazine in the management of the institutionalized and psychiatric patient with chronic brain syndrome. Dis. Nerv. Syst. 16, 336 – 369.

Lal, H. B. and Bahl, A. L. (1967) Treatment of myocardial infarction with phenothiazine derivatives. J. Assoc. Physicians India 15, 69 – 72.

Lamy, P. P. and Vestal, R. E. (1976) Drug prescribing for the elderly. Hosp. Pract. 11, 111 – 118.

Lehmann, H. E. and Ban, T. A. (1970) Thiothixene in geriatrics. Psychopharmacol. Bull. 6, 123 – 124.

Manos, N., Gkiouzepas, J. and Logothetis, J. (1981) The need for continuous use of antiparkinsonian medication with chronic schizophrenic patients receiving long-term neuroleptic therapy. Am. J. Psychiatry 138, 184 – 188.

Marler, E. E. J. (1967) Pharmacological and Chemical Synonyms, 4th edn. Excerpta Medica, Amsterdam.

Martensson, E. and Roos, B. E. (1973) Serum levels of thioridazine in psychiatric patients and healthy volunteers. Eur. J. Clin. Pharmacol. 6, 181 – 186.

Muusze, R. G. and Vanderheeren, F. A. J. (1977) Plasma levels and half lives of thioridazine and some of its metabolites. II. Low doses in older psychiatric patients. Eur. J. Clin. Pharmacol. 11, 141 – 147.

Novak, L. P. (1972) Aging, total body potassium, fat-free mass, and cell mass in males and females between ages 18 and 35 years. J. Gerontol. 27, 438 – 443.

Petrie, W. M. and Ban, T. A. (1981) Propranolol in organic agitation. Lancet I (8215), 324.

Petrie, W. M., Ban, T. A., Berney, S., Fujimori, M., Guy, W., Ragheb, M., Wilson, W. M. and Schaffer, J. D. (1982) Loxapine in psychogeriatrics: a placebo and standard-controlled clinical investigation. J. Clin. Psychopharacol. 2, 122 – 126.

Pollack, B. (1956) The addition of chlorpromazine to the treatment program for emotional behavioral disorders in the aged. Geriatrics 11, 253 – 259.

Prien, R. F. (1975) A survey of psychoactive drug use on the aged in Veterans Administration. In: S. Gerson and A. Raskin (Eds), Aging, Vol. 2: Genesis and Treatment of Psychologic Disorders in the Elderly. Raven Press, New York, pp. 143 – 154.

Prien, R. F. and Cole, J. O. (1978) The use of psychopharmacological drugs in the aged. In: W. G. Clark and J. DelGiudice (Eds), Principles of Pharmacology, 2nd edn. Academic Press, New York, pp. 695 – 705.

Proctor, R. C., Bailey, W. H. and Morehouse, W. G. (1958) An analeptic tranquilizer for senile psychosis. Report 8. Clinical and pharmacological studies of Nicozoi with Reserpine. J. Am. Geriatr. Soc. 6, 291 – 294.

Puls, R. J. (1976) Pulse-wave changes in aged patients during thyroglobulin-reserpine therapy. J. Am. Geriatr. Soc. 15, 759 – 779.

Rada, R. T. and Kellner, R. (1976) Thiothixene in the treatment of geriatric patients with chronic organic brain syndrome. J. Am. Geriatr. Soc. 24, 105 – 107.

Raskind, M., Alvarez, C. and Herlin, S. (1979) Fluphenazine enanthate in the outpatient treatment of late paraphrenia. J. Am. Geriatr. Soc. 10, 459 – 463.

Ray, W. A., Federspiel, C. F. and Shaffner, W. (1980) A study of antipsychotic drug use in nursing homes: epidemiologic evidence suggesting misuse. Am. J. Public Health 70, 485 – 491.

Reedy, W. J. (1967) An internist's observations on thioridazine in the elderly. J. Am. Geriatr. Soc. 15, 587 – 592.

Risch, S. C., Groom, G. P. and Janowsky, D. S. (1982) The effects of psychotropic drugs on the cardiovascular system. J. Clin. Psychiatry 43:5 (Sec. 2), 16 – 31.

Riss, E., Hemli, S. and Abinader, E. (1969) Neuroleptanalgesia in the treatment of acute myocardial infarction. Isr. J. Med. Sci. 5, 747 – 749.

Ritama, V., Vapaatalo, H. I., Neuvonen, P. J., Idanpaan-Heikkila, J. E. and Paasonen, M. K. (1969) Phenothiazines and intestinal dilation. Lancet 1, 470.

Rivera-Calimlim, L., Kerzher, B. and Karch, F. E. (1978) Effect of lithium on plasma chlorpromazine levels. Clin. Pharmacol. Ther. 23, 451 – 455.

Robinson, D. B. (1969) Evaluation of certain drugs in geriatric patients. Arch. Gen. Psychiatry 25, 41 – 46.

Rosen, H. J. (1979) Double-blind comparison of haloperidol and thioridazine in geriatric outpatients. J. Clin. Psychiatry 40, 24 – 31.

Scheline, R. R. (1973) Metabolism of foreign compounds by gastrointestinal microorganisms. Pharmacol. Rev. 25, 451 – 532.

Schooler, N. R. (1978) Antipsychotic drugs and psychological treatment in schizophrenia. In: M. A. Lipton, A. DiMascio and K. F. Killam (Eds), Psychopharmacology: A Generation of Progress. Raven Press, New York, pp. 1155 – 1168.

Seager, C. P. (1955) Chlorpromazine in the treatment of elderly psychotic women. Br. Med. J. i, 882 – 884.

Shanas, E. (1974) Health status of older people. Cross national implications. Am. J. Public Health 64, 261 – 264.

Sheppard, C., Bhattacharyya, A., DiGiacomo, M. et al. (1964) Effects of acetophenazine dimaleate on paranoid symptomatology in female geriatric patients. Double-blind study. J. Am. Geriatr. Soc. 12, 884 – 888.

Silverman, M., Parker, J. B. and Busse, E. W. (1959) A review of drugs in the elderly psychiatric patients. N.C. Med. J. 20, 428 – 432.

Singh, K. P. and Sharma, V. N. (1969) 10-N substituted phenothiazine derivatives in auricular arrhythmias. Arch. Int. Pharmacodyn. Ther. 177, 168 – 178.

Singh, K. P. and Sharma. V. N. (1970) Chemical constitution and drug action of N-substituted phenothiazine in ventricular ectopic tachycardia. Jpn. J. Pharmacol. 20, 173 – 178.

Sloane, R. B. (1978) Psychiatric problems of the aged. Cont. Educat. 11, 42 – 47.

Smith, G. R., Taylor, C. M. and Linkous, P. (1974) Haloperidol versus thioridazine for the treatment of psychogeriatric patients: a double-blind clinical trial. Psychosomatics 15, 134 – 138.

Smith, J. M. and Baldessarini, R. J. (1980) Changes in prevalence, severity, and recovery in tardive dyskinesia with age. Arch. Gen. Psychiatry, 37, 1368 – 1373.

Sovner, R. and DiMascio, A. (1978) Extrapyramidal syndromes and other neurological side effects of psychotropic drugs. In: M. A. Lipton, A. DiMascio and K. F. Killam (Eds), Psychopharmacology. A Generation of Progress. Raven Press, New York, pp. 1021 – 1032.

Stewart, R. B., May, F. E., Hale, W. E. and Marks, R. G. (1982) Psychotropic drug use in an ambulatory elderly population. Gerontology 28, 328 – 335.

Stotsky, B. A. (1972) Haloperidol in the treatment of geriatric patients. In: A. DiMascio and R. I. Shader (Eds), Butyrophenones in Psychiatry. Raven Press, New York, pp. 120 – 122.

Tsuang, M. M., Lu, L. M., Stotsky, B. A. et al (1971) Haloperidol versus thioridazine for hospitalized psychogeriatric patients. Double-blind study. J. Am. Geriatr. Soc. 19, 593 – 600.

Verwoerdt, A. (1976) Clinical Geropsychiatry. Williams and Wilkins, Baltimore, pp. 196 – 200.

Vincent, F. M. (1980) Phenothiazine-induced phenytoin intoxication. Ann. Intern. Med. 93, 56 – 57.

Yudofsky, S., Williams, D. and Gorman, J. (1981) Propanolol in the treatment of rage and violent behavior in patients with chronic brain syndromes. Am. J. Psychiatry 138, 218 – 220.

Burrows/Norman/Davies (eds) Antipsychotics

Chapter 18

Adverse effects, cardiotoxicity and drug interactions of antipsychotic drugs

TREVOR R. NORMAN[1], GRAEME J. SLOMAN[2]
and
GRAHAM D. BURROWS[1]

[1]Department of Psychiatry, University of Melbourne, Austin Hospital, Heidelberg 3084, Victoria, and [2]Department of Cardiology, Epworth Hospital, Richmond 3121, Victoria, Australia

INTRODUCTION

Antipsychotic drugs are indicated for a number of psychiatric disorders but find their major use in the treatment of the diverse group of disorders known as schizophrenia. Additionally, they may be used for the treatment of acute hypomanic episodes, late paraphrenia, organic brain syndromes, Huntington's disease and Gilles de la Tourette syndrome.

Chemically, a diverse group of compounds have been used in the treatment of psychoses and some are listed in Table 1. The phenothiazines are the oldest group of drugs used and they can be further subdivided into aliphatic, piperidine and piperazine types according to the side chain attached to the basic nucleus (see Fig. 1). Among the other chemical classes there are less compounds which have demonstrated clinical antipsychotic effects. Certain elements of chemical structure and three-dimensional conformation appear to be essential for antipsychotic activity (Pauling, 1976). For example, the phenothiazines have a three-carbon separation between the ring structure and the nitrogen attached to a side chain. A detailed discussion of structure-activity relationships is beyond the scope of this chapter and has been described elsewhere (Pauling, 1976; Schmutz and Picard, 1980).

Clinical studies have shown that all of the antipsychotics are superior to placebo and at least as effective as chlorpromazine in treating schizophrenia (Davis et al., 1983). Symptom clusters do not predict individual patient responses to individual drugs. All antipsychotics produce changes in common features of the disorder. The rationale for the choice of one drug over another has been discussed earlier by Hollister (Chapter 11).

Antipsychotics exert their therapeutic effects by their action on dopamine receptors (Enna and Coyle, 1983). It is held that a decrease in postsynaptic dopaminergic transmission has beneficial effects in schizophrenia. In addition, antipsychotics have effects on other neurotransmitter receptors including adrenergic, muscarinic-cholinergic, serotonergic and histamine H_1 and H_2 receptors. It is unlikely that these effects are related to their therapeutic action, since there is a poor correlation between clinical potency and receptor affinity (Peroutka and Snyder, 1980). Rather it is likely that side effects correlate better with these interactions. The more potent β-blockers, for example, are more sedative and more likely to cause postural hypotension.

ADVERSE EFFECTS OF ANTIPSYCHOTIC DRUGS

The majority of patients who receive psychotropic medications will experience side effects. In some cases these may be so troublesome to the patient that they will

TABLE 1

Chemical classes of antipsychotic drugs.

1. *Phenothiazines*	
a) Aliphatics	e.g. Chlorpromazine, triflupromazine
b) Piperidine	e.g. Thioridazine, mesoridazine
c) Piperazine	e.g. Trifluoperazine, fluphenazine, perphenazine
2. *Thioxanthenes*	
e.g. Thiothixene, chlorprothixene, flupenthixol	
3. *Butyrophenones*	
e.g. Haloperidol, droperidol	
4. *Other chemical classes*	
a) Dibenzoxazepines	e.g. Loxapine
b) Dibenzodiazepines	e.g. Clozapine
c) Dihydroindolone	e.g. Molindone
d) Diphenylbutyrylpiperidines	e.g. Penfluridol, pimozide

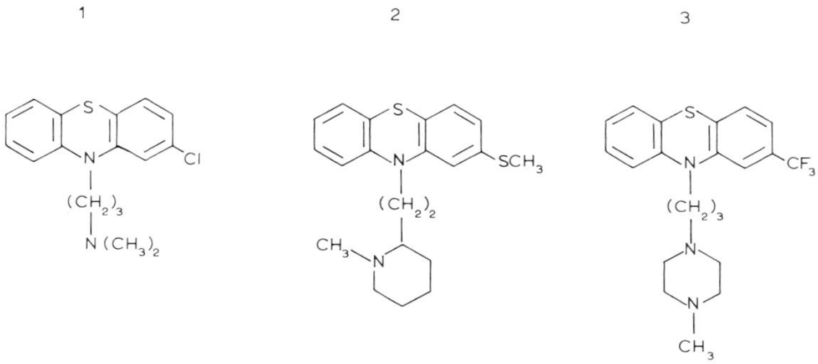

Fig. 1. The three classes of phenothiazines. 1) Chlorpromazine, an aliphatic compound; 2) thioridazine, a piperidine compound; and 3) trifluoperazine, a piperazine compound.

discontinue medication. This kind of problem can be circumvented by warning the patient beforehand that they may experience such effects. It should also be noted that many patients receiving placebos also experience side effects. In rare cases severe adverse effects, warranting the withdrawal of medication, are experienced. A discussion of the possible side effects of antipsychotic medications is presented with an emphasis on cardiotoxicity. Tardive dyskinesia is reviewed elsewhere in this volume and is not discussed. For convenience, effects are discussed by organ systems.

Autonomic effects

As noted above, antipsychotics have effects on both muscarinic-cholinergic and α-adrenergic receptors and these actions explain many of the common side effects. Dry mouth, blurred vision, diarrhoea, nasal congestion, urinary retention, dry skin, excessive perspiration have all been noted. Dry mouth usually diminishes during the course of treatment. Sucking on sweets is not generally recommended since this can lead to monilial infestation and may increase dental caries. Blurred vision is generally observed soon after commencing treatment and disappears a short time later. Urinary retention presents most often in males with prostatic hypertrophy and in severe cases may require catheterisation. Management of the symptoms, by lowering the dose of drug or changing to another drug if this were ineffective, should have been attempted before such a step was taken.

Dermatological effects

Skin reactions (dermatitis, urticaria) are often observed but are not serious. They usually disappear with continued treatment, but interruption of drug therapy may be necessary. Photosensitivity reactions occur with the phenothiazines which produce effects similar to severe sunburn on parts of the body which have been exposed. Avoiding prolonged exposure to direct sunlight and using a sun-screen lotion are advisable counteractive measures. Skin pigmentation may also occur with the phenothiazines, especially thioridazine and chlorpromazine, and may indicate possible pigmentation of the retina.

Cardiotoxic effects

Phenothiazines

Haemodynamic effects. Hypotension following administration of chlorpromazine or thioridazine is well recognized, and occurs in about 2 – 4% of patients (Klein and Davis, 1969). Swett (1975) noted only 15 cases of cardiovascular reactions in over 500 patients receiving chlorpromazine with 12 of these being cases of hypotension. Foster et al. (1954) showed that small doses (5 – 25 mg) of chlorpromazine intravenously (i.v.) caused systolic and diastolic falls in blood pressure of up to 15%. This was accompanied by rises in pulse rate. Falls in blood pressure of up to 25% were noted in patients over 60 years of age receiving doses as low as 5 – 10 mg i.v. These workers also demonstrated a vasodilator action of chlorpromazine. As a result of these observations, several workers have used low i.v. doses of chlorpromazine to reduce systemic vascular resistance and increase the cardiac index in patients with congestive heart failure and cardiogenic shock (Goldberg et al., 1969; Loeb et al., 1969; Gulotta, 1970; Elkayam et al., 1977). The mechanism of this action is probably related to peripheral α-adrenergic blockade as well as a central action.

Hypotension is not as common with piperazine derivatives (e.g. fluphenazine, trifluoperazine) as it is with the aliphatic or piperidine compounds. Small falls in systolic blood pressure accompanied by a slight fall in pulse rate have been noted following single intramuscular injections of 2.4 mg of trifluoperazine (Raiski, cited in Rudenko and Lepakhin 1979). Postural hypotension is of particular concern in the elderly.

Electrocardiographic effects. Thioridazine, a piperidine derivative, has most often been implicated in electrocardiographic changes observed in patients receiving antipsychotic drugs. Aliphatic compounds, such as chlorpromazine, cause ECG changes less often while the piperazine derivatives, e.g. trifluoperazine, are less often implicated. Nevertheless, ECG changes have been observed in patients receiving all classes of phenothiazine derivatives. Kelly et al. (1963) reported a quinidine-like effect of thioridazine on ventricular repolarization in doses as low as 200 mg/day. Changes observed in the ECG included depression, widening, notching, flattening and inversion of the T waves, prolongation of the QT interval and the presence of U waves. In Kelly et al.'s series of 28 patients, two patients receiving in excess of 1.5 g of thioridazine per day, on some occasions, died. No clear-cut relationship between thioridazine dosage and cardiac effects has been observed except that in doses above 800 mg/day their incidence increases sharply (Wendkos, 1964). Ban and St-Jean (1964) noted similar ECG changes in patients receiving thioridazine, chlorpromazine or trifluoperazine. The most pronounced effect was with thioridazine and the least with trifluoperazine. Huston and Bell (1966) recorded

TABLE 2

Electrocardiographic effects of some antipsychotic drugs.

Authors	Study	Abnormalities observed
Alexander and Nino (1969)	7 patients receiving chlorpromazine, thioridazine or fluphenazine with other drugs	Myocardial infarction; left bundle branch block; inverted T waves; sinus tachycardia; non-specific T-wave changes
Rasenack and Gattenlöhner (1976)	chlorprothixene overdose in 27-year-old female	Severe arrhythmias mainly ventricular tachycardia
Chouinard et al. (1975)	96 patients receiving chlorpromazine	34% of patients with some or all of blunting, broadening, notching of T waves; reduction of T-wave amplitude
Fletcher et al. (1969)	3 patients taking thioridazine	First degree atrioventricular block, conduction delays, atrial flutter
Giles and Modlin (1968)	19-year-old male taking 4 × 900 mg/d thioridazine	Ventricular tachycardia. Fatal outcome
Huston and Bell (1966)	random ECGs on 106 patients receiving thioridazine or chlorpromazine	Increased QT_c interval. Broadened or notched T waves. Abnormalities in 52% of patients examined
Levine and Marshall (1975)	thioridazine overdose in 30-year-old male	Ventricular tachycardia, bifid T waves
Aherwadkar et al. (1974)	one patient receiving chlorpromazine	Right bundle branch block, left anterior hemiblock
Raj and Benson (1975)	random ECGs on 140 patients receiving various phenothiazines mainly chlorpromazine, thioridazine, trifluoperazine, fluphenazine	T-wave changes, S-T depression, PR and QT prolongation, sinus tachycardia and right bundle branch block in 42% of patients
Axelsson and Aspenstrom (1982)	43 patients receiving thioridazine	Rounded, blunted, notched or biphasic T waves

electrocardiograms on 106 patients receiving thioridazine alone or in combination with another phenothiazine. The ECG was repeated 3 months later on 68 patients. About half the patients at each examination had abnormal recordings, with females exhibiting more abnormalities than males. The age of patients or their number of years on phenothiazine therapy was not related to the frequency of ECG changes observed. No instances of arrhythmia were noted. The fact that the changes observed were reversible on drug withdrawal and were variable at the repeat examination led these authors to suggest that the changes were benign. ECG effects reported in some other studies are summarized in Table 2.

According to Alexander (1968), the true prevalence of cardiotoxicity of phenothiazines is probably unknown due to the fact that large numbers of patients receive these drugs without any detailed evaluation of their cardiovascular status. He recommends periodic cardiological evaluation including chest X-ray and ECG. It is unlikely for the majority of patients that the appearance of abnormal ECG changes or evidence of cardiomegaly will justify discontinuation of phenothiazines, given the serious nature of their mental state. In patients with an already compromised cardiovascular status, consideration should be given to using drugs other than thioridazine.

Sudden unexpected death. Case reports of sudden unexpected deaths in patients receiving phenothiazines have appeared in the literature since these drugs were widely prescribed in man. Expert opinion is divided on whether or not such deaths are a consequence of drug administration. Leestma and Koenig (1968) reviewed 58 cases of sudden death in patients receiving phenothiazines and concluded that at least some of these cases were the result of drug administration. They proposed that the two predominant mechanisms responsible for death were aspiration and rapid asphyxiation and sudden cessation of cardiovascular competence. Earlier, Hollister and Kosek (1965) had reached similar conclusions in reviewing six cases of sudden death. Similarly, Moore and Book (1970) noted 12 cases of death in patients receiving phenothiazines which could not be explained at postmortem examination. Richardson et al. (1966) had also reported an identical series of 12 cases.

Contrary to the above reports, no increase in the number of sudden, unexplained deaths in psychiatric inpatients immediately before and after the introduction of phenothiazines has been noted (Brill and Patton, 1962; Hussar, 1962). Doubts about the existence of phenothiazine death have been raised in another study (Peele and von Loetzen, 1973). Cardiac side effects were evaluated in 1,932 psychiatric inpatients and in the 1,884 patients without co-existing cardiac disease occurred in 1.3% of patients (Swett and Shader, 1977). Sinus tachycardia was the most common reaction and two cases of sudden unexpected death occurred in patients not receiving phenothiazines. These studies suggest that sudden unexpected death in patients receiving phenothiazines does not occur more frequently than in the general population. Indeed, a more recent study suggested that hospitalised chronic schizophrenia patients may actually be at a decreased risk for death compared to age and sex matched general population (Craig and Lin, 1981). Leber (1981) has summarized the evidence for unexpected death and phenothiazine treatment and concluded that the relationship between the two is still unclear. This unsatisfactory situation is likely to continue, since cause and effect are difficult to prove unequivocally. For the physically healthy patient, it would appear that risk of sudden death is small, probably no more than that for the general population not receiving phenothiazines. For patients with impaired cardiovascular function there is an increased risk of sudden death albeit small. Common sense dictates a cautious approach to the treatment of such patients with frequent ECG monitoring.

Overdosage. A major concern with the use of all psychotropic medications is the possibility of their use in attempted and successful suicides. The phenothiazines are no exception to this and are often implicated in drug overdosage (Davis et al., 1968). All overdoses represent a potential hazard to the patient's well-being. The prevalence of serious complications or deaths from phenothiazine overdose is apparently quite low, but fatalities are recorded (Davis et al., 1968; Donlon and Tupin, 1977). In children, the risk of death is much higher.

Allen et al. (1980) reviewed 56 cases of self-poisoning with antipsychotic drugs (mainly chlorpromazine and thioridazine) and noted severe depression of the central nervous system leading to hypotension, respiratory failure, tachycardia and other cardiac arrhythmias. In the fatalities reported by Donlon and Tupin (1977), cardiac arrhythmia was suggested as the cause of death. Treatment of phenothiazine overdose should be directed to supportive management of the cardiovascular complications. Continuous cardiac monitoring should be implemented in patients who have taken a phenothiazine overdose. This is illustrated by the case of a thioridazine overdose who had brief unpredictable episodes of ventricular tachycardia and fibrillation up to 48 hours after drug ingestion (Hollow et al., 1974). Since these drugs have long plasma half-lives, cardiac monitoring for several days after the overdose is probably advisable. Ventricular arrhythmias can be managed by administration of lidocaine. Extrapyramidal symptoms can be managed with antiparkinsonian drugs, but since these are also anticholinergic they should be administered only if the symptoms are severe. Convulsions can be controlled with barbiturates, phenytoin or diazepam. Respiratory depression is often a problem and a clear airway must be maintained.

Another measure that may be used with effect is gastric lavage, even some time after ingestion this may remove considerable amounts of drug. If the patient is conscious, syrup of ipecacuanha can be used instead. Administration of activated charcoal may also slow drug absorption. Forced diuresis and haemodialysis are probably ineffective measures since these drugs are highly protein-bound. It should be stressed that there are no specific antidotes for phenothiazine poisoning.

Butyrophenones

Haloperidol, the most frequently prescribed butyrophenone, is apparently the safest antipsychotic drug with respect to the cardiovascular system (Paul et al., 1976). Gerle (1964) reviewed the side effect data for haloperidol and found relatively few cardiac side effects. A consistent small decrease in arterial blood pressure was noted. Mehta et al. (1979) reported cardiac arrythmias in a hypomanic patient undergoing rapid neuroleptization with haloperidol. On the third day of treatment (total dose of haloperidol 160 mg), the patient developed hypotension, rapid pulse and extrasystoles. An ECG confirmed premature ventricular beats and haloperidol was discontinued. The patient was later treated with thiothixene and the ECG returned to normal. Some cases of sudden death in patients receiving haloperidol have been reported (Ketai et al., 1979; Smith et al., 1980; Modestin et al., 1981; Mahutte et al., 1982). The problems of ascribing sudded death to drug treatment have been discussed above. In three of the above cases the patients were being treated by the rapid neuroleptization technique. Various explanations of the cause of death in these patients were offered: drug-induced laryngeal spasm; pulmonary oedema; myocardial infarction. Whatever the cause of death, they provide a clear warning of the complications that can arise in antipsychotic drug therapy.

Thioxanthenes and other antipsychotics

Compared to other antipsychotics, the thioxanthenes appear to have less effect on the cardiovascular system. Dillenkoffer et al. (1974) observed drug-related ECG changes in 1 of 13 patients receiving thiothixene compared to 11 of 13 patients receiving thioridazine. Haemodynamic changes have also been observed but were not regarded as being clinically significant (Carlsson et al., 1976). Sudded unexpected deaths in this class of antipsychotic have been reported in three patients receiving flupenthixol decanoate (Turbott and Smeeton, 1984). In each case, the patients had received other antipsychotic drugs but in two of the cases flupenthixol was the sole medication at the time of death. The sudden collapse of cardiovascular competence in these cases could not be entirely dismissed as the cause of death.

Clinical trials with pimozide have generally failed to show any adverse effects on the cardiovascular system, although in some studies changes in blood pressure, heart rate and ECG have been reported (Pinder et al., 1976). Three cases of sudden death possibly related to pimozide ingestion have been noted, but concomitant drug therapy may also have been involved (ADRAC, 1974).

In both low and high doses, clozapine did not have any significant effects on the ECG of the majority of patients. In some patients sinus tachycardia, shortened PQ interval and flattened T waves have been noted. These changes were reversible on the discontinuation of clozapine (Ayd, 1974). Agranulocytosis is a more prominent side effect of this drug.

Endocrine effects

Neuroendocrine effects of antipsychotic drugs have been reviewed elsewhere (Beumont and Bergen, 1982). Galactorrhoea, associated with chlorpromazine administration, was noted soon after the introduction of the drug into clinical practice. An association with other antipsychotic drugs has also been noted (Shader and DiMascio, 1970). The frequency of this side effect is uncertain due to inconsistency in the methods of gathering data. Galactorrhoea may also occur in men but not as frequently as in women. It is generally accepted that galactorrhoea is a consequence of hyperprolactinaemia arising from dopamine receptor antagonism by antipsychotic drugs. Gynaecomastia may also occur in patients receiving antipsychotics but according to Beumont and Bergen (1982) is probably unrelated to their administration.

Amenorrhoea and other menstrual disturbances have been attributed to antipsychotic administration, however irregularities of the menstrual cycle have been noted in schizophrenia before the advent of psychopharmaceuticals. If amenorrhoea is associated with galactorrhoea then this most probably represents an effect of drugs.

Small inconsistent effects on other hormones (e.g. growth hormone, ACTH, thyroid hormones) have been noted, but the clinical relevance is unclear. Weight gain sometimes associated with phenothiazine treatment lacks an explanation in terms of effects on the endocrine system.

Extrapyramidal effects

All currently marketed antipsychotic drugs cause extrapyramidal reactions. Differences in the propensity to cause these effects exist between drugs with high potency drugs more likely to induce a reaction. Interindividual differences in susceptibility are also an important consideration. Ayd (1983) surveyed extrapyramidal reactions over a 20-year period and noted four general types of effects: akinesia, acute dystonias, akathisia and Parkinsonism.

Akinesia is often mistaken for sedation although the patients may complain of weakness and fatigue rather than drowsiness (Rifkin et al., 1975). Ayd (1983) suggests that almost every patient receiving a clinically effective dose of antipsychotic drug experiences mild akinesia. Moderate and severe akinesia are probably part of Parkinsonism. Accordingly, symptoms can be managed by dose reduction, at least for mild akinesia, or by the administration of an antiparkinson drug, e.g. trihexyphenidyl or benztropine mesylate.

Acute dystonias occur in about 10% of patients receiving antipsychotics with the highest frequency in patients receiving haloperidol and the lowest in thioridazine-treated patients (Swett, 1975). The majority of reactions occur within the first 72 hours of treatment. They may involve spasms of the neck muscles (torticollis), the spine, and extremities or the eye muscles (oculogyric crisis). These reactions can be managed with diphenhydramine or antiparkinson agents. Intravenous diazepam has been used with success in treating oculogyric crisis (Korczyn and Goldberg, 1972).

Akathisia is a subjective state of motor restlessness characterized by an inability to sit still. There is constant movement of some part of the body even when the patient is sitting or standing. It may be alleviated by dosage reduction or the use of antiparkinson drugs.

Parkinsonism is characterized by tremor, slow movements, rigidity, drooling, mask-like face and slow mental activity. About 13 – 15% of patients may develop parkinsonism and usually this occurs most often in patients receiving high-potency drugs (Ayd, 1983). Drug-induced parkinsonism develops gradually with most patients having prodromal symptoms (e.g. weakness, paraesthesias, less spontaneity). Dosage reduction and antiparkinson agents are used for treatment. Antiparkinson drugs need not be continued indefinitely and may be discontinued after 6 – 8 weeks.

Neuroleptic malignant syndrome

Neuroleptic malignant syndrome (Delay and Deniker, 1968) is a potentially fatal complication of antipsychotic therapy. The essential features are unexplained hyperthermia, muscular rigidity, hypertension, and reduced consciousness. A number of other signs may also be noted (Henderson and Wooten, 1981). Relatively few cases are reported in the literature with all of the varous classes of antipsychotics being implicated. Symptoms may occur soon after therapy or after increasing the dose. Symptoms may resolve spontaneously but about 30% of reported cases have been fatal. Treatment includes cessation of antipsychotics, general supportive care, cooling, prevention of sepsis and physiotherapy. Specific treatments have included bromocriptine and dantrolene (see Zubenko and Pope, 1983).

Other effects

Decreased white blood cell counts occasionally producing agranulocytosis may occur in some patients. This is nearly always preceded by sore throat and fever and can be treated by drug withdrawal and administration of an antibiotic. Cholestatic jaundice usually appears soon after the drug is commenced and many cases are associated with chlorpromazine. Sexual dysfunction including loss of libido and impotence in men is a well-known effect. Pigmentary retinopathy leading to irreversible loss of visual acuity has often been noted with high-dose thioridazine administration. Chlorpromazine may also produce pigmentary deposits in the eye. Antipsychotics lower the seizure threshold and may provoke seizures in some patients, particularly those with a history of epilepsy.

ANTIPSYCHOTIC DRUG INTERACTIONS

When two or more drugs are coadministered, the possibility of an interaction between them arises. The important issue is not that such interactions occur but whether they are of clinical significance. In this respect, Curry (1977) has identified some circumstances which seem to lead to important interactions.

1) One or more of the drugs concerned has a narrow therapeutic index;
2) drug effects are closely related to plasma concentrations;
3) the effects of the drugs involved are similar;
4) the drugs involved affect delicately balanced physiological control mechanisms.

Drug interactions occur either as the result of a pharmacokinetic or pharmacodynamic mechanism. Some pharmacokinetic interactions have been summarized by Cooper (1978). Antacid preparations slow the absorption of chlorpromazine and probably other antipsychotics as well. Clinically, this is of minor significance and may even be beneficial by reducing peak plasma concentration and hence sedation. Barbiturates accelerate the metabolism of antipsychotics and could reduce their clinical efficacy. Several studies have investigated the effect of antiparkinson drugs on antipsychotic plasma concentrations. In general, the levels are decreased but it is doubtful if the clinical efficacy is seriously altered (Cooper, 1978). Lithium delays gastric emptying rate and slows the absorption of chlorpromazine (Rivera-Calimlim et al., 1978). This is of potential importance in the treatment of bipolar disorders where these two agents are sometimes coprescribed. Phenothiazines inhibit the metabolism and increase the activity of oral anticoagulants (Griffin and D'Arcy, 1979). They may inhibit phenytoin metabolism and so increase the risk of phenytoin intoxication (Kutt and McDowell, 1968).

Phenothiazines block a variety of actions of adrenaline and antagonize adrenaline-induced hypertension by their α-adrenergic blocking action. It has also been reported that the antihypertensive effects of guanethidine are antagonized by antipsychotics. On the other hand, potentiation of the effects of guanethidine and other hypotensive drugs has been reported. In either case, the patient should be observed for either inadequate control of hypertension or exaggerated hypotensive effects. Sedative effects of the antipsychotics are potentiated by alcohol and other CNS depressants and such combinations are best avoided. Antipsychotics reduce the effects of L-dopa and as noted above cause parkinsonism themselves. The combination of lithium and haloperidol may cause neurological complications – lithium appears to potentiate the effects of haloperidol. Often it is necessary to use haloperidol for the control of hypomanic episodes in bipolar patients being treated with lithium. In these cases the clinical state should be monitored frequently. The combination of a phenothiazine and monoamine oxidase inhibitor may lead to hypertension and increased extrapyramidal reactions. A more detailed guide to drug interactions is presented by Griffin and D'Arcy (1979).

SUMMARY

Clinically serious adverse effects with antipsychotic medications occur relatively infrequently. The major concerns are extrapyramidal symptoms, which occur in a substantial number of patients, and tardive dyskinesia as discussed in chapter 15.

Cardiovascular side effects of antipsychotic medications have been demonstrated in patients receiving antipsychotic drugs. The prevalence of these effects appears to be low though this may reflect an absence of systematic research rather than an absence of effect. Both the mechanical and electrical activity of the heart may be affected by antipsychotic administration and is not predictable. Dosage, length of time on drugs or age do not appear to be related to the development of cardiovascular problems. Clearly, a previously compromised cardiovascular status or undetected, asymptomatic cardiac disease will more likely lead to the development of abnormalities. Cases of sudden unexpected death occurring in patients receiving all classes of antipsychotic medication have been reported, but it is unclear whether they are related to drug ingestion. Cardiovascular problems with these agents are less problematic than extrapyramidal side effects or tardive dyskinesia.

Some clinically significant pharmacokinetic and pharmacodynamic drug interactions have been reported with the antipsychotics and should alert clinicians to the dangers of polypharmacy with these drugs.

REFERENCES

ADRAC (1974) Adverse Drug Reactions Advisory Committee Report for 1973. Med. J. Aust. 2, 875 – 880.

Aherwadkar, S. J., Efendigil, M. C. and Coulshed, N. (1974) Chlorpromazine therapy, and associated acute disturbances of cardiac rhythm. Br. Heart J. 36, 1251 – 1252.

Alexander, C. S. (1968) Cardiotoxic effects of phenothiazines and related drugs. Circulation 38, 1014 – 1015.

Alexander, C. S. and Nino, A. (1969) Cardiovascular complications in young patients taking psychotropic drugs. Am. Heart J. 78, 757 – 769.

Allen, M. D., Greenblatt, D. J. and Noel, B. J. (1980) Overdosage with antipsychotic agents. Am. J. Psychiatry 137, 234 – 236.

Axelsson, R. and Aspenstrom, G. (1982) Electrocardiographic changes and serum concentrations in thioridazine-treated patients. J. Clin. Psychiatry 43, 332 – 335.

Ayd, Jr., F. J. (1974) Clozapine, a unique new neuroleptic. Int. Drug Ther. Newsletter 9, (2 + 3), 1 – 12.

Ayd, Jr., F. J. (1983) Early-onset neuroleptic-induced extrapyramidal reactions: a second survey, 1961 – 1981. In: J. T. Coyle and S. J. Enna (Eds), Neuroleptics: Neurochemical, Behavioral and Clinical Perspectives. Raven Press, New York, pp. 75 – 92.

Ban, T. A. and St-Jean, A. (1964) The effect of phenothiazines on the electrocardiogram. Can. Med. Assoc. J. 91, 537 – 540.

Beumont, P. J. V. and Bergen, J. (1982) Neuroendocrine effects of neuroleptics. In: P. J. V. Beumont and G. D. Burrows (Eds), Handbook of Psychiatry and Endocrinology. Elsevier Biomedical Press, Amsterdam. pp. 157 – 181.

Brill, M. and Patton, R. E. (1962) Clinical and statistical analysis of population changes in New York State mental hospitals since the introduction of psychotropic drugs. Am. J. Psychiatry 119, 20 – 35.

Carlsson, C., Dencker, S. J., Grimsby, G., Haggendal, J. and Johnsson, G. (1976) Hemodynamic effects of thiothixene and chlorpromazine in schizophrenic patients at rest and during exercise. Int. J. Clin. Pharmacol. 13, 262 – 268.

Chouinard, G., Annable, L., Melançon, J. and Chabot, M. (1975) Chlorpromazine-induced electrocardiogram abnormalities. Int. J. Clin. Pharmacol. 11, 327 – 331.

Cooper, T. B. (1978) Plasma level monitoring of antipsychotic drugs. Clin. Pharmacokinetics 3, 14 – 38.

Craig, T. J. and Lin, S. P. (1981) Mortality among psychiatric inpatients. Age-adjusted comparison of populations before and after psychiatric drug era. Arch. Gen. Psychiatry 38, 935 – 938.

Curry, S. H. (1977) Drug Disposition and Pharmacokinetics. Blackwell Scientific Publications, Oxford – London – Edinburgh – Melbourne.

Davis, J. M., Bartlett, E. and Termini, B. A. (1968) Overdosage of psychotropic drugs: a review. Dis. Nerv. Syst. 29, 157 – 164.

Davis, J., Janicak, P, Linden, R., Moloney, J. and Parkovic, I. (1983) Neuroleptics and psychotic disorders. In: J. T. Coyle and S. J. Enna (Eds), Neuroleptics: Neurochemical, Behavioral and Clinical Perspectives. Raven Press, New York. pp. 15 – 64.

Delay, J. and Deniker, P. (1968) Drug-induced extrapyramidal syndromes. In: P. J. Vinken and G. W. Bruyn (Eds), Handbook of Clinical Neurology: Diseases of the Basal Ganglia, Vol. 6. North Holland Publishing Co., Amsterdam, pp. 248 – 266.

Dillenkoffer, R. L., George, R. B., Bishop, M. P. and Gallant, D. M. (1974) Electrocardiographic evaluation of thiothixene: a double-blind comparison with thioridazine. Adv. Biochem. Psychopharmacol. 9, 487 – 495.

Donlon, P. T. and Tupin, J. P. (1977) Successful suicides with Thioridazine and Mesoridazine. Arch. Gen. Psychiatry 34, 955 – 957.

Elkayam, U., Rotmensch, H. H., Terdiman, R., Geller, E. and Laniado, S. (1977) Hemodynamic effects of chlorpromazine in patients with acute myocardial infarction and pump failure. Chest 72, 623 – 627.

Enna, S. J. and Coyle, J. T. (1983) Neuroleptics. In: J. T. Coyle and S. J. Enna (Eds), Neuroleptics: Neurochemical, Behavioral and Clinical Perspectives. Raven Press, New York, pp. 1 – 14.

Fletcher, G. F., Kazamias, T. M. and Wenger, N. K. (1969) Cardiotoxic effects of Mellaril: conduction disturbance and supraventricular arrhythmias. Am. Heart J. 78, 135 – 138.

Foster, C. A., O'Mullane, E. J., Gaskell, P. and Churchill-Davidson, H. C. (1954) Chlorpromazine: a study of its action on the circulation in man. Lancet 2, 614 – 617.

Gerle, B. (1964) Clinical observations of the side effects of haloperidol. Acta Psychiatr. Scand. 40, 65 – 76.

Giles, T. D. and Modlin, R. K. (1968) Death associated with ventricular arrhythmia and thioridazine hydrochloride. J. Am. Med. Assoc. 205, 108 – 110.

Goldberg, S. J., Linde, L. M., Wolfe, R. R. Griswold, W. and Momma, K. (1969) The effects of meperidine, promethazine and chlorpromazine on pulmonary and systemic circulation. Am. Heart J. 77, 214 – 221.

Griffin, J. P. and D'Arcy, P. F. (1979) A Manual of Adverse Drug Interactions, 2 edn. John Wright and Son, Ltd, Bristol.

Gulotta, S. J. (1970) Chlorpromazine in the treatment of cardiogenic shock. Am. Heart J. 80, 570 – 573.

Henderson, V. W. and Wooten, G. F. (1981) Neuroleptic malignant syndrome: a pathogenetic role for dopamine receptor blockade? Neurology 31, 132 – 135.

Hollister, L. E. and Kosek, J. C. (1965) Sudden death during treatment with phenothiazine derivatives. J. Am. Med. Assoc. 192, 93 – 95.

Hollow, V. M., Clarke, G. M. and Weekes, J. W. (1974) Case report: thioridazine overdose. Anaesth. Intens. Care 2, 375 – 379.

Hussar, A. E. (1982) Effect of tranquillizers on medical morbidity and mortality in a mental hospital. J. Am. Med. Assoc. 179, 682.

Huston, J. R. and Bell, G. E. (1966) The effect of thioridazine hydrochloride and chlorpromazine on the electrocardiogram. J. Am. Med. Assoc. 198, 16 – 20.

Kelly, H. G., Fay, J. E. and Laverty, S. G. (1963) Thioridazine hydrochloride (Mellaril): its effect on the electrocardiogram and a report of two fatalities with electrocardiographic abnormalities. Can. Med. Assoc. J. 89, 546 – 554.

Ketai, R. I., Mathews, J. and Mozdzen, J. J. (1979) Sudden death in a patient taking haloperidol. Am. J. Psychiatry 136, 112 – 113.

Klein, D. F. and Davis, J. M. (1969) Diagnosis and Drug Treatment of Psychiatric Disorders. Waverly Press, Baltimore.

Korczyn, A. D. and Goldberg, G. J. (1972) Intravenous diazepam in drug-induced dystonic reactions. Br. J. Psychiatry 121, 75 – 77.

Kutt, H. and McDowell, F. (1968) Management of epilepsy with diphenylhydantoin sodium. Dosage regulation for problem patients. J. Am. Med. Assoc. 203, 969 – 972.

Leber, P. (1981) Sudden death as a risk of neuroleptic treatment (a continuing controversy). Psychopharmacol. Bull. 17, 6 – 9.

Leestma, J. E. and Koenig, K. L. (1968) Sudden death and phenothiazines. A current controversy. Arch. Gen. Psychiatry 18, 137 – 148.

Levine, D. F. and Marshall, A. J. (1975) Cardiac arrhythmia induced by phenothiazine. Lancet 2, 990.

Loeb, H. S., Pietras, R. J., Ninos, N. et al. (1969) Hemodynamic responses to chlorpromazine in patients in shock. Arch. Intern. Med. 124, 354 – 358.

Mahutte, C. K., Nakasato, S. K. and Light, R. W. (1982) Haloperidol and sudden death due to pulmonary edema. Arch. Intern. Med. 142, 1951 – 1952.

Mehta, D., Mehta, S., Petit, J. and Shriner, W. (1979) Cardiac arrhythmia and haloperidol. Am. J. Psychiatry 136, 1468 – 1469.

Modestin, J. Krapf, R. and Böker, W. (1981) A fatality during haloperidol treatment, mechanism of sudden death. Am. J. Psychiatry 138, 1616 – 1617.

Moore, M. T. and Book, M. H. (1970) Sudden death in phenothiazine therapy: clinicopathologic study of 12 cases. Psychiatry Q. 44, 389 – 402.

Paul, S. M., Gallant, D. and Mielke, D. H. (1976) Cardiotoxicity of commonly prescribed psychotherapeutic drugs: clinical implications. In: E. Usdin and I. Forrest (Eds), Psychotherapeutic Drugs, Part I. Marcel Dekker, New York. pp. 483 – 519.

Peele, R. and von Loetzen, I. S. (1973) Phenothiazine deaths, a critical review. Am. J. Psychiatry 130, 306.

Pauling, P. (1976) The significance of conformation. In: E. Usdin and I. Forrest (Eds), Psychotherapeutic Drugs. Marcel Dekker, New York. pp. 59 – 82.

Peroutka, S. J. and Snyder, S. H. (1980) Relationships of neuroleptic drug effects at brain dopamine, serotonin, α-adrenergic and histamine receptors to clinical potency. Am. J. Psychiatry 137, 1518 – 1519.

Pinder, R. M., Brogden, R. N., Sawyer, P. R., Speight, T. M., Spencer, R. and Avery, G. S. (1976) Pimozide: a review of its pharmacological properties and therapeutic uses in psychiatry. Drugs 12, 1 – 40.

Raiski, V. (1976) The influence of trifluoperazine on some indexes of hemodynamics, vessel tonus and electrophysiological process in the heart. In: Questions of Psychopharmacology, Moscow, p. 181. Quoted in Rudenko and Lepakhin q.v. p. 44.

Raj, M. V. J. and Benson, R. (1975) Phenothiazines and the electrocardiogram. Postgradr. Med. J. 51, 65 – 68.

Rasenack, U. and Gattenlöhner, W. (1976) Intoxicationen mit trizyklischen Psychopharmaka. Med. Klin. 71, 507 – 512.

Richardson, H. L. Graupner, K. E. and Richardson, M. E. (1966) Intramyocardial lesions in patients dying suddenly and unexpectedly. J. Am. Med. Assoc. 195, 254 – 260.

Rifkin, A., Quitkin, F. and Klein, D. F. (1975) Akinesia. A poorly recognized drug-induced extrapyramidal behavioral disorder. Arch. Gen. Psychiatry 32, 672 – 674.

Rivera-Calimlim, L., Kerzner, B. and Karch, F. E. (1978) Effect of lithium on plasma chlorpromazine levels. Clin. Pharmacol. Ther. 23, 451 – 455.

Rudenko, G. M. and Lepakhin, V. K. (1979) The major tranquillizers. In: M. N. G. Dukes (Ed.), Side Effects of Drugs, Annual 3. Elsevier, Amsterdam, pp. 39 – 58.

Schmutz, J. and Picard, C. W. (1980) Tricyclic neuroleptics: structure activity relationships. In: F. Hoffmeister and G. Stille (Eds), Handbook of Experimental Pharmacology, Vol. 55, Part I: Psychotropic Agents. Springer-Verlag, Heidelberg. pp. 3 – 26.

Shader, R. I. and Di Mascio, A. (Eds) (1970) Psychotropic Drugs and Side Effects. Clinical and Theoretical Perspectives. Williams and Wilkins Co, Baltimore.

Smith, R. E., Low, N. N. and Nasrallah, H. A. (1980) Haloperidol and an unrelated sudden death. Am. J. Psychiatry 137, 843 – 844.

Swett, Jr., C. (1975) Adverse reactions to chlorpromazine in medical patients. A report from the Boston Collaborative Drug Surveillance Program. Boston University Medical Center. Curr. Ther. Res. 18, 199 – 206.

Swett, C. P. and Shader, R. I. (1977) Cardiac side effects and sudden death in hospitalized psychiatric patients. Dis. Nerv. Syst. 38, 69 – 72.

Turbott, J. and Smeeton, W. I. (1984) Sudden death and flupenthixol decanoate. Aust. N. Z. J. Psychiatry 18, 91 – 94.

Wendkos, M. H. (1964) The significance of electrocardiographic changes produced by thioridazine. J. New Drugs 4, 322 – 332.

Zubenko, G. and Pope, H. G. (1983) Management of a case of neuroleptic malignant syndrome with bromocriptine. Am. J. Psychiatry 140, 1619 – 1620.

Subject index

Abnormal Involuntary Movements Scale (AIMS) 188, 230
Absorption 106
Absorption processes, models of 85
Acetophenazine 142, 241, 248
Acetylcholine 118, 202
Achalasia 247
ACTH *see* Adrenocorticotrophic hormone
Administration, routes of 87 – 88, 134, 144 – 145, 174
Adolescents 215, 217, 220, 227 – 229, 231
Adrenal cortex and enkephalins 28
Adrenergic agents 118
α-Adreneric blockade 246, 263
β-Adreneric blockade *see* Beta-blockers
Adrenocorticotrophic hormone (ACTH) 30, 261
Adverse effects *see* Side effects
Aged *see* Elderly
Aggressiveness 169, 244
  in children 214 – 219, 223 – 228
Agitation 243
Agranulocytosis 131, 245, 248, 262
Akathisia 51, 143, 163, 179, 219, 231, 244, 261
  with haloperidol 109
Akinesia 261, 262
Alcohol 263
Alpha-adrenergic effects 4
Amenorrhea 11, 20, 261
Amine metabolites
  in CSF 38
Aminergic effects of drugs 119
Amoxapine 129, 133, 134
  and tardive dyskinesia 191
c-AMP 198
Amphetamine 43, 217 – 219
  see also Dextroamphetamine
Amygdala 12
Antacid preparations 263
Anticholinergic drugs 14 – 15
Anticholinergic effects 178, 247
  of antiparkinson drugs 244
  of clozapine 130
  of thioxanthenes 118 – 120
Anticholinergics
  and tardive dyskinesia 187, 191
Anticoagulants, oral 263
Anticonvulsants 245
Antidepressants
  and tardive dyskinesia 191
Antihistamines 119
  and tardive dyskinesia 191
Antihistaminic effect
  of thioxanthenes 120
Antiparkinsonian drugs 7, 51, 176, 179, 180, 244, 247
  for dystonias 261
  and fluphenazine level 92
  and haloperidol level 111

in overdose 259
plasma level effects 92, 263
Antipsychotic drugs
adverse effects 253 – 267
atypical 131
cardiovascular effects 253 – 260
in children 213 – 238
dosage regulation 230 – 232
growth effect 230, 231
indications 213 – 215
long-term effects 224 – 230
overmedication 228, 231, 233
short-term effects 216 – 224, 228 – 229
choice of 141 – 145, 244
classification 142
efficacy 254
in the elderly 239 – 242
adverse effects 244 – 247
autonomic effects 247
indications for 239
pharmacokinetics 240 – 241
sedation 247
equal efficacy 144
high dose 110
hormonal effects 12
interactions 263
neurotransmitter effects 254
newer agents 147 – 161
non-specific receptor effects 13, 58
prediction of response 47 – 54
prolactin effects 12 – 21
structure-activity relationships 253 – 254
tardive dyskinesia suppression 200, 205 – 206
withdrawal symptoms 207
Anxiety 51, 124, 163, 164, 166, 186, 243
Anxiety, severe 3, 4
Apomorphine 36, 43, 118, 130, 154, 155, 197, 200, 201
Arcuate nucleus 12, 28
Area under the curve 88
Arrhythmias *see* Cardiovascular effects
Ascorbic acid 76
Assay methods 72 – 77
sensitivity and accuracy 72
Attention deficit disorder 214
Autism 214 – 230 *passim*
Autonomic effects 247, 261

Baclofen 154, 203
Barbiturates 111, 205, 259, 263
Basal ganglia 12
Benadryl 229
Benzamide 142
Benzamides
newer agents 149 – 152
Benzhexol 7
Benzodiazepines 4, 154, 163 – 172
enhancement of neuroleptics 166 – 168
in tardive dyskinesia 203
Benztropine 7, 14, 179, 244, 261
Beta-adrenergic blockers *see* Beta-blockers
Beta-blockers 153, 243
Bioavailability 240
Biofeedback 205
Bipolar disorder
in children 214
Blood-brain barrier 13, 82, 84, 240
Blood concentration-clinical response 225, 232
Blood concentrations
applications of 99 – 100
and clinical response 106
Blood dyscrasias 178
Brain stem 28
Brain syndromes, acute or chronic 3
Breast-feeding 180
Bromperidol 142
blood concentrations 100
Bruegel's syndrome 194
Butaclamol 152
Butaperazine 92, 142
blood concentration-clinical response 106
plasma level studies 64
Butyrophenones 3, 6, 7, 142, 254
cardiovascular effects 260
in children 217, 220, 222 – 223
in the elderly 242 – 243
long-acting forms 174
newer agents 148 – 149
plasma level and clinical response 99 – 114
prolactin effects 13
tardive dyskinesia 191

Camazepam 168
Cancer, breast 21
Cardiovascular effects 7
antipsychotic drugs 253 – 260
butyrophenones 260
elderly 246, 248
phenothiazines 256 – 259

therapeutic, of chlorpromazine 246, 256
thioridazine 246, 256 – 260
thioxanthenes 260
CAT *see* Computerized axial tomography
Catatonia 31
Catecholamine
effects of thioxanthenes 118 – 120
Caudate nucleus 35
Cerebellar stimulation 205
Cerebrospinal fluid (CSF)
amine metabolites 38
chlorpromazine concentration 66, 89
endorphin studies 30, 31
Cessation of drugs 176
Child studies 213 – 238
methodological issues 215 – 216
Children
aggressiveness 214 – 217 *passim*
antipsychotic drugs 213 – 238
indications for 214 – 215
see also main entry
chlorpromazine 216 – 219, 221, 223, 225, 226, 229, 232
conduct disorder 214, 220 – 223, 226
haloperidol 214, 217, 219 – 228, 230, 232
mental retardation 215, 219, 223, 224, 227 – 229
overmedication 228, 231, 233
pimozide 214
stereotypies 220 – 221, 224, 229 – 230
tardive dyskinesia 188, 229 – 230
thioridazine 215, 216 – 218, 224, 225, 227 – 229
Chlordiazepoxide 164 – 167
Chlorpromazine 3, 141 – 142, 144, 150, 153, 155, 156, 164 – 167, 180
for acute treatment 6, 7
children 216 – 219, 221, 223, 225, 226, 229, 232
classification 6, 254
CSF studies 66
dosage 4
dysphoric response 50
elderly 241 – 242, 245 – 247
equivalents 74
GH effects 17
i.v. contraindication 6
lithium effect 263
long-term retention 91
metabolites 80 – 84
activity 84
polarity 81 – 83
non-specificity 141 – 142
pharmacokinetics 85 – 90
plasma levels 15, 62, 66
prediction of response 48, 50 – 51
PRL effects 13
saliva levels 52 – 53
side effects 142, 262
steady state concentration 88
stereotypies 197
thioxanthene analogue 117
TSH effects 18
unbound fraction 92
Chlorprothixene 142, 165 – 166, 247
classification 254
clinically available forms 121
ECG effects 257
formula dosage and analogues 116 – 117
pharmacology 118
Choice of drug 141 – 145, 244
Cholecystokinin 41
Cholestatic jaundice 262
Choline 202
Cholinergic effects 4, 6
tardive dyskinesia 200, 202 – 203, 206
Chorea, choreathetoses 196
Chorea gravidarum 196
Chronobiological effects 15 – 16
Cingulate gyrus 12
Clinics, depot neuroleptic 175 – 176
Clonazepam 154
Clonidine 205
Clopenthixol 243
clinically available forms 121
decanoate 174
dosage and duration 175
formula dosage and analogues 116 – 117
long-acting esters 121
pharmacology 118
Clozapine 129 – 132, 142, 197
agranulocytosis with 131
cardiac effects 260
classification 254
EPS absence 130 – 131
formula 130
half-life 131
metabolism 131 – 132
pharmacokinetics 131
pharmacology 129 – 131

plasma levels 131 – 132
PRL effect 130
tardive dyskinesia effect 131, 197, 200, 206
Cognitive effects of antipsychotic drugs 215, 225 – 230, 244
Compliance 6, 73, 125, 144, 173
and subjective response 51
Computerized axial tomography scans (CAT) 198
Conduct disorder
children 214, 220 – 223, 226
Confusional states 247
Confusional states, acute 242
Corpus callosum 12
Corpus striatum 120
clozapine effect 130
Cortisol 17 – 18
antipsychotic drug effects 12
Cross-reactivity of metabolites 73
CSF *see* Cerebrospinal fluid
Cyclazocine 31
Cyproheptadine 204

Deanol 202
Death, sudden unexpected 258 – 260
Delirium 130, 247
Delusions 31, 37
Dementia 242, 244
Denervation, chemical 196
Denture problems
in tardive dyskinesia 205
Depot neuroleptics 107, 122 – 123, 144, 243
see also Long-acting neuroleptics
Depression 3, 51, 122, 124 – 125, 149, 176, 178
elderly 242
Derivatisation 74
Dermatological effects 255 – 256
Des-Tyr-α-endorphin 34
Des-Tyr-γ-endorphin (DTγE) 30, 34 – 39, 206
Desenkephalin-γ-endorphin (DEγE) 34 – 38
Dextroamphetamine 216, 218
see also Amphetamine
Diazepam 124, 154, 165, 166, 242, 259, 261
high dose 164, 168 – 169
and tardive dyskinesia 206
Dibenzepine 129
Dibenzodiazepine 142
Dibenzoxazepine 142
Dibenzoxazepines 13, 129, 142
Dihydroindolone 142, 148
prolactin effects 13
Diphenhydramine 180, 261
Diphenylbutylpiperidines 142, 151
long-acting forms 174
Distribution of drug 103, 119, 133, 240
Disulfiram 204
Domperidone
prolactin effects 13
L-Dopa 155, 263
L-Dopa carbidopa 155
Dopamine (DA) 11 – 13, 18, 74, 118, 120, 130, 149 – 150
agonist 118, 154, 201
antagonist 187, 200
blockade 17 – 18
and γ-endorphin 35
gonadotropin effects 18
receptor binding and lipophilicity 82, 83
receptor sites 197
receptors 155, 225, 254
supersensitivity 154, 196 – 197, 206
Dopamine-beta-hydroxylase inhibitors 204
Dopamine metabolites 120, 131
CSF 197 – 198, 204
thioxanthenes 120
Dopaminergic effects
of antipsychotic drugs 4
Dopaminergic pathways 11 – 14
Dosage preparations 144
Droperidol 142
classification 254
Drug holidays 191
Drug interactions
and haloperidol plasma concentrations 111
DTγE *see* Des-Tyr-γ-endorphin
Dynorphins 28, 31
Dyskinesia *see* Tardive dyskinesia
Dysphagia 247
Dysphoric response 50 – 51, 228
Dystonia 179, 194, 244, 261
in children 217, 220, 222, 223, 229, 231
with haloperidol 7, 109
musculorum deformans 194
Dystonic reaction, acute (Pisa syndrome) 195

ECG changes 149
with long-acting neuroleptics 178
with phenothiazines 256 – 258
Elderly
antipsychotic drugs 239 – 252

adverse effects 244 – 247
pharmacokinetics 240 – 241
cognitive effects 244
depression 242
extrapyramidal side effects 244
hypotension 246, 248, 256
paranoia 239, 243
physical illness 240
side effects 244 – 248
tardive dyskinesia 244, 248
thioridazine 239, 241 – 248
Electroconvulsive therapy (ECT) 205
tardive dyskinesia 192
Electroencephalogram (EEG) 122
B-mitten dysrhythmia 193
Electron-capture detection 71, 72, 75, 76
Elimination 85 – 87
α-Endorphin 30, 34
β-Endorphin 28 – 34, 206
antidepressant effect 33
γ-Endorphin 28 – 30, 33 – 41
actions 30
amine metabolite effects 38
animal studies 33
brain dopamine 35 – 36
clinical trials 37 – 41
hormonal effects 38
Endorphins 27 – 46
Enkephalins 28, 31
analogue (FK33 824) 205
Enzyme induction 85, 88
barbiturates 112
fluphenazine 91
Epilepsy 178
Estazolam 154, 168
Estrogens 14, 20, 205
Extrapyramidal side effects 51, 123, 150, 178, 261 – 262
in children 217
clozapine absence 130
correlation with haloperidol concentration 108 – 111
and dopamine blockade 4
elderly 244
of haloperidol 7
with parkinsonism 194 – 195
of piperidine phenothiazines 6
thioridazine 261
treatment of 179

Family of schizophrenic patient 7, 8, 175, 177
First-pass effect 84, 85
and intramuscular injection 67
FK33-824 33
Flupenthixol 142, 145, 149
classification 254
clinically available forms 121
decanoate 120, 122 – 123, 174, 179
in depression 123 – 124
dosage and duration 175
sudden unexpected death 260
in depression 124 – 125
dosage formula and analogues 116 – 117
long-acting esters 121
plasma level studies 65
Fluphenazine 142, 144, 166, 167, 207
advantages 143
cardiovascular effects 256 – 257
children 217, 219, 232
classification 254
decanoate 5, 6, 8, 67, 91, 122 – 123, 145, 152, 174, 179
dosage and duration 5, 175
elderly 242
half-life 174
plasma levels 179 – 181
elderly 242
enanthate 67, 91, 174
dosage and duration 175
enzyme induction, lack of 91
esters and tardive dyskinesia 191
first-pass effect 85, 91
formula 81
half-life 91
hydrochloride
half-life 174
metabolism 82
plasma level studies 64
Fluspirilene 142, 151, 174
dosage and duration 175
Follicle-stimulating hormone (FSH) 11, 12
Fusaric acid 204

GABA, gamma-acetylenic 203
GABA, gamma-vinyl 203 – 204
GABA (gamma aminobutyric acid) 170, 200, 203, 204, 206
GABA agonists 153
Galactorrhea 11, 19, 20, 261
Gas chromatography 71 – 76

of haloperidol 100
Gas-liquid chromatography 133
Genetic factor in schizophrenia 40
Glaucoma 247
Glutamate decarboxylase 203
Gonadotropins 18
Grandiosity 243
Growth hormone (GH) 11, 12, 17, 261
Growth in children 230, 231
Guanethidine 263
Gynecomastia 261

Haemodialysis 32, 259
Half-life
of chlorpromazine 90 – 91
of drug 86
Hallucinations 31, 32, 37, 164, 168, 220, 243
Hallucinations, auditory 3
Haloperidol 6, 15, 35, 123, 142, 144, 150, 155, 165
acute and long-term management 7
advantages 143
assay methods 99 – 101
blood level correlations
with EPS 108 – 111
with side effects 108
cardiovascular safety 260
children 214, 217, 219 – 228, 230
classification 254
decanoate 145, 149, 174
dosage and duration 175
plasma levels 107 – 108
dosage 5
dysphoric response 50
dystonias 261
elderly 241, 242, 247, 248
high-dose 110
hormonal effects 13, 19
intravenous 166
with lithium 263
metabolic pathway 99
in non-responders 104 – 107
oral bioavailability 103
plasma level studies 65, 100 – 104
prediction of response 49 – 51
red blood cell concentrations 103
reduced 75, 76
stereotypies 197
High performance liquid chromatography 71, 74 – 77
Hippocampus 28
Homovanillic acid (HVA) 198, 204
see also Dopamine metabolites
Hostility 242, 243
Huntington's chorea 195
5-Hydroxy indoleacetic acid (5-HIAA) 198, 204
see also Amine metabolites
5-Hydroxy tryptamine 198
Hyperactivity in children 214 – 217 *passim*
Hyperprolactinemia 4, 11, 19, 261
Hypertonia
in neonate 180
Hypotension 178
elderly 246, 256
Hypothalamo-pituitary axis 11, 16

Imipramine 165
Impulsivity 215
Interindividual variation
in plasma levels 59 – 60, 62, 68, 85, 108
Interpeduncular nucleus 12
Interview procedure 181
Intestinal mucosa, metabolism in 84
Intramuscular dosage 88, 108, 120, 174
Intravenous dosage 87 – 88
chlorpromazine 6
haloperidol 7, 166

Largactil 3
Lecithin 202
Lenperon 149
Lethargy in children 228
Leu5-β-endorphin 32
Levodopa 197, 201
dyskinesia 194
see also L-dopa
Levomepromazine 111
pharmacokinetics 93
Libido 178
Lidocaine 259
Limbic system 28
clozapine effect 130
Lipophilicity 174
of metabolites 82
β-Lipotropin (LPH) 30
Lithium 155, 156, 263
in children 217, 219, 223
in tardive dyskinesia 204
Long-acting neuroleptics 107, 173 – 183, 177

adverse side effects 178
classification 174
contraindications 178
duration of treatment 176
follow-up system 177
interview procedure 181
special indications for 173
see also Depot neuroleptics
Lorazepam 167 – 168
Loxapine 129, 130, 132 – 136, 142, 197
advantages 143
in children 221, 222
classification 254
dosage 132
elderly 242, 248
enterohepatic circulation 135
measurement 133 – 134
metabolism 133 – 134
pharmacokinetics 133 – 136
in schizophrenia 132 – 133
Luteinizing hormone (LH) 11, 12
Lymphocytes 40

Manganese 205
Mania 3, 123 – 124, 155 – 156
Mass fragmentography 71, 73, 75, 76
Median eminence 12
Meige syndrome 194
Melanin affinity
of thioxanthenes 119
Melanocyte stimulating hormone release
inhibiting factor 205
Memory effects 225, 247
Menstrual disturbance 178
Mental retardation 215, 219, 223, 224,
227 – 229
Meprobamate 164
Mesolimbic system 13
Mesolimbic tardive dyskinesia 206 – 207
Mesoridazine 142, 242
classification 254
Metabisulfite sodium 76
Metabolites, active 82, 84, 92, 99
3-Methoxy-4-hydroxyphenyl glycol (MHPG)
198, 204
see also Amine metabolites
Methylphenidate 197, 200, 216, 218, 222, 243
Metiapine 129, 130
Metoclopramide 13, 150 – 151
Molindone 142, 148
advantages 143
in children 220 – 221, 232
classification 254
Monitoring
see Blood concentrations; Plasma levels
Monoamine oxidase inhibitors 263
Morphine 205
Muscimol 203

Naloxone 30 – 32, 205
Naltrexone 30 – 32
Neonate 180
Neuroendocrine effects 11 – 25, 261
Neuroleptic malignant syndrome 262
Neuroleptics *see* Antipsychotic drugs
Neuropeptides 24
Niacinamide 205
Nicotinic acid 243
Nigrostriatum 196 – 197, 200, 203
Nitrogen-sensitive detection 71, 72, 75, 76
Non-compliance 7 – 8, 17, 243
see also Compliance
Non-responders to treatment
in plasma level studies 62, 66
Non-response
and absorption 106
and drug concentration 104 – 107
Noradrenaline 130
see also Norepinephrine
Norepinephrine
in tardive dyskinesia 204
see also Noradrenaline
Nortriptyline 124
Nucleus accumbens 12
Nursing homes 239

Ocular effects 262
Oculogyric crisis 261
Olfactory tubercle 12
Opiate mixed agonist-antagonist 31
Opioid peptides 28, 29
Optical effects of drugs 245
Oral contraceptive-induced chorea 196
Oral dosage 88
Organic brain disease
and tardive dyskinesia 192
Organic brain syndromes 125, 241 – 243
Organic psychoses 243, 244
Orofacial dyskinesia, spontaneous 189, 193,
245

Orofacial dystonia (Meige syndrome) 194
Orthostatic hypotension
246, 248, 256
see also Hypotension
Outpatient management
with long-acting neuroleptics 176
Overdose 73, 259
of loxapine 135 – 136
Overmedication 228, 231, 233
Oxyprothepine 174
decanoate 175

Pain 30
Paralytic ileus 247
Paranoia
and problems of compliance 6
Paranoid symptoms 32, 169, 239, 243
Parenteral dosage 119, 144, 245
Parkinsonism 143, 244
with haloperidol 109
Parkinson's disease 194, 196, 199, 244
Partition ratios 81, 83
Penfluridol 14, 17, 142, 151, 174
advantages 143
in children 224
classification 254
dosage and duration 175
Pentazocine 31
Perazine pharmacokinetics 93
Perphenazine 111, 142, 150, 242
classification 254
enanthate 174
dosage and duration 175
pharmacokinetics 93
PETT 199
Pharmacokinetic data
and clinical response 52 – 53
Pharmacokinetics
of phenothiazines 85 – 94
Phenothiazines 142
α-adrenergic blocking action 263
agranulocytosis with 245
aliphatic 141 – 142, 246, 247, 253 – 256
formula 255
cardiovascular effects 256 – 259
in children 216 – 217
classification 253 – 255
elderly 241 – 243, 247 – 248
free fraction 92
hormonal effects 13, 19
long-acting forms 174
metabolic reactions 79 – 85
optical effects 245
pharmacokinetics 85 – 97
piperazine 6, 7, 142, 253 – 256
formula 255
piperidine 6, 142, 246, 247, 253 – 256
formula 255
sites of metabolism 84
tardive dyskinesia 191
Phenytoin 245, 259, 263
chorea 196
tardive dyskinesia 191
Phosphatidyl choline (lecithin) 202
Physical illness 240
Physostigmine 195, 202
Pimozide 18, 142, 151 – 152
blood concentrations 100
cardiovascular effects 260
children 214
classification 254
dosage 5
growth hormone effects 17
Piperacetazine 142
Piperazine phenothiazines 6, 7, 142
Piperidine phenothiazines 6, 142
Pipothiazine
palmitate 174
dosage and duration 175
pharmacokinetics 93
undecylenate 174
dosage and duration 175
Pisa syndrome 195
Pituitary 12
hormones 11 – 25, 27 – 46
prolactin reserve 16
Plasma level-age correlation 240 – 241
Plasma level-dose relationship
within patient 89
Plasma level measurement 71 – 78
analytical techniques 72 – 75
butyrophenones 72 – 76
phenothiazines 71 – 76
plasma extraction 75
requirements 72
sample collection and storage 76
stability of samples 76
Plasma levels
antiparkinson drug effects 263
clozapine 131 – 132

individual variation 85
thioridazine 240
Plasma levels and clinical response 52, 57 – 70
butaperazine 64, 75
chlorpromazine 52 – 53, 62 – 63
in chronic schizophrenics 66 – 67
fluphenazine, fluphenazine decanoate 64, 73, 75, 76
haloperidol 65, 73, 75, 76
interindividual differences 59 – 60, 62, 68
perphenazine 73
of prolactin 63
studies 61 – 65
theoretical basis 58
thiothixene 52, 120 – 121
trifluoperazine 73, 75, 76
value of monitoring 59 – 60
Plasma levels and side effects 66
Pneumonitis, aspiration 186
Polarity of metabolites 81 – 82
Polypharmacy 240
tardive dyskinesia 193
Positron emission transaxial tomography (PETT) 199
Post mortem studies
endorphins 31
tardive dyskinesia 198
Pregnancy 179 – 180
Pro-opiomelanocortico system 28
Procyclidine 244
Progesterone 20
Prolactin
antipsychotic drug effects 12 – 21
clozapine effect 130
CSF levels 17
gender effects 14
plasma level and clinical response to drugs 63, 65
psychosis correlation 16
Promazine
classification 6
dosage 4
Promethazine
metabolism 84
Propranolol 153, 205, 206
Protein binding 119, 259
Psychosis, supersensitivity 207
Puerperium 180
Pyridoxine 205

Quinidine-like effects 246

Rabbit syndrome 195, 229
Radioimmunoassay 71, 73, 75, 76, 101, 133
of haloperidol 101
Radioreceptor assay 71, 74, 75, 77, 101
of haloperidol 101
Rapid neuroleptization 260
Red blood cell concentrations 64 – 66, 103
Red cell binding of drug 240
Relapse 176, 179, 243
Relapse and prolactin level 17
Reserpine 13, 144, 200, 243
Response to antipsychotic drugs, prediction 47 – 54
Retinitis pigmentosa 245
Rigidity 179, 244, 262
Rockland Research Institute Dyskinesia Rating Scale 230

Saliva levels and clinical response 52 – 53
Schizoaffective psychosis 124, 156, 168, 169
Schizophrenia
in children and adolescents 214, 217, 220 – 222
and endorphins 30 – 41
management 3 – 8
with long-acting neuroleptics 175 – 181
prediction of response 47 – 54
refractory 106, 156
elderly 243
types I and II 41
School Phobia 228
Sedation 6, 118, 137, 150, 216 – 223, 225, 229, 243, 247, 263
Seizures 125, 132, 216, 229, 245, 259, 262
Septal nucleus 12
Serotonin 118, 204
in tardive dyskinesia 204
see also 5-Hydroxy tryptamine
Sexual dysfunction 20, 143, 247
Side effects
in children 218 – 219, 222 – 223, 228 – 230, 231
correlation with blood levels 108 – 111
in the elderly 244 – 248
of long-acting neuroleptics 178 – 179
and neurotransmitter action 254
see also Individual effects, e.g. Akathisia; Dystonia, etc

Sleep
movement disorders 195
tardive dyskinesia in 186
Social help 8
Spiroperidol 204
in radioreceptor assay 74
Stability of plasma samples 76
Steady state concentration 88
of long-acting haloperidol 107
Stereotaxic surgery 205
Stereotypies 197
children 220 – 221, 224, 229 – 230
of schizophrenia 195 – 196
Stria terminalis 12
Substance P 203
Substantia nigra 12, 203
Suicide 259
Sulpiride 13, 35, 142, 149 – 150
Sundowner syndrome 242
Syntonic response 50

Tardive dyskinesia 8, 111, 125, 131, 151, 153, 154, 155, 163, 176, 179, 185 – 212
age and sex effects 190, 245
amine effects 187
atypical 187, 198
children 188, 229 – 230, 233
cholinergic effects 200, 202 – 203, 206
clozapine 197, 200, 206
cortical neurons 199
DA supersensitivity 196 – 197
differential diagnosis 193 – 196, 199
disappearance in sleep 186
drug liability 191
elderly 244, 248
electroconvulsive therapy (ECT) 192
extrapyramidal side effects sensitivity 192
future research 205 – 207
manifestations 186
mesolimbic 206 – 207
nigrostriatum 196 – 197
non-pharmacological treatments 205
organic brain disease 192
pathophysiology 196 – 199
pharmacology 199 – 206
polypharmacy 193
post-mortem studies 198
prevalence and risk factors 188 – 193, 245
reversibility 187
spontaneous remission 188
sub-types 186 – 187
Tardive dysmentia 207
Testosterone 12, 19
Tetrabenazine 167, 200
Tetrahydroacridine (tacrine, THA) 202
Therapeutic range 85
Therapeutic window 58
of haloperidol 102 – 103
Thioproperazine 142
Thioridazine 92, 124, 142, 165, 166, 167
advantages 143
blood concentration-clinical response 106
cardiovascular effects 246, 256 – 260
children 215, 216 – 218, 224, 225, 227 – 229
classification 254
dosage 232
elderly 239, 241 – 248
extrapyramidal side effects 261
formula 81
hormonal effects 17 – 19
plasma levels 240
unbound fraction 92
Thiothixene 142, 144, 242, 244, 248, 260
advantages 143
anxiolytic properties 124
in children 220, 232
classification 254
clinically available forms 121
dysphoric response 50
formula dosage and analogues 116 – 117
metabolism 119 – 120
pharmacology 118
plasma level and clinical response 52
plasma levels 119
prediction of response 48 – 51
Thioxanthenes 3, 6, 7, 115 – 128, 142, 254
adverse drug reactions 125 – 126
animal studies 118
antihistaminic effects 120
cardiovascular effects 260
in children 220
clinical studies 121
DA receptor blockade 120
dopamine metabolites 120
EEG effects 122
elderly 242, 247
extrapyramidal side effects 122
formulae 117
isomers 115
long-acting forms 174

measurement 120 – 121
mood elevating effect 122
in neurotic disorders 124 – 125
newer agents 149
in organic brain syndrome 125
pharmacokinetics 119 – 120
pharmacology 118 – 119
phenothiazine analogues 117
plasma level-clinical response 120 – 121
prolactin effects 13
protein binding 119
safety margin 118
treatment schedules 125
Thorazine 3
Thought disturbance 3
Thyroglobulin 243
Thyroid hormones 18, 261
Thyrotropin-releasing hormone 206
Tics 221, 225
Tissue retention of phenothiazines 85, 123
Torticollis 7, 261
Tourette's disorder 214, 220, 221, 224, 225, 227, 228, 229, 231
Toxicity
behavioural 221, 228, 231
cardiovascular
see Cardiovascular effects
Tranquillization 3
Transcutaneous stimulation 205
Trebenzomine 152
Tremor 179, 244, 262
Trifluoperazine 142, 148, 150, 197, 241
in children 217, 219, 222, 232
classification 254
ECG effects 256 – 257
formula 81
half-life 93
pharmacokinetics 93
Trifluperidol
in children 217, 221, 222, 232
Triflupromazine 142
classification 254
Trihexyphenidyl 244, 261
Tryptaminergic effects 4
Tryptophan
in tardive dyskinesia 204
TSH
antipsychotic drug effects 12
Tuberoinfundibular DA system 11, 13, 14
tolerance development 14
Tumors 21, 151, 224
Tyrosine hydroxylase 154

Urinary retention 247

Valproate sodium 154, 203
Vanilmandelic acid (VMA) 120
Ventricular size 16
and response to drugs 52
Violent behaviour 244

Weight gain 178, 261
Weight reduction with molindone 148